ORTHOPAEDIC

Examination, Evaluation, & Intervention

Notice

Medicine is an ever-changing science. As new research and clinical experience broaden our knowledge, changes in treatment and drug therapy are required. The authors and the publisher of this work have checked with sources believed to be reliable in their efforts to provide information that is complete and generally in accord with the standards accepted at the time of publication. However, in view of the possibility of human error changes in medical sciences, neither the editors nor the publisher nor any other party who has been involved in the preparation or publication of this work warrants that the information contained herein is in every respect accurate or complete, and they disclaim all responsibility for any errors or omissions or for the results obtained from use of the information contained in this work. Readers are encouraged to confirm the information contained herein with other sources. For example and in particular, readers are advised to check the product information sheet included in the package of each drug they plan to administer to be certain that the information contained in this work is accurate and that changes have not been made in the recommended dose or in the contraindications for administration. This recommendation is of particular importance in connection with new or infrequently used drugs.

ORTHOPAEDIC
Examination, Evaluation, & Intervention

A Pocket Handbook

Mark Dutton, PT
West Penn Allegheny Health System (WPAHS)
Adjunct Clinical Assistant Professor
Duquesne University
Pittsburgh, Pennsylvania

McGRAW-HILL
Medical Publishing Division

New York   Chicago   San Francisco   Lisbon   London   Madrid   Mexico City
Milan   New Delhi   San Juan   Seoul   Singapore   Sydney   Toronto

Orthopaedic Examination, Evaluation, & Intervention: A Pocket Handbook

1 2 3 4 5 6 7 8 9 0   DOC/DOC   0 9 8 7 6 5

ISBN: 0-07-144786-5

This book was set in Times Roman by International Typesetting and Composition.
The editors were Michael Brown and Karen G. Edmonson.
The production supervisor was Catherine Saggese.
Project management was provided by International Typesetting and Composition.
The cover was designed by Mary McKeon.
The indexer was Susan G. Hunter.
RR Donnelley was printer and binder.

This book is printed on acid-free paper.

Cataloging-in-Publication data for this title is on file with the Library of Congress.

*To my long-suffering wife, Beth,
and the other lights of my life, Leah and Lauren*

Contents

Preface

This handbook was designed with the outpatient orthopaedic student and novice clinician in mind. The amount of information needed to perform a thorough orthopaedic examination continues to grow; indeed, it has now become impossible to completely memorize. Although all of this information is available in the parent book for this handbook, *Orthopaedic Examination, Evaluation, and Intervention*, it is neither feasible nor practical for the clinician to carry the larger text around the clinic. What is needed is a quick reference source that summarizes the most pertinent and frequently used information from the main text.

This handbook has been designed to provide guidelines to steer the clinician through the complex progression of the clinical examination, evaluation, and intervention of the outpatient orthopaedic patient using a number of simple tools. One such tool is the flow diagram. The flow diagrams in this handbook follow a logical and biomechanical approach and are based on the clinical findings. In addition, to assist the clinician with differential diagnosis, quick-reference tables and illustrations are provided to highlight those joints and regions that are capable of referring symptoms to the various areas of the body.

The first section of the handbook provides an overview of the neuromusculoskeletal system. Chapter 1 outlines the pertinent anatomy, physiology, and biomechanics. Chapter 2 describes the components of the nervous system. Chapters 3 through 5 cover the principles behind an orthopaedic examination, systems review, and evaluation respectively. The initiation and progression of the intervention is a difficult concept for the student and novice clinician to grasp. Chapter 6 outlines the key principles to use when formulating ideas for appropriate intervention beyond the use of electrotherapeutic modalities.

Subsequent chapters are arranged to cover each body area in turn. To help direct the student and novice clinician during the examination, tables and flow diagrams for each of the joints are provided. Separate tables include information to assist the student with the complex task of differential diagnosis.

It is hoped that this handbook will prove to be a valuable guide and resource.

Mark Dutton, PT

Acknowledgments

I would like to give special thanks to my family for their continued support during the times I have to spend away from them.

Thanks also to Neha Rathor of ITC, and the exceptional team at McGraw-Hill, especially Mike Brown who continues to provide me with support and guidance.

To Bill McGowan, whose hidden creative talents provided most of the artwork, and to Bob Davis for his excellent photography.

Finally, my thanks go to the staff at Human Motion Rehabilitation of Allegheny General Hospital for their continued dedication and for the inspiration they provide me.

1 | Functional Anatomy and Biomechanics of the Musculoskeletal System

The musculoskeletal system, working intimately with the nervous system, functions to produce coordinated movement and to provide adequate joint stabilization and feedback during both sustained positions and movements. The musculoskeletal structures involved with human motion include the muscles and tendons, which produce the movement, and the joints, around which the motions occur. For the physical therapist designing and supervising rehabilitation programs, a working knowledge of functional anatomy and biomechanics is essential: a fundamental skill of the physical therapist is to identify, analyze, and solve problems related to human movement.

TERMINOLOGY

Anatomic knowledge provides the framework on which understanding of physiologic processes, clinical evaluations of pathology and trauma, and interventions are based.[1] Recently, many of the more traditional anatomic names for structures have undergone some modification. These modifications are outlined in the book *Terminologia Anatomica*.[2] These changes in terminology have already been widely incorporated in health science educational programs and publications. Table 1-1 outlines some of the terminology changes to terms commonly used in physical therapy. In order to facilitate the transition, and to help integrate the new anatomic terminology, the new terms are used within this text followed by the old term in parentheses. For example, the common fibular nerve is written as common fibular (peroneal) nerve. Other tables outlining commonly used terminology can be found in the Appendix.

Muscle

Muscle (Figure 1-1) is a very specialized tissue that has both the ability to contract and the ability to conduct electrical impulses. Muscles are classified both functionally as either voluntary or involuntary, and structurally as either smooth, striated (skeletal), or cardiac (Table 1-2). There are approximately 430 skeletal muscles in the body, each of which can be considered anatomically as a separate organ. Of these 430 muscles, about 75 pairs provide the majority of body movements and postures.[3] Various terms are used to describe the functions of these paired muscles:

1. *Agonist muscle.* An agonist muscle contracts to produce the desired movement.
2. *Synergist muscle.* Synergist muscles are muscle groups that work together to produce a desired movement.[4] In essence, synergist muscles can be viewed as the agonist's helper muscles since the force generated by the synergists works in the same direction as the agonist.
3. *Antagonist muscle.* Antagonists resist the agonist movement by relaxing and lengthening in a gradual manner to ensure that the desired motion occurs, and that it does so in a coordinated and controlled fashion.

1

TABLE 1-1 Abridged List of New Terms from Terminologia Anatomica

New terminology (from list of English equivalents)	Traditional terminology
General anatomy	
Median plane	Midsagittal plane, median sagittal plane
Lateral cervical region	Posterior triangle of neck
Posterior cervical region	Nuchal region
Skeletal system	
Cranium	Skull
Articular system	
Ulnar collateral ligament of (the) wrist	Medial collateral ligament of wrist
Radial collateral ligament of (the) wrist	Lateral collateral ligament of wrist
Tibial collateral ligament	Medial collateral ligament
Fibular collateral ligament	Lateral collateral ligament
Medial ligament of ankle	Deltoid ligament
Muscular system	
Extensor digitorum (muscle)	Extensor digitorum communis muscle
Extensor indicis (muscle)	Extensor indicis proprius muscle
Flexor digitorum superficialis (muscle)	Flexor digitorum sublimis muscle
Adductor minimus (muscle)	Horizontal (pubic) component of adductor magnus muscle
External oblique (muscle)	External abdominal oblique muscle
Internal oblique (muscle)	Internal abdominal oblique muscle
Transverse abdominal (muscle)	Transverse abdominis muscle
Tensor of (the) fascia lata (muscle)	Tensor fasciae latae muscle
Fibularis longus (muscle)	Peroneus longus muscle
Fibularis brevis (muscle)	Peroneus brevis muscle
Fibularis tertius (muscle)	Peroneus tertius muscle
Nervous system, spinal nerves	
Anterior rami	Ventral primary rami
Posterior rami	Dorsal primary rami
Spinal (sensory) ganglion	Dorsal root ganglion
Superior trunk of brachial plexus	Upper trunk of brachial plexus
Inferior trunk of brachial plexus	Lower trunk of brachial plexus
Fibular nerve	Peroneal nerve
Medial cutaneous nerve of (the) arm	Medial brachial cutaneous nerve
Medial cutaneous nerve of (the) forearm	Medial antebrachial cutaneous nerve
Lateral cutaneous nerve of (the) forearm	Lateral antebrachial cutaneous nerve
Lateral cutaneous nerve of (the) thigh	Lateral femoral cutaneous nerve
Posterior cutaneous nerve of (the) thigh	Posterior femoral cutaneous nerve
Anterior cutaneous nerve of (the) thigh	Anterior femoral cutaneous nerve
Common fibular nerve	Common peroneal nerve
Deep fibular nerve	Deep peroneal nerve
Superficial fibular nerve	Superficial peroneal nerve
Integumentary system	
Subcutaneous tissue	Superficial fascia

Source: Greathouse DG, Halle JS, Dalley AF: Terminologia anatomica: Revised anatomical terminology. J Orthop Sports Phys Ther 2004;34:363–367.

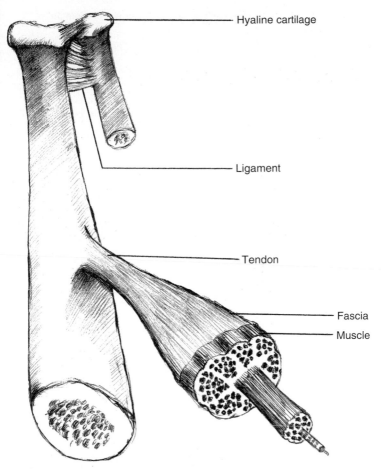

FIG. 1-1   Illustration depicting the relationship between muscle, tendon, ligament, fascia, and hyaline cartilage.

Most skeletal muscles span only one joint. However, some skeletal muscles cross two or more joints (Table 1-3). A two-joint muscle is more prone to adaptive shortening than a one-joint muscle.

Based on contractile properties, four different types of skeletal muscle fibers have been recognized:

TABLE 1-2 Muscle Structure Types

Muscle type	Example
Striated (Skeletal)	Spanning joints and attached to bones via tendons
Smooth	Walls of hollow internal organs
Cardiac	Heart muscle

TABLE 1-3 Examples of Skeletal Muscles that Cross Two or More Joints

Erector spinae
Biceps brachii
Long head of the triceps brachii
The hamstring muscle group
The iliopsoas
Rectus femoris
Gastrocnemius
A number of muscles crossing the wrist/finger and foot/ankle joints

1. Type I (slow-twitch red oxidative) (Table 1-4)
2. Type IIa (fast-twitch red oxidative) (Table 1-4)
3. Type IIb (fast-twitch white glycolytic) (Table 1-4)
4. Type IIc (fast-twitch intermediate)

Human muscles contain a genetically determined mixture of both slow and fast fiber types. In humans, most limb muscles contain a relatively equal distribution of each muscle fiber type, while the back and trunk demonstrate a predominance of slow-twitch fibers. The use of specific muscle fibers is dependent on the desired activity. Although, the two fiber types generally produce the same amount of force per contraction, the fast-twitch fibers produce that force at a higher rate (they fire more rapidly—hence their name). Thus, activities that require a limited amount of time to generate maximal force use a predominance of fast-twitch fiber recruitment. Activities that involve repeated and extended muscle contractions such as those required for endurance events entail more involvement of the slow-twitch fibers.

Based on function, Janda[5] further subdivided skeletal muscles into two groups: postural or tonic muscles (Table 1-5).

Bone

The function of bone is to provide support, enhance leverage, protect vital structures, provide attachments for both tendons and ligaments, and store minerals, particularly calcium (see *Orthopaedic Examination, Evaluation, and Intervention*, p 9). Bones also may serve as useful landmarks during the palpation phase of the examination.

Tendons

Tendons (see Figure 1-1) are cordlike structures that function to attach muscle to bone and to transmit the forces generated by muscles to bone in order to

TABLE 1-4 Muscle Fiber Types

Type	Type I	Type IIa	Type IIb
Diameter	Small	Intermediate	Large
Capillaries	Many	Many	Few
Resistance to fatigue	High	Intermediate	Low
Glycogen content	Low	Intermediate	High
Respiration	Aerobic	Aerobic	Anaerobic
Twitch rate	Slow	Fast	Fast
Myosin ATPase content	Low	High	High

TABLE 1-5 Functional Division of Muscle Groups

Tonic (movers) group	Postural (stabilizers) group
Examples:	*Examples:*
Gastrocnemius/Soleus	Peronei
Tibialis posterior	Tibialis anterior
Short hip adductors	Vastus medialis and lateralis
Hamstrings	Gluteus maximus, medius, minimus
Rectus femoris	Serratus anterior
Tensor fascia lata	Rhomboids
Erector spinae	Lower portion trapezius
Quadratus lumborum	Short/deep cervical flexors
Pectoralis major	Upper limb extensors
Upper portion of trapezius	Rectus abdominis
Levator scapulae	
Sternocleidomastoid	
Scalenes	
Upper limb flexors	
• Primarily Type IIa muscle fibers	• Primarily Type I muscle fibers
• Prone to adaptive shortening	• Prone to develop weakness and
• Prone to develop hypertonicity	muscle inhibition
• Dominate in new movement	• Dominate in postural or sustained
situations	activities
• Generally cross two or more joints	• Primarily cross one joint

Source: Jull GA, Janda V: Muscle and motor control in low back pain. In Twomey LT, Taylor JR (eds): Physical Therapy of the Low Back: Clinics in Physical Therapy, p 258. New York, Churchill Livingstone, 1987.

achieve movement or stability of the body in space (see *Orthopaedic Examination, Evaluation, and Intervention*, p 9).[6] The thickness of each tendon varies and is proportional to the size of the muscle from which they originate.

Ligaments

Ligaments (see Figure 1-1) are densely packed connective tissue structures that consist largely of directionally oriented, high tensile-strength collagen (see *Orthopaedic Examination, Evaluation, and Intervention*, p 9). Ligaments contribute to the stability of joint function by preventing excessive motion, acting as guides to direct motion, and providing proprioceptive information for joint function (Table 1-6). Because of their function as supporting cables in an environment of high tensile forces, ligaments must be relatively inextensible to minimize transmission loss of energy.

Fascia

Fascia (see Figure 1-1) is viewed as the connective tissue that provides support and protection to the joint, and acts as an interconnection between tendons, aponeuroses, ligaments, capsules, nerves, and the intrinsic components of muscle.

Cartilage Tissue

The development of bone is usually preceded by the formation of cartilage tissue. Cartilage tissue exists in three forms: hyaline (see Figure 1-1), elastic, and fibrocartilage (see *Orthopaedic Examination, Evaluation, and Intervention*, p 9).

TABLE 1-6 Major Ligaments of the Upper and Lower Quadrants

Joint	Ligament	Function
Upper quadrant		
Shoulder complex	Coracoclavicular	Fixes the clavicle to the coracoid process
	Costoclavicular	Fixes the clavicle to the costal cartilage of the first rib
Glenohumeral	Coracohumeral	Reinforces the upper portion of the joint capsule
	Glenohumeral ("Z")	Reinforces the anterior and inferior aspect of the joint capsule
	Coracoacromial	Protects the superior aspect of the joint
Elbow	Annular	Maintains the relationship between the head of the radius and the humerus and ulna
	Ulnar (medial) collateral	Provides stability against valgus (medial) stress, particularly in the range of 20–130° of flexion and extension
	Radial (lateral) collateral	Provides stability against varus (lateral) stress and functions to maintain the ulnohumeral and radiohumeral joints in a reduced position when the elbow is loaded in supination
Wrist	Extrinsic palmar	Provide the majority of the wrist stability
	Intrinsic	Serves as rotational restraints, binding the proximal carpal row into a unit of rotational stability
Fingers	Interosseous	Bind the carpal bones together
	Volar and collateral interphalangeal	Prevent displacement of the interphalangeal joints
Lower quadrant		
Spine	Anterior longitudinal ligament	Functions as a minor assistant in limiting anterior translation, and vertical separation of the vertebral body
	Posterior longitudinal ligament	Resists vertebral distraction of the vertebral body
		Resists posterior shearing of the vertebral body
		Acts to limit flexion over a number of segments
		Provides some protection against intervertebral disk protrusions
	Ligamentum flavum	Resists separation of the lamina during flexion
	Interspinous	Resists separation of the spinous processes during flexion
	Iliolumbar (lower lumbar)	Resists flexion, extension, axial rotation, and side bending of the L5 vertebra on the sacrum

6

Joint	Ligament	Function
Sacroiliac	Sacrospinous	Creates greater sciatic foramen Resists forward tilting of the sacrum on the hip bone during weight bearing of the vertebral column
	Sacrotuberous	Creates lesser sciatic foramen Resists forward tilting of the sacrum on the hip bone during weight bearing of the vertebral column
	Interosseous	Resists anterior and inferior movement of the sacrum
	Dorsal sacroiliac (long)	Resists backward tilting of the sacrum on the hip bone during weight bearing of the vertebral column
Hip	Ligamentum teres	Transports nutrient vessels to the femoral head
	Iliofemoral	Limits hip extension
	Ischiofemoral	Limits anterior displacement of the femoral head
	Pubofemoral	Limits hip extension
Knee	Medial collateral	Stabilizes medial aspect of tibiofemoral joint against valgus stress
	Lateral collateral	Stabilizes lateral aspect of tibiofemoral joint against varus stress
	Anterior cruciate	Resists anterior translation of the tibia and posterior translation of the femur
	Posterior cruciate	Resists posterior translation of the tibia and anterior translation of the femur
Ankle	Medial collaterals (deltoid)	Provides stability between the medial malleolus, navicular, talus, and calcaneus against eversion
	Lateral collaterals	Stabilizes the lateral ankle especially against inversion
Foot	Long plantar	Provides indirect plantar support to the calcaneocuboid joint by limiting the amount of flattening of the lateral longitudinal arch of the foot
	Bifurcate	Supports the medial and lateral aspects of the foot when weight bearing in a plantar flexed position
	Calcaneocuboid	Provides plantar support to the calcaneocuboid joint and possibly helps to limit flattening of the lateral longitudinal arch

Joints

Joints are bone regions that are capped and surrounded by connective tissues that hold the bones together and determine the type and degree of movement between them. Joints may be classified as *diarthrosis*, which permit free bone movement, and *synarthrosis*, in which very limited or no motion occurs (Table 1-7).

Synovial Fluid

Articular cartilage is subject to a great variation of loading conditions, and joint lubrication through synovial fluid is necessary to minimize frictional resistance between the weight-bearing surfaces. Fortunately, synovial joints are blessed with a very superior lubricating system, which permits a remarkably frictionless interaction at the joint surfaces (see *Orthopaedic Examination, Evaluation, and Intervention*, p 12).

Bursae

Closely associated with some synovial joints are flattened, saclike structures called *bursae* that are lined with a synovial membrane and filled with synovial fluid. The bursa produces small amounts of fluid, allowing for smooth and almost frictionless motion between contiguous muscles, tendons, bones, ligaments, and skin (Box 1-1).

Mechanoreceptors

All synovial joints of the body are provided with an array of corpuscular (mechanoreceptors) and noncorpuscular (nociceptors) receptor endings. These receptor endings have varying characteristic behaviors and distributions depending on the articular tissue (Table 1-8). Freeman and Wyke categorized the mechanoreceptors into four different types (Table 1-9).[7,8]

The articular mechanoreceptors (Types I, II, and III) are stimulated by mechanical forces (soft tissue elongation, relaxation, compression, and fluid tension) and mediate proprioception.[7,9,10] The type IV variety is a nociceptor.[10]

Other receptors found in the joint include proprioceptors (Table 1-10). Proprioception is considered a specialized variation of the sensory modality of touch, which plays an important role in coordinating muscle activity, involves

TABLE 1-7   Joint Types

Type	Characteristics	Examples
Diarthrosis	Fibroelastic joint capsule, which is filled with a lubricating substance called *synovial fluid*	Hip, knee, shoulder, and elbow joints
Synarthrosis Synostosis joints Synchondrosis	United by bone tissue Joined by either hyaline or fibrocartilage	Sutures and gomphoses The epiphyseal plates of growing bones and the articulations between the first rib and the sternum
Syndesmosis	Joined together by an interosseous membrane	The symphysis pubis

---

BOX 1-1 Musculoskeletal Tissues

For the purpose of an orthopaedic examination, Cyriax subdivided musculoskeletal tissues into those considered to be "contractile" and those considered as "inert" (noncontractile).[11]

- *Contractile.* Contractile tissue as defined by Cyriax, is a bit of a misnomer, as the only true contractile tissue in the body is the muscle fiber. However, included under this term are the muscle belly, the tendon, the tenoperiosteal junction, the submuscular/tendinous bursa, and bone (tenoosseous junction), as all are stressed to some degree with a muscle contraction.
- *Inert tissue.* Inert tissue as defined by Cyriax includes the joint capsule, the ligaments, the bursa, the articular surfaces of the joint, and the synovium, the dura, bone, and fascia.

The tenoosseous junction and the bursae are placed in each of the subdivisions due to their close proximity to contractile tissue, and their capacity to be compressed or stretched during movement.

---

the integration of sensory input concerning static joint position (joint position sensibility), joint movement (kinesthetic sensibility), velocity of movement, and force of muscular contraction, from the skin, muscles, and joints (see *Orthopaedic Examination, Evaluation, and Intervention*, pp 55–57).[12,13] Proprioception can be both conscious, as occurs in the accurate placement of a limb, and unconscious, as occurs in the modulation of muscle function.[13,14]

JOINT MOVEMENT

Terminology

When describing joint movements, it is necessary to have a starting position as the reference position. This starting position is referred to as the *anatomic reference position*. The anatomic reference position for the human body is

TABLE 1-8 Characteristics of Mechanoreceptors and Nocioceptors

Type of sensory receptors	Stimulus		Receptor	
	General term	Specific nature	Term	Location
Mechano-receptors	Pressure	Movement of hair in a hair follicle	Afferent nerve fiber	Base of hair follicles
		Light pressure	Meissner's corpuscle	Skin
		Deep pressure	Pacinian corpuscle	Skin
		Touch	Merkel's corpuscle	Skin
Nociceptors	Pain	Distension (stretch)	Free nerve endings	Wall of gastrointestinal tract, pharynx, and skin

Source: Previte JJ: Human Physiology. New York, McGraw-Hill, 1983.

TABLE 1-9 Mechanoreceptor Types

Type	Location	Function
I. Small Ruffini endings. Slow-adapting, low threshold stretch receptors	The joint capsule, and in ligaments	Important in signaling actual joint position or changes in joint positions Contribute to reflex regulation of postural tone, to coordination of muscle activity, and to a perceptional awareness of joint position An increase in joint capsule tension by active or passive motion, posture, or by mobilization or manipulation, causes these receptors to discharge at a higher frequency.[a,b]
II. Pacinian corpuscles. Rapidly adapting, low threshold receptors	In adipose tissue, the cruciate ligaments, the anulus fibrosus, ligaments, and the fibrous capsule	Sense joint motion and regulate motor-unit activity of the prime movers of the joint. Type II receptors are entirely inactive in immobile joints and become active for brief periods at the onset of movement and during rapid changes in tension. The Type II receptors fire during active or passive motion of a joint, or with the application of traction.
III. Large Ruffini. Slowly adapting, high threshold receptors	Ligaments and the fibrous capsule.	Detect large amounts of tension. These receptors only become active in the extremes of motion or when strong manual techniques are applied to the joint.
IV. Nociceptors. Slowly adapting, high threshold free nerve endings		Inactive in normal circumstances but become active with marked mechanical deformation or tension Also active in response to direct mechanical or chemical irritation

[a]Wyke BD: The neurology of joints: A review of general principles. Clin Rheum Dis 1981;7:223–239.
[b]Wyke BD: Articular neurology and manipulative therapy. In Glasgow EF, et al. (eds): Aspects of Manipulative Therapy, pp 72–77. New York: Churchill Livingstone, 1985.

described as the erect standing position with the feet just slightly separated and the arms hanging by the side, the elbows straight and with the palms of the hand facing forward (Figure 1-2).

Directional Terms

Directional terms are used to describe the relationship of body parts or the location of an external object with respect to the body (Table 1-11).[15]

Movements of Body Segments

Movements of body segments occur in three dimensions along imaginary planes and around various axes of the body.

TABLE 1-10 Characteristics of the Propioceptors

Type of sensory receptors	Stimulus		Receptor	
	General term	Specific nature	Term	Location
Proprio-ceptors	Tension	Distension	Corpuscles of Ruffini	Skin and capsules in joints and ligaments
		Length changes	Muscle spindles	Skeletal muscles
		Tension changes	Golgi tendon organs	Between muscles and tendons

Source: Previte JJ: Human Physiology. New York, McGraw-Hill, 1983.

TABLE 1-11 Directional Terms

Term	Explanation
Superior or cranial	Closer to the head
Inferior or caudal	Closer to the feet
Anterior (ventral)	Toward the front of the body
Posterior (dorsal)	Toward the back of the body
Medial	Toward the midline of the body
Lateral	Away from the midline of the body
Proximal	Closer to the trunk
Distal	Away from the trunk
Superficial	Toward the surface of the body
Deep	Away from the surface of the body in the direction of the inside of the body

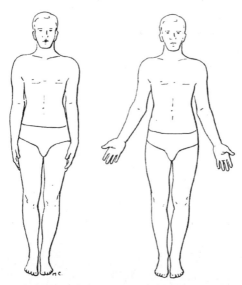

FIG. 1-2 The anatomic reference position of the body. (*Reproduced with permission from Luttgens K, Hamilton N: Kinesiology, p 40 (Fig. 2.9), 9th ed. New York, McGraw-Hill, 1997.*)

Planes of the Body

There are three traditional planes of the body corresponding to the three dimensions of space: sagittal, frontal, and transverse (Figure 1-3).[15]

- *Sagittal.* The sagittal plane (Figure 1-3a), also known as the anterior-posterior or median plane, divides the body vertically into left and right halves of equal size.
- *Frontal.* The frontal plane (Figure 1-3b), also known as the lateral or coronal plane, divides the body equally into front and back halves.
- *Transverse.* The transverse plane (Figure 1-3c), also known as the horizontal plane, divides the body equally into top and bottom halves.

If movement occurs in a plane that passes through the center of gravity, that movement is deemed to have occurred in a *cardinal* plane. Few movements involved with functional activities occur in pure cardinal planes. Instead, most movements occur in an infinite number of vertical and horizontal planes parallel to the cardinal planes (see below).

Axes of the Body

Three reference axes are used to describe human motion: frontal, sagittal, and longitudinal. The axis around which the movement takes place is always perpendicular to the plane in which it occurs.

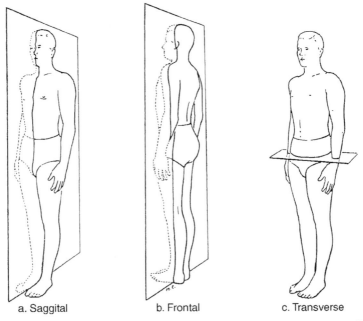

a. Saggital   b. Frontal   c. Transverse

FIG. 1-3   Planes of the body. (*Reproduced with permission from Luttgens K, Hamilton N: Kinesiology, p 31 (Fig. 2.1), 9th ed. New York, McGraw-Hill, 1997.*)

- *Frontal.* The frontal axis, also known as the transverse axis, is perpendicular to the sagittal plane.
- *Sagittal.* The sagittal axis is perpendicular to the frontal plane.
- *Longitudinal.* The longitudinal axis, also known as the vertical axis, is perpendicular to the transverse plane.

The planes and axes for the more common planar movements are outlined in Table 1-12.

Both the configuration of a joint and the line of pull of the muscle acting at a joint determine the motion that occurs at a joint:

- A muscle whose line of pull is lateral to the joint is a potential abductor.
- A muscle whose line of pull is medial to the joint is a potential adductor.
- A muscle whose line of pull is anterior to a joint has the potential to extend or flex the joint. At the knee, an anterior line of pull may cause the knee to extend, whereas at the elbow joint, an anterior line of pull, may cause flexion of the elbow.
- A muscle whose line of pull is posterior to the joint has the potential to extend or flex a joint (refer to example above).

Joint Kinematics

Kinematics is the study of motion. In studying joint kinematics, two major types of motion are involved: (1) the osteokinematic and (2) the arthrokinematic.

Osteokinematic Motion

Osteokinematic motion occurs when any object forms the radius of an imaginary circle about a fixed point. All human body segment motions involve osteokinematic motions. Examples of osteokinematic motion include abduction or adduction of the arm, flexion of the hip or knee, and side flexion of the trunk.

TABLE 1-12 Planar Motions and Their Respective Planes and Axes of Motion

Planar motion	Plane and axis of motion
Flexion, extension, hyperextension, dorsiflexion, and plantar flexion	In a sagittal plane around a frontal-horizontal axis
Abduction, adduction; side flexion of the trunk; elevation, and depression of the shoulder girdle; radial and ulnar deviation of the wrist; eversion and inversion of the foot	In the frontal plane around a sagittal-horizontal axis
Rotation of the head, neck, and trunk; internal and external rotation of the arm or leg; horizontal adduction and abduction of the arm or thigh; pronation and supination of the forearm	In the transverse plane around the longitudinal axis
Arm circling and trunk circling (circumduction)	Involve an orderly sequence of circular movements that occur in the sagittal, frontal, and intermediate oblique planes, so that segment as a whole incorporates a combination of flexion, extension, abduction, and adduction

Arthrokinematic Motion

The motions occurring at the joint surfaces are termed *arthrokinematic* movements. For the sake of simplicity, the shapes of these articulating surfaces in synovial joints are described as being *ovoid* or *sellar* in shape. Under this concept, an articulating surface can be either concave (female) or convex (male) in shape or a combination of both shapes (sellar). An example of an ovoid joint is the glenohumeral joint—the humeral head is the convex surface and the glenoid fossa is the concave surface. An example of a sellar joint is the first carpometacarpal joint.

Normal arthrokinematic motions must occur for full-range physiologic motion to take place. A restriction of arthrokinematic motion results in a decrease in osteokinematic motion. The three types of movement that occur at the articulating surfaces include:[16]

- *Roll.* A roll occurs when the points of contact on each joint surface are constantly changing (Figure 1-4). This type of movement is analogous to a tire on a car as the car rolls forward. The term *rock* is often used to describe small rolling motions.
- *Slide.* A slide is a pure translation. It occurs if only one point on the moving surface makes contact with varying points on the opposing surface (see Figure 1-4). This type of movement is analogous to a car tire skidding when the brakes are applied suddenly on a wet road. This type of motion is also referred to as *translatory* or *accessory* motion. The roll of a joint always occurs in the same direction as the swing of a bone, whereas the shapes of the articulating surfaces determine the direction of the joint glide (Figure 1-5). This rule is often referred to as the *concave-convex rule*: If the joint surface

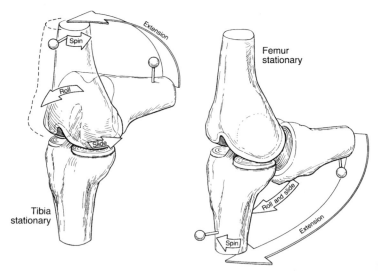

FIG. 1-4 Joint movements. (*Reproduced with permission from Dutton M: Manual Therapy of the Spine, p 43 (Fig. 3.1). New York, McGraw-Hill, 2001.*)

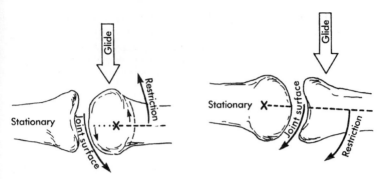

FIG. 1-5   Gliding motions according to joint surface shapes. (*Reproduced with permission from Dutton M: Manual Therapy of the Spine, p 44 (Fig. 3.2). New York, McGraw-Hill, 2001.*)

is convex relative to the other surface, the slide occurs in the opposite direction to the osteokinematic motion (see Figure 1-5). If, on the other hand, the joint surface is concave, the slide occurs in the same direction as the osteokinematic motion.

- *Spin.* A spin is defined as any movement in which the bone moves but the mechanical axis remains stationary. A spin involves a rotation of one surface on an opposing surface around a longitudinal axis (see Figure 1-4). This type of motion is analogous to the pirouette performed in ballet. Spin motions in the body include internal and external rotation of the glenohumeral joint when the humerus is abducted to 90°, and at the radial head during forearm pronation and supination.

Osteokinematic and arthrokinematic motions are directly proportional to each other and one cannot occur completely without the other. It therefore follows that if a joint is not functioning correctly, one, or both, of these motions is at fault. When examining a patient with movement impairment, it is critical that the clinician determines whether the osteokinematic motion or the arthrokinematic motion is restricted so that the intervention can be made as specific as possible.

Degrees of Freedom

The number of independent modes of motion at a joint is called the *degrees of freedom* (DOF) (Table 1-13). If a joint can swing in one direction or can only spin, it is said to have 1 DOF.[4,17–19] If a joint can spin and swing in one way only or it can swing in two completely distinct ways, but not spin, it is said to have 2 DOF.[4,17–19] If the bone can spin and also swing in two distinct directions then it is said to have 3 DOF.[4,17–19]

Most habitual movements, or those movements that occur most frequently at a joint, involve a conjunct rotation. However, the conjunct rotations are not always under volitional control. In fact, the conjunct rotation is only under volitional control in joints with 3 DOF (glenohumeral, and hip joints). In those joints with fewer than 3 DOF (hinge joints such as the tibiofemoral and ulnohumeral joints), the conjunct rotation occurs as part of the movement but

TABLE 1-13 Degrees of Freedom and Joint Examples

Degrees of freedom	Joint examples
1	The proximal interphalangeal joint
2	The tibiofemoral joint, temporomandibular joint, proximal and distal radioulnar joints, subtalar joint, and talocalcaneal joint
3	Glenohumeral joint and hip

is not under voluntary control. Joint mobilizing techniques must take into consideration both the relative shapes of the articulating surfaces, in addition to the conjunct rotation that is associated with a particular motion.

Close-Packed and Open-Packed Positions of the Joint

Joint movements are usually accompanied by a relative compression (approximation) or distraction (separation) of the opposing joint surfaces. These relative compressions or distractions affect the level of *congruity* of the opposing surfaces. The position of maximum congruity of the opposing joint surfaces is termed the *close-packed* position of the joint. The close-packed positions for the various joints are depicted in Table 1-14. The position of least congruity is termed the *open-packed* position. The open-packed positions for the various joints are depicted in Table 1-15. Movements toward the close-packed position of a joint involve an element of compression, whereas movements out of this position involve an element of distraction.

TABLE 1-14 The Close-Packed Position of the Major Joints

Joint	Position
Zygapophysial (spine)	Extension
Temporomandibular	Teeth clenched
Glenohumeral	Abduction and external rotation
Acromioclavicular	Arm abducted to 90°
Sternoclavicular	Maximum shoulder elevation
Ulnohumeral	Extension
Radiohumeral	Elbow flexed 90°, Forearm supinated 5°
Proximal radioulnar	5° supination
Distal radioulnar	5° supination
Radiocarpal (wrist)	Extension with radial deviation
Metacarpophalangeal	Full flexion
Metacarpophalangeal	Full opposition
Interphalangeal	Full extension
Hip	Full extension, internal rotation, abduction
Tibiofemoral	Full extension, external rotation of tibia
Talocrural (ankle)	Maximum dorsiflexion
Subtalar	Supination
Midtarsal	Supination
Tarsometatarsal	Supination
Metatarsophalangeal	Full extension
Interphalangeal	Full extension

TABLE 1-15 The Open-Packed (Resting) Position of the Major Joints

Joint	Position
Zygapophysial (spine)	Midway between flexion and extension
Temporomandibular	Mouth slightly open (freeway space)
Glenohumeral	55° abduction, 30° horizontal adduction
Acromioclavicular	Arm resting by side
Sternoclavicular	Arm resting by side
Ulnohumeral	70° flexion, 10° supination
Radiohumeral	Full extension, full supination
Proximal radioulnar	70° flexion, 35° supination
Distal radioulnar	10° supination
Radiocarpal (wrist)	Neutral with slight ulnar deviation
Carpometacarpal	Midway between abduction-adduction and flexion-extension
Metacarpophalangeal	Slight flexion
Interphalangeal	Slight flexion
Hip	30° flexion, 30° abduction, slight lateral rotation
Knee	25° flexion
Talocrural (ankle)	10° plantar flexion, midway between maximum inversion and eversion
Subtalar	Midway between extremes of range of movement
Midtarsal	Midway between extremes of range of movement
Tarsometatarsal	Midway between extremes of range of movement
Metatarsophalangeal	Neutral
Interphalangeal	Slight flexion

Hypomobility, Hypermobility, and Instability

If a joint moves less than what is considered normal, or when compared to the same joint on the opposite extremity, it may be deemed *hypomobile*. A joint that moves more than considered normal when compared to the same joint on the opposite extremity may be deemed *hypermobile*. Hypermobility may occur as a generalized phenomenon or be localized to just one direction of movement.

The term *stability*, specifically related to the joint, has been the subject of much research.[20–35] In contrast to a hypermobile joint, an unstable joint involves a disruption of the osseous and ligamentous structures of that joint, and results in a loss of function. Joint stability may be viewed as a factor of joint integrity, elastic energy, passive stiffness, and muscle activation.

- *Joint integrity.* Joint integrity is enhanced in those ball and socket joints with deeper sockets, or steeper sides as opposed to those with planar sockets and shallower sides. Joint integrity is also dependent on the attributes of the supporting structures around the joint, and the extent of joint disease.
- *Elastic energy.* Connective tissues are elastic structures and as such, are capable of storing elastic energy when stretched. This stored elastic energy may then be used to help return the joint to its original position when the stresses are removed.
- *Passive stiffness.* Individual joints have passive stiffness that increases toward the joint end range. An injury to these passive structures causing inherent loss in the passive stiffness, results in joint laxity.[36]
- *Muscle activation.* Muscle activation increases stiffness, both within the muscle and within the joint(s) it crosses.[37] However, the synergists and

antagonist muscles that cross the joint must be activated with the correct and appropriate activation in terms of magnitude or timing. A faulty motor control system can lead to inappropriate magnitudes of muscle force and stiffness, allowing for a joint to buckle or undergo shear translation.[37]

Pathologic breakdown of the above factors may result in *instability*. Two types of instability are recognized: articular and ligamentous. Articular instability can lead to abnormal patterns of coupled and translational movements.[38] Ligamentous instability may lead to multiple planes of aberrant joint motion.[39]

REFERENCES

1. Greathouse DG, Halle JS, Dalley AF: Terminologia anatomica: revised anatomical terminology. J Orthop Sports Phys Ther 2004;34:363–367.
2. Federative Committee on Anatomical Terminology: Terminologia Anatomica. Stuttgart, Germany, Georg Thieme Verlag, 1998.
3. Hall SJ: The biomechanics of human skeletal muscle. In Hall SJ (ed): Basic Biomechanics, pp 146–185. New York, McGraw-Hill, 1999.
4. MacConnail MA, Basmajian JV: Muscles and Movements: A Basis for Human Kinesiology. New York, Robert Krieger, 1977.
5. Janda V: Muscle Function Testing, pp 163–167. London, Butterworths, 1983.
6. Teitz CC, et al.: Tendon problems in athletic individuals. J Bone Joint Surg 1997;79-A:138–152.
7. Freeman MAR, Wyke BD: An experimental study of articular neurology. J Bone Joint Surg 1967;49B:185.
8. Wyke BD: The neurology of joints. Ann R Coll Surg Engl 1967;41:25–50.
9. Chusid JG: Correlative Neuroanatomy & Functional Neurology, pp 144–148. Norwalk, CT, Appleton-Century-Crofts, 1985.
10. Wyke BD: The neurology of joints: a review of general principles. Clin Rheum Dis 1981;7:223–239.
11. Cyriax J: Textbook of Orthopaedic Medicine, Diagnosis of Soft Tissue Lesions, 8th ed. London, Bailliere Tindall, 1982.
12. McCloskey DI: Kinesthetic sensibility. Physiol Rev 1978;58:763–820.
13. Borsa PA, et al.: Functional assessment and rehabilitation of shoulder proprioception for glenohumeral instability. J Sport Rehab 1994;3:84–104.
14. Lephart SM, et al.: Proprioception of the shoulder joint in healthy, unstable and surgically repaired shoulders. J Shoulder Elbow Surg 1994;3:371–380.
15. Hall SJ: Kinematic concepts for analyzing human motion. In Hall SJ (ed): Basic Biomechanics, pp 28–89. New York, McGraw-Hill, 1999.
16. MacConaill MA: Arthrology. In Warwick R, Williams PL (eds): Gray's Anatomy. Philadelphia, PA, WB Saunders, 1975.
17. Lehmkuhl LD, Smith LK: Brunnstrom's Clinical Kinesiology, pp 361–390. Philadelphia, PA, FA Davis, 1983.
18. Rasch PJ, Burke RK: Kinesiology and Applied Anatomy. Philadelphia, PA, Lea and Febiger, 1971.
19. Steindler A: Kinesiology of the Human Body under Normal and Pathological Conditions. Springfield, IL, Charles C Thomas, 1955.
20. Answorth AA, Warner JJP: Shoulder instability in the athlete. Orthop Clin N Am 1995;26:487–504.
21. Bergmark A: Stability of the lumbar spine. Acta Orthop Scand 1989;60:1–54.
22. Boden BP, et al.: Patellofemoral instability: evaluation and management. J Am Acad Orthop Surg 1997;5:47–57.
23. Callanan M, et al.: Shoulder instability. Diagnosis and management. Aust Family Phys 2001;30:655–661.
24. Cass JR, Morrey BF: Ankle instability: current concepts, diagnosis, and treatment. Mayo Clin Proc 1984;59(3):165–170.

25. Clanton TO: Instability of the subtalar joint. Orthop Clin N Am 1989;20:583–592.
26. Cox JS, Cooper PS: Patellofemoral instability. In Fu FH, Harner CD, Vince KG (eds): Knee Surgery, pp 959–962. Baltimore, MD, Williams & Wilkins, 1994.
27. Freeman MAR, Dean MRE, Hanham IWF: The etiology and prevention of functional instability of the foot. J Bone Joint Surg 1965;47B:678–685.
28. Friberg O: Lumbar instability: a dynamic approach by traction-compression radiography. Spine 1987;12:119–129.
29. Grieve GP: Lumbar instability. Physiotherapy 1982;68:2.
30. Hotchkiss RN, Weiland AJ: Valgus stability of the elbow. J Orthop Res 1987;5:372–377.
31. Kaigle A, Holm S, Hansson T: Experimental instability in the lumbar spine. Spine 1995;20:421–430.
32. Kuhlmann JN, et al.: Stability of the normal wrist. In Tubiana R (ed): The Hand, pp 934–944. Philadelphia, PA, WB Saunders, 1985.
33. Landeros O, Frost HM, Higgins CC: Post traumatic anterior ankle instability. Clin Orthop 1968;56:169–178.
34. Luttgens K, Hamilton N: The center of gravity and stability. In Luttgens K, Hamilton N (eds): Kinesiology: Scientific Basis of Human Motion, pp 415–442. Dubuque, IA, McGraw-Hill, 1997.
35. Wilke H, et al.: Stability of the lumbar spine with different muscle groups: a biomechanical in vitro study. Spine 1995;20:192–198.
36. Panjabi MM: The stabilizing system of the spine. Part 1. Function, dysfunction adaption, and enhancement. J Spinal Disord, 1992;5:383–389.
37. McGill SM, Cholewicki J: Biomechanical basis for stability: an explanation to enhance clinical utility. J Orthop Sports Phys Ther 2001;31:96–100.
38. Gertzbein SD, et al.: Centrode patterns and segmental instability in degenerative disc disease. Spine 1985;10:257–261.
39. Cholewicki J, McGill S: Mechanical stability of the in vivo lumbar spine: implications for injury and chronic low back pain. Clin Biomech 1996;11:1–15.

2 | The Nervous System

OVERVIEW

The nervous system can be divided into two anatomic divisions, each with their own subdivisions:

- Central nervous system
  - Brain
  - Spinal cord
- Peripheral nervous system
  - Cranial nerves (with the exception of the second cranial nerve)
  - Spinal nerve roots
  - Dorsal root ganglia
  - Peripheral nerve trunks and their terminal branches
  - Peripheral autonomic nervous system

CENTRAL NERVOUS SYSTEM

The central nervous system (CNS) consists of the brain and an elongated spinal cord. The spinal cord participates directly with the transmission of motor information that controls body movements, the processing and transmission of sensory information from the trunk and limbs, and the regulation of visceral functions.[1]

The spinal cord also provides a conduit for the two-way transmission of messages between the brain and the body. These messages may descend, or ascend along pathways, or tracts, which are fiber bundles of similar groups of neurons, each with specific functions (Boxes 2-1 to 2-3).[2–15]

Three membranes, or meninges, envelop the structures of the CNS: the dura, the arachnoid, and the pia (see *Orthopaedic Examination, Evaluation, and Intervention*, p 22). The meninges, and related spaces, are important to both the nutrition and protection of the spinal cord. The cerebrospinal fluid that flows through the meningeal spaces, and within the ventricles of the brain, provides a cushion for the spinal cord. The meninges also form barriers that resist the entrance of a variety of noxious organisms.

The spinal cord has an external segmental organization (Figure 2-1). Each of the 31 pairs of spinal nerves that arise from the spinal cord has a ventral root and a dorsal root, with each root made up of one to eight rootlets, and each root consisting of bundles of nerve fibers.[16] In the dorsal root of a typical spinal nerve, lies a dorsal root ganglion, a swelling that contains nerve cell bodies.[16]

PERIPHERAL NERVOUS SYSTEM—SOMATIC NERVES

The somatic divisions of the peripheral nervous system consist of the cranial nerves and the spinal nerves.

Cranial Nerves

The cranial nerves (CN) are typically described as comprising 12 pairs, which are referred to by the Roman numerals I through XII (Table 2-1). The cranial

BOX 2-1 The Dorsal Medial Lemniscus Tract

- Conveys impulses concerned with well-localized touch and with the sense of movement and position (kinesthesis)
- Important in moment-to-moment (temporal) and point-to-point (spatial) discrimination
- Makes it possible for you to put a key in a door lock without light or visualize the position of any part of your body without looking
- Lesions to the tract from destructive tumors, hemorrhage, scar tissue, swelling, infections, direct trauma, etc., abolish or diminish tactile sensations and movement or position sense
- The cell bodies of the primary neurons in the dorsal column pathway are in the spinal ganglion; the peripheral processes of these neurons begin at receptors in the joint capsule, muscles, and skin (tactile and pressure receptors)

BOX 2-2 The Spinothalamic Tract

The spinothalamic tract helps mediate the sensations of pain, cold, warmth, and touch from receptors throughout the body (except the face) to the brain.[2–5]

- Laterally projecting spinothalamic neurons are more likely to be situated in laminae I and V.
- Medially projecting cells are more likely to be situated in the deep dorsal horn and in the ventral horn.

Most of the cells project to the contralateral thalamus, although a small fraction projects ipsilaterally.[6]

Spinothalamic axons in the anterior-lateral quadrant of the spinal cord are arranged somatotopically—at cervical levels, spinothalamic axons representing the lower extremity and caudal body are placed more laterally, and those representing the upper extremity and anterior body, more anterior-medially.[7,8]

Most of the neurons show their best responses when the skin is stimulated mechanically at a noxious intensity. However, many spinothalamic tract cells also respond, although less effectively, to innocuous mechanical stimuli, and some respond best to innocuous mechanical stimuli.[9]

A large fraction of spinothalamic tract cells also respond to a noxious heating of the skin,[10] while others respond to stimulation of the receptors in muscles,[11] joints, or viscera.[12]

Spinothalamic tract cells can be inhibited effectively by repetitive electrical stimulation of peripheral nerves,[13] with the inhibition outlasting the stimulation by 20–30 minutes.

Some inhibition can be evoked by stimulation of the large myelinated axons of a peripheral nerve, but the inhibition is much more powerful if small myelinated or unmyelinated afferents, are included in the volleys.[14] The best inhibition is produced by stimulation of a peripheral nerve in the same limb as the excitatory receptive field, but some inhibition occurs when nerves in other limbs are stimulated. A similar inhibition results when high-intensity stimuli are applied to the skin with a clinical transcutaneous electrical nerve stimulator (TENS) unit in place of direct stimulation of a peripheral nerve.[15]

As the spinothalamic tract ascends, it migrates from a lateral position to a posterior-lateral position. In the midbrain, the tract lies adjacent to the medial lemniscus. The axons of the secondary neurons terminate in one of a number of centers in the thalamus.

BOX 2-3 The Spinocerebellar Tract

- Conducts impulses related to the position and movement of muscles to the cerebellum, enabling the cerebellum to add smoothness and precision to patterns of movement initiated in the cerebral hemispheres.
- Spinocerebellar impulses do not reach the cerebrum directly and therefore have no conscious representation.
- Four tracts constitute the spinocerebellar pathway: posterior spinocerebellar and cuneocerebellar, and anterior and rostral spinocerebellar tracts. The posterior spinocerebellar tract conveys muscle spindle- or tendon organ-related impulses from the lower half of the body (below the level of the T6 spinal cord segment). The cuneocerebellar tract is concerned with such impulses from the body above T6.
- The axons conducting impulses from muscle spindles, tendon organs, and skin in the lower half of the body are large type Ia, Ib, and type II fibers, the cell bodies of which are in the spinal ganglia of spinal nerves T6 and below.
- Primary neurons below L3 send their central processes into the posterior columns. These processes then ascend in the columns to the L3 level. From L3 up to T6, incoming central processes and those in the posterior columns project to the medial part of lamina VII, called Clarke's column. Here the central processes of the primary neurons synapse with secondary neurons, the axons of which are directed to the lateral funiculi as the posterior spinocerebellar tracts.

---

nerve roots enter and exit the brain stem to provide sensory and motor innervation to the head and muscles of the face. CN I (olfactory) and II (optic) are not true nerves but are fiber tracts of the brain (see *Orthopaedic Examination, Evaluation, and Intervention*, pp 23–25).

The Spinal Nerves

A total of 31 symmetrically arranged pairs of spinal nerves exit from all levels of the vertebral column, except for those of C1 and C2,[17] each derived from the spinal cord. The spinal nerves are divided topographically into 8 cervical pairs (C1-8), 12 thoracic pairs (T1-12), 5 lumbar pairs (L1-5), 5 sacral pairs (S1-5), and a coccygeal pair (see Figure 2-1). Nerve fibers can be categorized according to function: sensory, motor, or mixed (Table 2-2). The dorsal and ventral roots of the spinal nerves are located within the vertebral canal. The portion of the spinal nerve that is not within the vertebral canal, and which usually occupies the intervertebral foramen, is referred to as a peripheral nerve. Spinal nerves and peripheral nerves can be injured anywhere along their distribution, although some sites are more commonly injured than others. Compression and/or irritation of cervical or lumbar nerve roots can cause radiculopathy, a common cause of symptoms. Peripheral nerve injuries can occur at the level of the axon (i.e., axonopathy), the motor neuron or dorsal root ganglion (i.e., neuronopathies). Because motor and sensory axons run in the same nerves, disorders of the peripheral nerves (neuropathies) usually affect both motor and sensory functions. Peripheral symptoms can manifest as abnormal, frequently unpleasant sensations, which are variously described by the patient as numbness, pins and needles, and tingling, but more correctly termed *paresthesias*.[18] Paresthesias can occur anywhere within

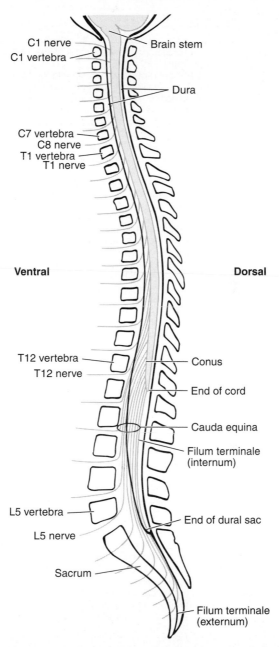

FIG. 2-1 Schematic illustration of the spinal cord. (*Reproduced with permission from Waxman: Corrective Neuroanatomy, p 71, 24th ed., New York, McGraw-Hill, 2000.*)

TABLE 2-1 Cranial Nerves and Their Functions

	Cranial nerve	Function
I.	Olfactory	The olfactory nerve is responsible for the sense of smell.
II.	Optic	The optic nerve is responsible for vision.
III.	Oculomotor	The somatic portion of the oculomotor nerve supplies the levator palpebrae superioris muscle, the superior, medial and inferior rectus muscles, and the inferior oblique muscles. These muscles are responsible for some eye movements.
		The visceral efferent portion of this nerve innervates two smooth intraocular muscles: the ciliary and the constrictor pupillae. These muscles are responsible for papillary constriction.
IV.	Trochlear	The trochlear nerve supplies the superior oblique muscle.
V.	Trigeminal	All three of these branches contain sensory cells.
		The ophthalmic and maxillary are exclusively sensory, the latter supplying the soft and hard palate, maxillary sinuses, upper teeth and upper lip and the mucous membrane of the pharynx.
		The mandibular branch carries sensory information but also represents the motor component of the nerve, supplying the muscles of mastication, both pterygoids, the anterior belly of digastric, tensor tympani, tensor veli palatini, and mylohyoid.
VI.	Abducens	The abducens nerve innervates the lateral rectus muscle.
VII.	Facial	The facial nerve comprises a sensory (intermediate) root, which conveys taste; a motor root; the facial nerve proper, which supplies the muscles of facial expression; the platysma muscle; and the stapedius muscle of the inner ear.
VIII.	Vestibulocochlear	The cochlear portion is concerned with the sense of hearing.
		The vestibular portion is part of the system of equilibrium, the vestibular system.
IX.	Glossopharyngeal	The glossopharyngeal nerve serves a number of functions, including supplying taste fibers for the posterior third of the tongue.
X.	Vagus	The vagus nerve contains somatic motor, visceral efferent, visceral sensory, and somatic sensory fibers. The functions of the vagus nerve are numerous.
XI.	Accessory	The cranial root is often viewed as an aberrant portion of the vagus nerve.
		The spinal portion of the nerve supplies the sternocleidomastoid and the trapezius muscles.
XII.	Hypoglossal	The hypoglossal nerve is the motor nerve of the tongue, innervating the ipsilateral side of the tongue, as well as forming the descendens hypoglossi, which anastomoses with other cervical branches to form the ansa hypoglossi, which in turn innervates the infrahyoid muscles.

TABLE 2-2 Nerve Fiber Types and Their Functions

Nerve fiber type	Function	Example
Sensory	Carry afferents from a portion of the skin. Carry efferents to the skin structures. This area of distribution is called a dermatome, which is a well-defined segmental portion of the skin (Figure 2-2), and generally follows the segmental distribution of the underlying muscle innervation.[2]	Lateral femoral cutaneous nerve Saphenous nerve Interdigital nerves
Motor	Carry efferents to muscles, and return sensation from muscles and associated ligamentous structures. Any nerve that innervates a muscle, also mediates the sensation from the joint on which that muscle acts.	Ulnar nerve Suprascapular nerve Dorsal scapular nerve
Mixed	Combination of skin, sensory, and motor functions	Median nerve Ulnar nerve (at the elbow as it enters the tunnel of Guyon) Common peroneal nerve Ilioinguinal nerve

a dermatomal distribution, or within a peripheral nerve distribution (Figure 2-2). The basic pathophysiology of paresthesias is some form of alteration in nerve or nerve pathway function. Paresthesias are thought to represent abnormal showers of impulses generated from an ectopic focus[19] and can arise from an abnormality anywhere along the sensory pathway, from the peripheral nerves to the sensory cortex of the CNS.[20]

The Cervical Nerves

The eight pairs of cervical nerves are derived from cord segments between the level of the foramen magnum and the middle of the seventh cervical vertebra.[21] Each nerve joins with a gray communicating ramus from the sympathetic trunk, and sends a small recurrent meningeal branch back into the spinal canal to supply the dura with sensory and vasomotor innervation. It also branches into anterior and posterior primary divisions, which are mixed nerves that pass to their respective peripheral distributions. The motor branches carry a few sensory fibers that convey proprioceptive impulses from the neck muscles.

Posterior Primary Divisions

The C1 (suboccipital) nerve serves the muscles of the suboccipital triangle, with very few sensory fibers.[21]

Anterior Primary Divisions

The anterior primary divisions of the first four cervical nerves (C1-4) form the cervical plexus.

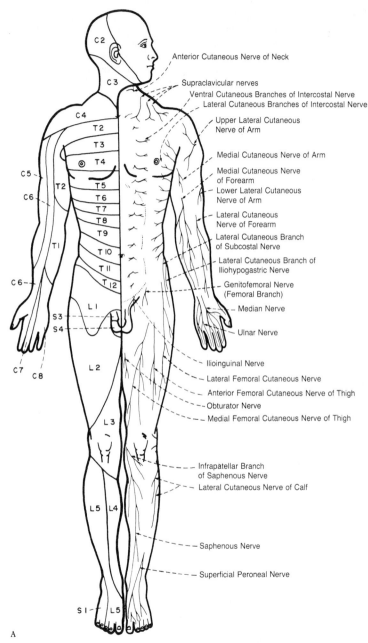

FIG. 2-2 Segmental distribution of the body. (*Reproduced with permission from Wilkins, Rengachary: Neurosurgery, vol 1, New York, McGraw-Hill, 1996.*) (*Continued*)

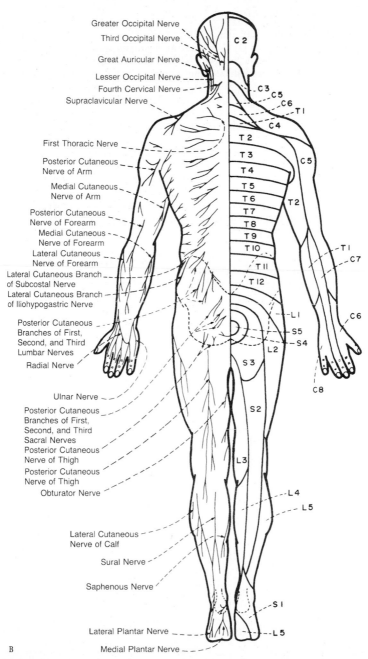

Greater Occipital Nerve
Third Occipital Nerve
Great Auricular Nerve
Lesser Occipital Nerve
Fourth Cervical Nerve
Supraclavicular Nerve
First Thoracic Nerve
Posterior Cutaneous Nerve of Arm
Medial Cutaneous Nerve of Arm
Posterior Cutaneous Nerve of Forearm
Medial Cutaneous Nerve of Forearm
Lateral Cutaneous Nerve of Forearm
Lateral Cutaneous Branch of Subcostal Nerve
Lateral Cutaneous Branch of Iliohypogastric Nerve
Posterior Cutaneous Branches of First, Second, and Third Lumbar Nerves
Radial Nerve
Ulnar Nerve
Posterior Cutaneous Branches of First, Second, and Third Sacral Nerves
Posterior Cutaneous Nerve of Thigh
Posterior Cutaneous Nerve of Thigh
Obturator Nerve
Lateral Cutaneous Nerve of Calf
Sural Nerve
Saphenous Nerve
Lateral Plantar Nerve
Medial Plantar Nerve

C 2
C 3
C 5
C 6
T 1
C 4
T 2
T 3
T 4
T 5
T 6
T 7
T 8
T 9
T 10
T 11
T 12
C 5
T 2
T 1
C 7
C 6
L 1
S 5
S 4
L 2
S 3
C 8
S 2
L 3
L 4
L 5
S 1
L 5

B

FIG. 2-2 (Continued)

The Cervical Plexus (C1-4) (Table 2-3)

Muscular branches (Figure 2-3) (see *Orthopaedic Examination, Evaluation, and Intervention*, p 31) Communication with the hypoglossal nerve from C1-2 carries motor fibers to the geniohyoid and thyrohyoid muscles, and to the sternohyoid and sternothyroid muscles by way of the superior root of the ansa cervicalis. The nerve to the superior belly of the omohyoid branches from the superior root. The nerve to the inferior belly of the omohyoid also branches from the loop of the ansa cervicalis. There is a branch to the sternocleidomastoid muscle from C2, and branches to the trapezius muscles (C3-4) via the subtrapezial plexus. Smaller branches to the adjacent vertebral musculature supply the rectus capitis lateralis and rectus capitis anterior (C1), the longus capitis (C2, 4) and longus coli (C1-4), the scalenus medius (C3, 4) and scalenus anterior (C4), and the levator scapulae (C3-5). The phrenic nerve (C3-5) consists of motor and sensory branches.[21] The motor branches supply the diaphragm. Sensory branches supply the pericardium, the diaphragm, and part of the costal and mediastinal pleurae.

The Brachial Plexus

The brachial plexus (Figure 2-4) arises from the anterior primary divisions of the fifth cervical through the first thoracic nerve roots, with occasional contributions from the fourth cervical and second thoracic roots. The roots of the plexus, which consist of C5 and C6, join to form the upper trunk, C7 becomes the middle trunk, and C8 and T1 join to form the lower trunks. Each of the trunks divides into anterior and posterior divisions, which then form cords (see Figure 2-4).

The anterior divisions of the upper and middle trunk form the lateral cord; the anterior division of the lower trunk forms the medial cord; and all three posterior divisions unite to form the posterior cord. The three cords, named for their relationship to the axillary artery, split to form the main branches of the plexus. These branches give rise to the peripheral nerves (Table 2-4): musculocutaneous (lateral cord) (Figure 2-5), axillary and radial (posterior cord) (Figure 2-6), median (medial and lateral cords) (Figure 2-7), and ulnar (medial cord) (Figure 2-8).[22] Numerous smaller nerves arise from the roots (Table 2-5), trunks (Table 2-6), and cords (Table 2-7) of the plexus (see *Orthopaedic Examination, Evaluation, and Intervention*, pp 31–34).

TABLE 2-3 Sensory Branches of the Cervical Plexus

Nerve	Supply
The small occipital nerve (C2, 3)	The skin of the lateral occipital portion of the scalp, the upper median part of the auricle, and the area over the mastoid process
The great auricular nerve (C2, 3)	Sensation to the ear and face over the ascending ramus of the mandible
The cervical cutaneous nerve (cutaneous coli) (C2, 3)	Supplies the skin over the anterior portion of the neck
Supraclavicular branches (C3, 4)	Supply the skin over the clavicle and the upper deltoid and pectoral regions, as low as the third rib

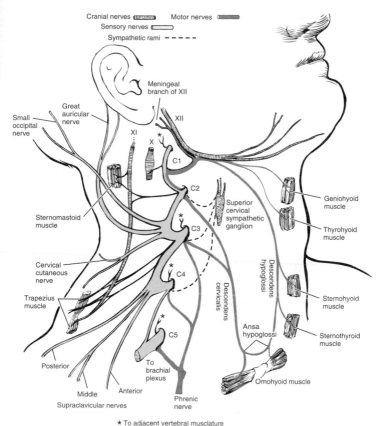

FIG. 2-3   The cervical plexus. (*Reproduced with permission from Waxman: Corrective Neuroanatomy, p 347, New York, McGraw-Hill, 2000.*)

The Thoracic Nerves

Dorsal Rami

The thoracic dorsal rami travel posteriorly, close to the vertebral zygapophyseal joints, before dividing into medial and lateral branches (Table 2-8).

The recurrent meningeal or sinuvertebral nerve, a branch of the spinal nerve, passes back into the vertebral canal through the intervertebral foramen. This nerve supplies the anterior aspect of the dura mater, outer third of the annular fibers of the intervertebral disks, vertebral body, and the epidural blood vessel walls, as well as the posterior longitudinal ligament.[23]

Ventral Rami

There are 12 pairs of thoracic ventral rami, and all but the twelfth are located between the ribs serving as intercostal nerves. All of the intercostal nerves

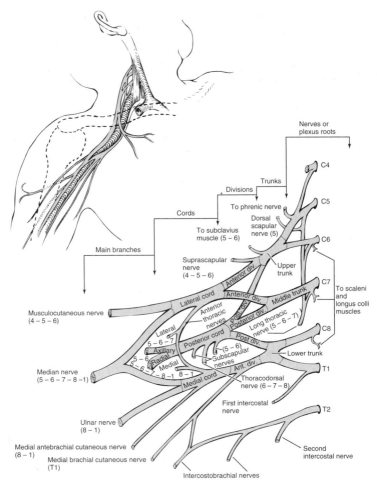

Nerves or
plexus roots

Trunks

Divisions

To phrenic nerve

Cords

Dorsal
scapular
nerve (5)

To subclavius
muscle (5 – 6)

Main branches

Suprascapular
nerve
(4 – 5 – 6)

Upper
trunk

C4

C5

C6

C7

To scaleni
and
longus colli
muscles

Anterior div.

Lateral cord

Anterior div.

Middle trunk

Musculocutaneous nerve
(4 – 5 – 6)

Anterior
thoracic
nerves

Post div.

Posterior div.

Long thoracic
nerve (5 – 6 – 7)

C8

Lateral
5 – 6 – 7

Posterior cord

Axillary
5 – 6

Radial

Medial
5 – 6 – 7 – 8 – 1

(5 – 6)
Subscapular
nerves

8 – 1

Post. div.

Ant. div.

Lower trunk

T1

Median nerve
(5 – 6 – 7 – 8 –1)

Medial cord

Thoracodorsal
nerve (6 – 7 – 8)

First intercostal
nerve

T2

Ulnar nerve
(8 – 1)

Medial antebrachial cutaneous nerve
(8 – 1)

Medial brachial cutaneous nerve
(T1)

Intercostobrachial nerves

Second
intercostal nerve

> Splitting of the plexus into anterior and posterior divisions is one of the most significant features
> in the redistribution of nerve fibers, because it is here that fibers supplying the flexor and
> extensor groups of muscles of the upper extremity are separated. Similar splitting is noted
> in the lumbar and sacral plexuses for the supply of muscles of the lower extremity.

FIG. 2-4 The brachial plexus. (*Reproduced with permission from Waxman: Corrective Neuroanatomy, p 348, New York, McGraw-Hill, 2000.*)

mainly supply the thoracic and abdominal walls with the upper two also supplying the upper limb. The thoracic ventral rami of T3-6 supply only the thoracic wall, while the lower five rami supply both the thoracic and abdominal walls. The subcostal nerve supplies both the abdominal wall and the gluteal skin.

Each of the ventral rami is connected with an adjacent sympathetic ganglion by gray and white rami communicantes. The communicating rami are branches of the spinal nerves that transmit sympathetic autonomic fibers to and from the sympathetic chain of ganglia. The fibers pass from spinal nerve to chain ganglia through the white ramus, and the reverse direction through the gray.

TABLE 2-4 Peripheral Nerves of the Upper Quadrant

Nerves	Nerve root	Muscles	Action
Musculocutaneous (Figure 2-5)	C5-6	Biceps, brachialis	Flexion of elbow
		Coracobrachialis	Shoulder flexion
Lateral brachial cutaneous nerve of the arm	C5-6	Sensory	Figure 2-5
Median (Figure 2-6)	C5-T1	Flexor carpi radialis	Radial flexion of wrist
		Flexor digitorum sublimis	Flexion of middle phalanges (digiti II-V)
		Flexor digitorum profundus (lateral half)	Flexion of distal phalanges (digiti II, III)
		Pronator teres, pronator quadratus	Pronation of forearm
		Abductor pollicis brevis	Abduction of thumb
		Opponens pollicis brevis	Opposition of thumb
		Flexor pollicis longus	Flexion of distal phalanx of thumb
		Flexor pollicis brevis	Flexion of proximal phalanx of thumb
Axillary (Figure 2-5)	C5-6	Deltoid	Shoulder abduction
		Teres minor	
Radial (Figure 2-7)	C5-T1	Triceps	Extension at elbow
		Brachioradialis	Flexion of forearm
		Extensor carpi radialis/ulnaris	Extension at wrist with radial/ulnar deviation
		Supinator	Supination of forearm
		Extensor pollicis brevis	Extension of thumb (proximal)
		Extensor pollicis longus	Extension of thumb (distal)
		Extensor indicis proprius	Extension of index (proximal)
		Extensor digiti V proprius	Extension of little finger (proximal)
		Extensor digiti communis	Extension of digits (II-V, proximal)

(*Continued*)

TABLE 2-4 Peripheral Nerves of the Upper Quadrant (*Continued*)

Nerves	Nerve root	Muscles	Action
Medial (dorsal) cutaneous (antebrachial) nerve of the forearm	C6-T1	Sensory	Figure 2-7
Lateral cutaneous (antebrachial) nerve of the forearm	C5-6	Sensory	Figure 2-5
Ulnar (Figure 2-8)	C8-T1	Flexor carpi ulnaris Flexor digitorum profundus (medial half) Abductor digiti minimi All other intrinsic muscles of hand	Ulnar flexion of wrist Flexion of distal phalanges (digiti IV, V) Abduction of digiti V Finger abduction/adduction

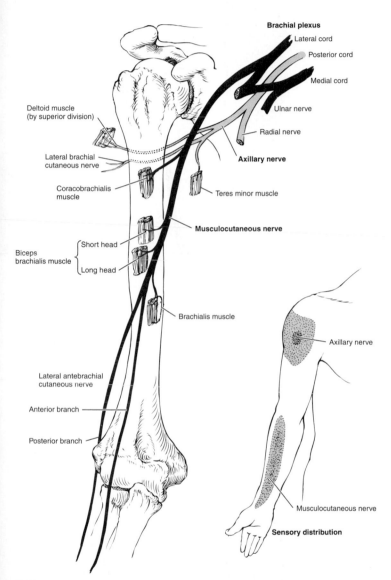

FIG. 2-5   The musculocutaneous (C5-6) and axillary (C5-6) nerves. (*Reproduced with permission from Waxman: Corrective Neuroanatomy, p 350, New York, McGraw-Hill, 2000.*)

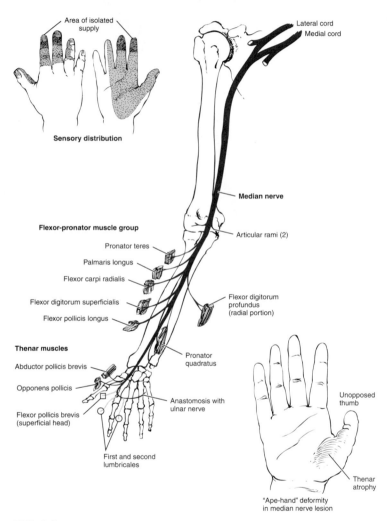

FIG. 2-6   The median nerve (C6-8; T1). (*Reproduced with permission from Waxman: Corrective Neuroanatomy, p 352, New York, McGraw-Hill, 2000.*)

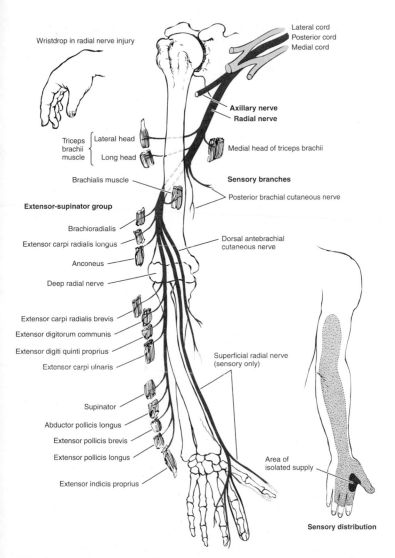

FIG. 2-7   The radial nerve (C6-8; T1). (*Reproduced with permission from Waxman: Corrective Neuroanatomy, p 351, New York, McGraw-Hill, 2000.*)

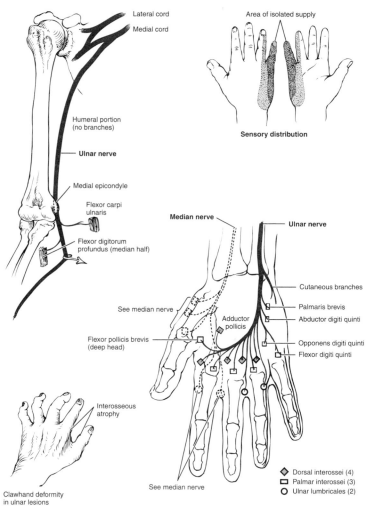

FIG. 2-8 The ulnar nerve (C8, T1). (*Reproduced with permission from Waxman: Corrective Neuroanatomy, p 353, New York, McGraw-Hill, 2000.*)

TABLE 2-5 Roots of the Brachial Plexus

Nerve	Supply	Action
The dorsal scapular nerve (C5)	Rhomboids	Scapular adduction
	Levator scapulae	Scapular elevation
The long thoracic nerve (C5, C6, and C7)	Serratus anterior (sole innervation)	Scapular abduction
		Scapular upward rotation
		Scapular elevation (weak)
Phrenic nerve (C3, C4, and C5)	Diaphragm	Increases vertical dimension of the chest cavity
		Increases abdominal pressure
Smaller branches from C6, C7, and C8	Scaleni	Rib elevation
	Longus coli	Neck side bending
		Neck rotation
		Neck flexion
		Flexes and rotates the cervical spine
The first intercostal nerve (T1)	Cutaneous	Sensation to anterior chest

TABLE 2-6 From the Trunks

Nerves	Nerve root	Muscles	Action
Subclavius	C5 and C6	Subclavius	Depresses the clavicle
			Fixates the clavicle during shoulder movements
Suprascapular	C5 and C6	Supraspinatus	Abducts the arm and stabilizes the glenohumeral joint
		Infraspinatus	Externally rotates the arm and stabilizes the glenohumeral joint

TABLE 2-7 From the Cords

Nerves	Nerve root	Muscles	Action
Lateral pectoral	C5, C6, and C7	Pectoralis major	Clavicular head: flexes and adducts arm Sternal head: adducts and internally rotates arm Accessory muscle of inspiration
Medial pectoral	C8 and T1	Pectoralis minor	Elevates ribs if the scapula is fixed Protracts scapula (assists the serratus anterior)
Upper subscapular	C7 and C8	Sub-scapularis	Internally rotates the arm Stabilizes the glenohumeral joint
Middle subscapular (Thoracodorsal)	C6, C7, and C8	Latissimus dorsi	Extends, adducts, and internally rotates arm Costal attachment helps with deep inspiration and forced expiration.
Lower subscapular	C5 and C6	Teres major	Internally rotates arm Adducts arm Stabilizes the glenohumeral joint
Medial antebrachial cutaneous	C8 and T1	Sensory	—
Medial brachial cutaneous	C8 and T1	Sensory	—

TABLE 2-8 The Thoracic Dorsal Rami

Medial branches	Lateral branches
Supply the short, medially placed back muscles (the iliocostalis thoracis, spinalis thoracis, semi-spinalis thoracis, thoracic multifidi, rotatores thoracis, and intertrans-versarii muscles) and the skin of the back as far as the midscapular line. The medial branches of the upper six thoracic dorsal rami pierce the rhomboids and trapezius, reaching the skin in close proximity to the vertebral spines, which they occasionally supply.	Supply smaller branches to the sacrospinalis muscles. The lateral branches increase in size the more inferior they are. They penetrate, or pass, the longissimus thoracis to the space between it and the iliocostalis cervicis, supplying both of these muscles, as well as the levatores costarum. The twelfth thoracic lateral branch sends a filament medially along the iliac crest, which then passes down to the anterior gluteal skin.

The Lumbar Plexus

The lumbar plexus (Figure 2-9) is formed from the ventral nerve roots of the second, third, and fourth lumbar nerves (in approximately 50% of cases, the plexus also receives a contribution from the last thoracic nerve) (Table 2-9) (see *Orthopaedic Examination, Evaluation, and Intervention*, pp 42–46). Table 2-10 outlines the peripheral nerves of the lumbar plexus.

The Sacral Plexus

The L4 and L5 nerves join medial to the sacral promontory, becoming the lumbosacral trunk. The lumbosacral trunk (L4, 5) descends into the pelvis, where it enters the formation of the sacral plexus. The S1-4 nerves converge with the lumbosacral trunk in front of the piriformis muscle, forming the

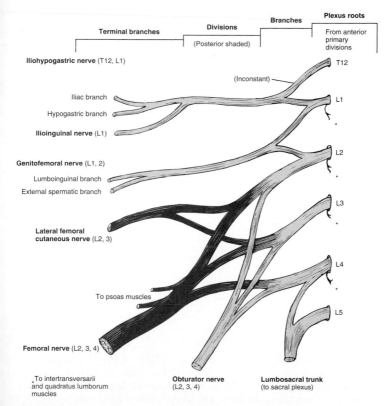

FIG. 2-9 The lumbar plexus. (*Reproduced with permission from Waxman: Corrective Neuroanatomy, p 354, New York, McGraw-Hill, 2000.*)

TABLE 2-9 Major Nerves of the Lumbosacral Plexus

Nerves	Nerve root	Muscles	Action
Femoral	L2-4	Iliopsoas	Flexion of hip
		Quadriceps	Extension of knee
Obturator	L2-4	Adductor longus, adductor brevis, adductor magnus	Adduction of hip
Superior gluteal	L4, L5, and S1	Gluteus medius, gluteus minimus, gluteus maximus	Abduction of hip
Sciatic	L4-S3	Biceps femoris, semitendinosus, semimembranosus	Flexion of leg at knee
Sciatic branches: Deep peroneal	L4-S2	Tibialis anterior	Dorsiflexion of foot
		Extensor digitorum longus	Extension of toes
		Extensor hallucis longus	Extension of great toe
Sciatic branches: Superficial peroneal	L4-S1	Peroneus	Eversion of foot
Sciatic branches: Tibial	L4-S3	Gastrocnemius, soleus	Plantar flexion of foot
		Flexor digitorum longus	Flexion of distal phalanges (II-IV)
		Flexor hallucis longus	Flexion of distal phalanges (I)
		Flexor digitorum brevis	Flexion of middle phalanges (II-V)
		Flexor hallucis brevis	Flexion of middle phalanges (I)
Lateral cutaneous nerve of the leg	L4-S2	Sensory	—
Medial plantar	L4-5	—	—
Sural	S1-2	—	—
Lateral plantar	S1-2	—	—
Pudendal	S2-4	Perineal and sphincters	Closure of sphincters, contraction of pelvic floor

broad triangular band of the sacral plexus (Figure 2-10). The upper three nerves of the plexus divide into two sets of branches; the medial branches, which are distributed to the multifidi muscles, and the lateral branches, which become the medial cluneal nerves. The medial cluneal nerves supply the skin over the medial part of the gluteus maximus. The lower two posterior primary divisions, with the posterior division of the coccygeal nerve, supply the skin over the coccyx.

TABLE 2-10 Peripheral Nerves of the Lumbar Plexus

Nerves	Nerve root	Muscles	Action
The iliohypogastric nerve (Figure 2-9)	T12, L1	Sensory	The lateral (iliac) branch supplies the skin of the upper lateral part of the thigh. The anterior (hypogastric) branch supplies the skin over the symphysis.
The ilioinguinal nerve (Figure 2-9)	L1	Sensory	Supplies the skin of the upper medial part of the thigh and the root of the penis and scrotum or mons pubis and labium majores.
The genitofemoral nerve (Figure 2-9)	L1, 2	Sensory	The genital branch supplies the cremasteric muscle and the skin of the scrotum or labia. The femoral branch supplies the skin of the middle upper part of the thigh and the femoral artery.
Femoral (Figure 2-9)	L2-4	Iliopsoas Quadriceps	Flexion of hip Extension of knee
Saphenous	L3-4	—	—
Obturator (Figure 2-9)	L2-4	Adductor longus, adductor brevis, adductor magnus	Adduction of hip
Lateral cutaneous (femoral) nerve of the thigh	L2-3	Sensory	—
Posterior cutaneous nerve of the thigh	L2-3	Sensory	—
Anterior cutaneous (femoral) nerve of the thigh	L2-3	Sensory	—

Collateral Branches of the Posterior Division

(See *Orthopaedic Examination, Evaluation, and Intervention*, p 46)

- Superior gluteal nerve (see Table 2-11; Figure 2-10)
- Inferior gluteal nerve (see Table 2-11; Figure 2-10)
- Superior cluneal nerve
- Posterior cutaneous (femoral) nerve

Collateral Branches of the Anterior Division

Collateral branches from the anterior divisions extend to the quadratus femoris and gemellus inferior muscles (from L4, 5 and S1) and to the obturator internus and gemellus superior muscles (from L5 and S1, 2) (see Figure 2-10).

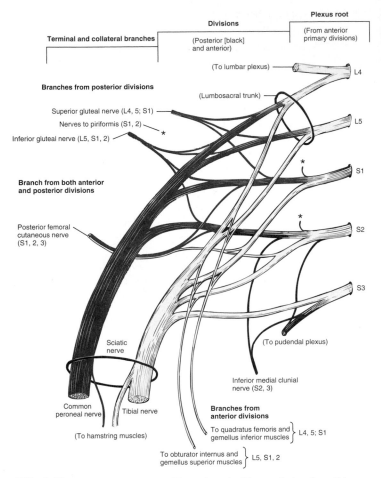

FIG. 2-10 The sacral plexus. (*Reproduced with permission from Waxman: Corrective Neuroanatomy, p 356, New York, McGraw-Hill, 2000.*)

Sciatic Nerve

The sciatic nerve (Figure 2-11) is the largest nerve in the body (see *Orthopaedic Examination, Evaluation, and Intervention*, pp 46–49). It arises from the L4, L5, and S1-3 nerve roots as a continuation of the lumbosacral plexus. The nerve is composed of the independent tibial (medial) (Figure 2-12) and common fibular (peroneal) (lateral) (Figure 2-13) divisions, which are usually united as a single nerve down to the lower portion of the thigh. The common fibular nerve is formed by the upper four posterior divisions (L4, 5 and S1, 2) of the sacral plexus, and the tibial nerve, is formed from all five anterior divisions (L4, 5 and S1, 2, 3). The tibial division is the larger of the two divisions (see Table 2-11).

TABLE 2-11 Nerves of the Sacral Plexus

Nerves	Nerve root	Muscles	Action
Superior gluteal (Figure 2-11)	L4, L5, and S1	Gluteus medius Gluteus minimus Tensor of the fascia latae	Abduction of hip
Inferior gluteal	L5-S2	Gluteus maximus	Extension of the hip
Sciatic (Figure 2-11)	L4-S3	Biceps femoris, semitendinosus, semimembranosus	Flexion of leg at knee
Sciatic branches:			
Deep fibular (peroneal) (Figure 2-11)	L4-S2	Tibialis anterior Extensor digitorum longus Extensor hallucis longus	Dorsiflexion of foot Extension of toes Extension of great toe
Sciatic branches:			
Superficial fibular (peroneal) (Figure 2-11)	L4-S1	Fibularis (peroneus) muscles	Eversion of foot
Sciatic branches:			
Tibial (Figure 2-11)	L4-S3	Gastrocnemius, soleus Flexor digitorum longus Flexor hallucis longus Flexor digitorum brevis Flexor hallucis brevis	Plantar flexion of foot Flexion of distal phalanges (II-IV) Flexion of distal phalanges (I) Flexion of middle phalanges (II-V) Flexion of middle phalanges (I)
Lateral cutaneous nerve of the leg	L4-S2	Sensory	Figure 2-13
Medial plantar	L4-5	—	Figure 2-12
Sural	S1-2	—	Figure 2-12
Lateral plantar	S1-2	—	Figure 2-12

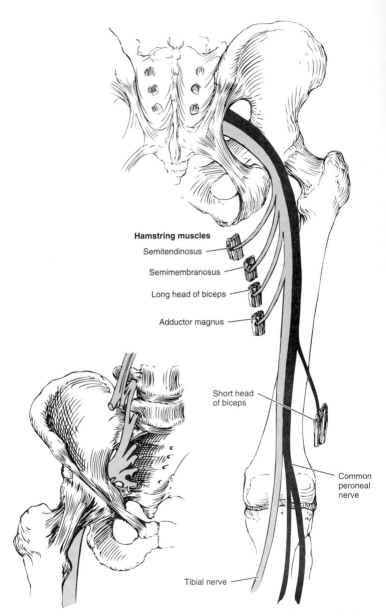

FIG. 2-11 The sciatic nerve (L4, 5; S1-3). (*Reproduced with permission from Waxman: Corrective Neuroanatomy, p 358, New York, McGraw-Hill, 2000.*)

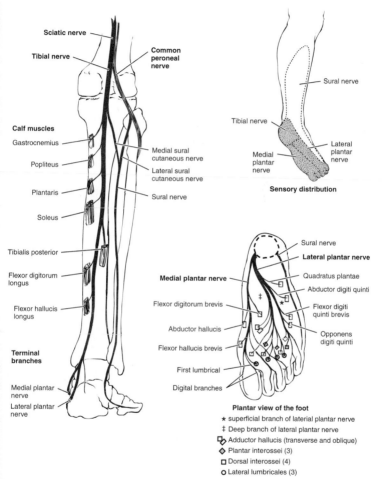

FIG. 2-12   The tibial nerve (L4, 5; S1-3). (*Reproduced with permission from Waxman: Corrective Neuroanatomy, p 360, New York, McGraw-Hill, 2000.*)

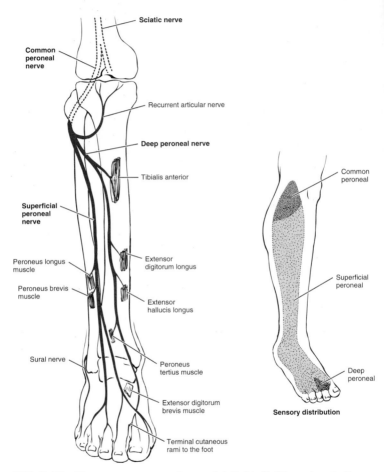

FIG. 2-13   The common peroneal nerve (L4, 5; S1, 2). (*Reproduced with permission from Waxman: Corrective Neuroanatomy, p 359, New York, McGraw-Hill, 2000.*)

Pudendal and Coccygeal Plexuses

The pudendal and coccygeal plexuses are the most caudal portions of the lumbosacral plexus and supply nerves to the perineal structures (Figure 2-14).

The pudendal plexus supplies the coccygeus, levator ani, and sphincter ani externus muscles. The pudendal nerve divides into:

- The inferior hemorrhoidal nerves to the external anal sphincter and adjacent skin
- The perineal nerve
- The dorsal nerve of the penis

The nerves of the coccygeal plexus are the small sensory anococcygeal nerves derived from the last three segments (S4, 5, C [coccyx]). They pierce the sacrotuberous ligament and supply the skin in the region of the coccyx.

PERIPHERAL NERVOUS SYSTEM—AUTONOMIC NERVES

The autonomic system (ANS) is the division of the peripheral nervous system that is responsible for the innervation of smooth muscle, cardiac muscle, and glands of the body, and functions primarily at a subconscious level.

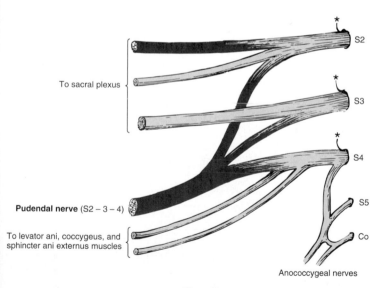

★ Visceral branches

FIG. 2-14   The pudendal and coccygeal plexuses. (*Reproduced with permission from Waxman: Corrective Neuroanatomy, p 361, New York, McGraw-Hill, 2000.*)

The ANS has two components: sympathetic (Figure 2-15) and parasympathetic (Figure 2-16), each of which is differentiated by its site of origin as well as the transmitters it releases (Table 2-12).[24] In general, these two systems have antagonist effects on their end organs.

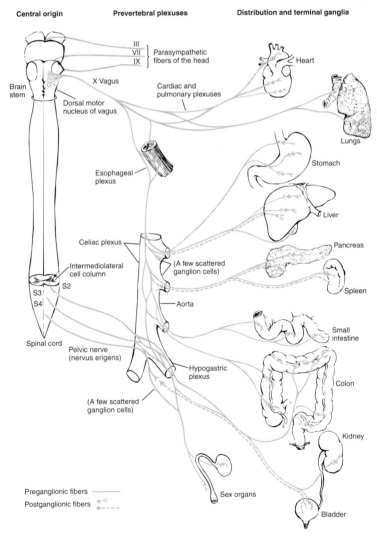

FIG. 2-15 Sympathetic division of the autonomic nervous system (left half). (*Reproduced with permission from Waxman: Corrective Neuroanatomy, p 252, New York, McGraw-Hill, 2000.*)

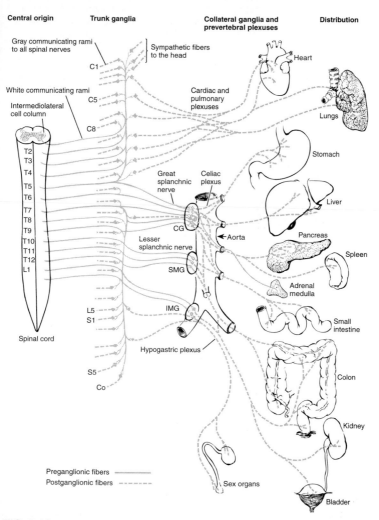

FIG. 2-16 Parasympathetic division of the autonomic nervous system (left half). (*Reproduced with permission from Waxman: Corrective Neuroanatomy, p 255, New York, McGraw-Hill, 2000.*)

TABLE 2-12 Autonomic Nervous System Divisions

	Sympathetic	Parasympathetic
General location	Thoracolumbar	Craniosacral
Specific location	Intermediolateral and medial gray T1-L 2	Cranial nerves III, VII, IX, X, and sacral segments S2-4
Pathway characteristics	Short preganglionic fibers	Long preganglionic fibers
	Long postganglionic fibers	Short postganglionic fibers
Principal neurotransmitter	Norepinephrine (except sweat glands)	Acetycholine

Source: Morgenlander JC: The autonomic nervous system. In Gilman S (ed): Clinical Examination of the Nervous System, pp 213–225. New York, McGraw-Hill, 2000.

REFERENCES

1. Martin J (ed): Introduction to the central nervous system. In Neuroanatomy: Text and Atlas, pp 1–32. New York, McGraw-Hill, 1996.
2. Willis WD: The Pain System. Basel, Karger, 1985.
3. Spiller WG, Martin E: The treatment of persistent pain of organic origin in the lower part of the body by division of the anterior-lateral column of the spinal cord. JAMA 1912;58:1489–1490.
4. Gowers WR: A case of unilateral gunshot injury to the spinal cord. Trans Clin Lond 1878;11:24–32.
5. Vierck CJ, Greenspan JD, Ritz LA: Long-term changes in purposive and reflexive responses to nociceptive stimulation following anterior-lateral chordotomy. J Neurosci 1990;10:2077–2095.
6. Willis WD, Coggeshall RE: Sensory Mechanisms of the Spinal Cord, 2nd ed. New York, Plenum, 1991.
7. Willis WD, et al.: Responses of primate spinothalamic tract neurons to natural stimulation of hindlimb. J Neurophysiol 1974;37:358–372.
8. Hyndman R, Van Epps C: Possibility of differential section of the spinothalamic tract. Arch Surg 1939;38:1036–1053.
9. Ferrington DG, Sorkin LS, Willis WD: Responses of spinothalamic tract cells in the superficial dorsal horn of the primate lumbar spinal cord. J Physiol 1987;388:681–703.
10. Kenshalo DR, et al.: Responses of primate spinothalamic neurons to graded and to repeated noxious heat stimuli. J Neurophysiol 1979;42:1370–1389.
11. Foreman RD, Schmidt RF, Willis WD: Effects of mechanical and chemical stimulation of fine muscle afferents upon primate spinothalamic tract cells. J Physiol 1979;286:215–231.
12. Milne RJ, et al.: Convergence of cutaneous and pelvic visceral nociceptive inputs onto primate spinothalamic neurons. Pain 1981;11:163–183.
13. Chung JM, et al.: Prolonged inhibition of primate spinothalamic tract cells by peripheral nerve stimulation. Pain 1984;19:259–275.
14. Chung JM, et al.: Factors influencing peripheral nerve stimulation produced inhibition of primate spinothalamic tract cells. Pain 1984;19:277–293.
15. Lee KH, Chung JM, Willis WD: Inhibition of primate spinothalamic tract cells by TENS. J Neurosurg 1985;62:276–287.
16. Waxman SG: Correlative Neuroanatomy, 24th ed. New York, McGraw-Hill, 1996.
17. Bogduk N: Innervation and pain patterns of the cervical spine. In Grant R (ed): Physical Therapy of the Cervical and Thoracic Spine. New York, Churchill Livingstone, 1988.
18. Rowland LP: Diseases of the motor unit. In Kandel ER, Schwartz JH, Jessell TM (eds): Principles of Neural Science, pp 695–712. New York, McGraw-Hill, 2000.

19. Asbury AK: Numbness, tingling, and sensory loss. In Isselbacher KJ, et al. (eds): Harrison's Principles of Internal Medicine, pp 133–136. New York, McGraw-Hill, 1994.
20. Thompson HG, Rowland LP: Pain and paresthesias. In Rowland LP (ed): Merritt's Textbook of Neurology, pp 28–31. Philadelphia, PA, Lea and Febiger, 1989.
21. Chusid JG: Correlative Neuroanatomy & Functional Neurology, pp 144–148. Norwalk, CT, Appleton-Century-Crofts, 1985.
22. Jenkins DB: Hollinshead's Functional Anatomy of the Limbs and Back, 7th ed. Philadelphia, PA, WB Saunders, 1998.
23. Mannheimer JS, Lampe GN: Clinical Transcutaneous Electrical Nerve Stimulation, pp 440–445. Philadelphia, PA, FA Davis, 1984.
24. Morgenlander JC: The autonomic nervous system. In Gilman S (ed): Clinical Examination of the Nervous System, pp 213–225. New York, McGraw-Hill, 2000.

3 | **The Examination**

An examination refers to the gathering of data and information concerning a topic.[1] The purpose of the examination is to obtain information that identifies and measures a change from normal. This is determined using information related by the patient in conjunction with clinical findings.

The examination consists of three components of equal importance: the history, the systems review, and the tests and measures (Figure 3-1).[1] The history, systems review (refer to Chapter 4), and tests and measures are closely related, in that they often occur concurrently. One further element, observation, occurs throughout.

OBSERVATION

Much can be learned from a thorough observation. Throughout the history, systems review, and tests and measures, collective observations form the basis for diagnostic deductions. The observation includes but is not limited to, an analysis of posture, structural alignment or deformity, scars, color changes, swelling, muscle atrophy, and the presence of any asymmetry.

Posture

Posture describes the relative positions of different joints at any given moment.[2] It is not clear what constitutes good or normal posture. Like gait, posture is a personal identifier—it is the reflection of the sum total of previous abrasions to the body and spirit (see *Orthopaedic Examination, Evaluation, and Intervention*, pp 189–190).

THE HISTORY

The history (Table 3-1) usually precedes the systems review and the tests and measures components of the examination, but it may also occur concurrently (see *Orthopaedic Examination, Evaluation, and Intervention*, pp 152–163). It is estimated that 80% of the necessary information to explain the presenting patient problem can be provided by a thorough history.[3]

Typically, the history taking begins with open-ended questions, such as, "Tell me why you are here" to encourage the patient to provide narrative information and to decrease the opportunity for biasing on the part of the clinician.[3] Questions that are more specific are asked as the examination proceeds (Table 3-2). The specific questions help to focus the examination and deter irrelevant information. *Neutral* questions should be used whenever possible. These questions are structured in such a way so as not to lead the patient into giving a particular response.

History of Current Condition

Onset of Symptoms

The clinician should determine the circumstances and manner in which the symptoms began, and the progression of those symptoms.[4] The mode of onset, or mechanism of injury can give clues as to the extent and nature of damage caused. Symptoms of pain or limitations of movement, with no apparent

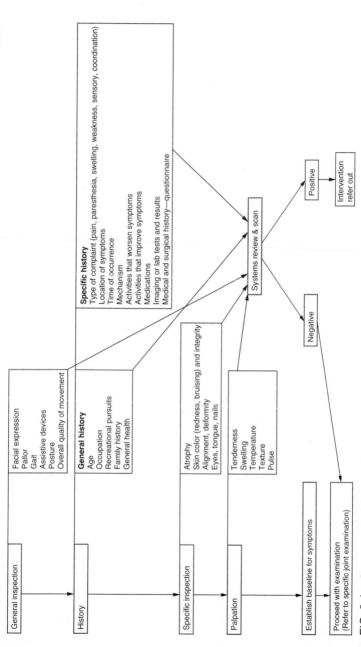

FIG. 3-1 Components of the examination and their interrelationships.

General inspection
- Facial expression
- Pallor
- Gait
- Assistive devices
- Posture
- Overall quality of movement

History

General history
- Age
- Occupation
- Recreational pursuits
- Family history
- General health

Specific history
- Type of complaint (pain, paresthesia, swelling, weakness, sensory, coordination)
- Location of symptoms
- Time of occurrence
- Mechanism
- Activities that worsen symptoms
- Activities that improve symptoms
- Medications
- Imaging or lab tests and results
- Medical and surgical history—questionnaire

Specific inspection
- Atrophy
- Skin color (redness, bruising) and integrity
- Alignment, deformity
- Eyes, tongue, nails

Palpation
- Tenderness
- Swelling
- Temperature
- Texture
- Pulse

Systems review & scan

Positive → Intervention refer out

Negative

Establish baseline for symptoms

Proceed with examination
(Refer to specific joint examination)

53

TABLE 3-1 Data Generated from the Patient History

- General demographics
- Social history and social habits
- Occupation/employment
- Growth and development
- Living environment
- History of current condition
- Functional status and activity level
- Medications
- Other test and measures
- Past history of current condition
- Past medical/surgical history
- Family history
- Health status

reason, are usually a result of inflammation, early degeneration, repetitive activity (microtrauma), or sustained positioning and postures.[5] However, such symptoms may also be associated with something more insidious.

If the injury is traumatic, the clinician should determine the specific mechanism, in terms of both the direction and force, and relate the mechanism to the presenting symptoms. If the injury is recent, an inflammatory source of pain is likely. A sudden onset of pain, associated with trauma, could indicate the presence of an acute injury such as a tear or fracture, whereas immediate pain and "locking" is most likely to result from an intra-articular block (Table 3-3).

If the onset is gradual or insidious, the clinician must determine if there are any predisposing factors, such as changes in the patient's daily routines or exercise programs. If there are no such factors, a more serious cause should be suspected until otherwise ruled out.

Because motor and sensory axons run in the same nerves, disorders of the peripheral nerves (neuropathies) usually affect both motor and sensory functions (Table 3-4). Peripheral symptoms can manifest as abnormal, frequently unpleasant sensations, which are variously described by the patient as numbness, pins and needles, and tingling.[6]

When these sensations occur spontaneously without an external sensory stimulus, they are called *paresthesias* (Tables 3-5 and 3-6).[6] Causalgia is an intense, burning type of paresthesia caused by trauma to a nerve (e.g., the median, ulnar, posterior tibial or fibular nerves). *Complex Regional Pain Syndrome*, traditionally termed *reflex sympathetic dystrophy*, is an unusual cause of paresthesias, pain, and autonomic dysfunction occurring after minor soft tissue injuries or fractures and usually affecting the distal extremities.[7] Myelinopathies occur at the level of the myelin sheath and can be inflammatory or hereditary.[8]

Central nervous system (CNS) causes of paresthesia include ischemia, obstruction, compression, infection, inflammation, and degenerative conditions (Table 3-7).[8] Correct diagnosis of the source of the paresthesias can be elicited by a thorough history and physical examination. Paresthesias that persist are likely to be associated with a serious medical problem and may require appropriate laboratory, radiographic, and special studies to confirm the diagnosis. Electromyographic (EMG) and nerve conduction studies (NCS) are often the most useful initial laboratory studies.[7]

TABLE 3-2 Contents of the Subjective History

The history of the current condition
- Did the condition begin insidiously, or was trauma involved?
- How long has the patient had the symptoms?
- Where are the symptoms?
- How does the patient describe the symptoms? Reports about numbness and tingling suggest a neurologic compromise. Reports of pain suggest a chemical or mechanical irritant. Pain needs to be carefully evaluated in terms of its site, distribution, quality, onset, frequency, nocturnal occurrence, aggravating factors, and relieving factors.
- Past history of current condition
- Has the patient had a similar injury in the past?
- Was it treated or did it resolve on its own? If it was treated, how was it treated and did the intervention help?
- How long did the last episode last?
- Past medical/surgery history
- How is the patient's general health?
- Does the patient have any allergies?
- Medications the patient is presently taking.
- Other tests and measures
- Has the patient had any imaging tests such as x-ray, MRI, CT scan, bone scan?
- Has the patient had an electromyographic (EMG) test, or a nerve conduction velocity test, which would suggest a compromise to the muscle tissue and/or neurologic system?
- Social habits (past and present)
- Does the patient smoke? If so, how many packs per day?
- Does the patient drink alcohol? If so, how often and how much?
- Is the patient active or sedentary?
- Social history
- Is the patient married, living with a partner, single, divorced, or widowed?
- Is the patient a parent or a single parent?
- Family history
- Is there a family history of the present condition?
- Growth and development
- Is the patient right or left handed?
- Were there any congenital problems?
- Living environment
- What type of home does the patient live in with reference to accessibility?
- Is there any support at home?
- Does the patient use any extra pillows or special chairs in order to sleep?
- Occupation/employment/school
- What does the patient do for work?
- How long has he or she worked there?
- What does the job entail in terms of physical requirements?
- What level of education did the patient achieve?
- Functional status/activity level
- How does the present condition affect the patient's ability to perform their activities of daily living?
- How does the present condition affect the patient at work?
- How does the patient's condition affect sleep?
- Is the patient able to drive? If so, for how long?

Source: Clarnette RG, Miniaci A: Clinical exam of the shoulder. Med Sci Sports Exerc 1998;30:1–6.

TABLE 3-3 Pain Descriptions and Potentially Related Structures

Type of pain	Potential source
Cramping, dull, sore, aching	Muscle
Dull, aching	Ligament, joint capsule
Sharp, shooting, pinching, gnawing	Nerve root
Sharp, burning, shooting	Nerve
Burning, pressure like, sting, smarting	Sympathetic nerve
Deep, nagging, dull	Bone
Sharp, severe, incapacitating	Fracture
Throbbing, pulsing, beating, diffuse	Vasculature

TABLE 3-4 Signs and Symptoms of Lower Motor Neuron (LMN) Lesions

Motor	Sensory	Sympathetic
Flaccid paralysis	Loss of or abnormal sensation	Loss of sweat glands (dryness)
Loss of reflexes	Loss of vasomotor tone: warm, flushed (early); cold, white (later)	Loss of pilomotor response
Muscle wasting and atrophy		
Lost synergistic action of muscles	Skin may be scaly (early); thin, smooth, and shiny (later)	
Fibrosis, contractures, and adhesions	Shallower skin creases	
Joint weakness and instability	Nail changes (striations, ridges, dry, brittle, abnormal curving, luster lost)	
Decreased range of motion and stiffness		
Disuse osteoporosis of bone	Ulceration	
Growth affected		

Source: Magee DJ (ed): Orthopedic Physical Assessment. Philadelphia, PA, WB Saunders, 2002.

TABLE 3-5 Types of Paresthesia[8]

Central	Peripheral
Ischemic	Neuropathy (see Table 3-8)
Cerebrovascular accident	
Transient ischemic attack	
Structural	
Tumor	
Trauma	
Infectious	
Brain abscess	
Encephalitis	

TABLE 3-6 Location and Probable Causes of Paresthesia

Paresthesia location	Probable cause
Lip (perioral)	Vertebral artery occlusion
Bilateral lower or bilateral upper extremities	Central protrusion of disk impinging on the spine
All extremities simultaneously	Spinal cord compression
One half of the body	Cerebral hemisphere
Segmental (in a dermatomal pattern)	Disk/nerve root involvement
Glove/stocking distribution	Diabetes mellitus neuropathy, lead/mercury poisoning
Half of face and opposite half of body	Brainstem impairment

The differential diagnosis of paresthesias and peripheral neuropathy is difficult. Peripheral neuropathies can be caused by entrapment syndromes, trauma, diabetes, hypothyroidism, vitamin B_{12} deficiency, alcoholism, inflammatory conditions, connective tissue disorders, toxic injury, hereditary conditions, malignancy, infections, and miscellaneous causes (see Table 3-7).[8] Peripheral neuropathy can also be mimicked by myelopathy, syringomyelia or dorsal column disorders, such as tabes dorsalis.[7] Hysteric symptoms can

TABLE 3-7 Selected Causes of Peripheral Neuropathy[8]

Metabolic/nutritional disturbances	Connective tissue disorders	Malignancy
Diabetes	Polyarteritis nodosa	Tumor compression
Hypothyroidism	Autoimmune vasculitis	Paraneoplastic syndromes
Vitamin B_{12} deficiency	Rheumatoid arthritis	
Alcoholism	Systemic lupus erythematosus	Lymphomas
Uremia		Cancer of the lung, stomach, breast, or ovary
Amyloidosis	Systemic sclerosis	
Porphyria	Sjögren's syndrome	

Entrapment syndromes	Toxins	Plasma cell dyscrasias
Carpal tunnel syndrome	Chemotherapy	Multiple myeloma
Ulnar entrapment syndrome	Heavy metals	Osteoclastic myeloma
Thoracic outlet syndrome	Medications (didanosine [Videx], zalcitabine [Hivid], stavudine [Zerit])	Monoclonal gammopathy
Lateral femoral cutaneous syndrome		Waldenstrom's macroglobulinemia
	Industrial exposures	Miscellaneous
Peroneal palsy	Chronic overdosage of pyridoxine	sarcoidosis
Tarsal tunnel syndrome		Malnutrition
Trauma	Hereditary conditions	Infections
Inflammation	Charcot-Marie-Tooth disease	Lyme disease
Acute idiopathic polyneuritis	Denny-Brown's syndrome	HIV infection
Chronic relapsing polyneuropathy	Familial amyloidotic polyneuropathy	Leprosy

HIV = human immunodeficiency virus.

sometimes mimic a neuropathy. It is useful to determine the pattern of involvement (Table 3-8).[7]

The patient history should determine time of onset, duration, and location of the symptoms; any accompanying pain or motor dysfunction; past medical history; current medical problems; current and past medications; recreational drug use; trauma; and toxic exposure.[8] Family history may reveal a relative with peripheral neuropathy, malignancy, diabetes, thyroid disease, or connective tissue disease. An occupational history of repetitive movement, use of vibratory tools, or toxin exposure may be important. The history will also help the physician determine if the condition is symmetric and primarily motor or sensory. A cranial nerve examination (see next section) can provide evidence of mononeuropathies or proximal involvement. In a patient with a distal symmetric sensorimotor neuropathy, the sensory examination shows reduced sensitivity to light touch, pinprick, and temperature in a stocking-and-glove distribution.[7] Deep tendon reflexes (DTRs) are reduced or absent. Severe, longstanding neuropathy can result in trophic changes including pes cavus, kyphoscoliosis, and a loss of hair in affected areas or ulceration.

Many medications can cause a peripheral neuropathy (Table 3-9), typically a distal symmetric axonal sensorimotor neuropathy.[7] Although the dispensing of medications is out of the scope of practice for a physical therapist, questioning the patient about prescribed medications can also reveal medical conditions that the patient might not have considered important to relate (Table 3-10).[9] Medications can also have an impact on clinical findings, and the success of an intervention.[10]

Questions about tobacco use and alcohol consumption give the clinician information about the general health of the patient as well as highlighting comorbidities. Although caffeine intake may appear to have little bearing on signs and symptoms, caffeine can have both behavioral and physical affects on the body. The behavioral effects of caffeine include increased arousal and vigilance and decreased fatigue and reaction time. With higher doses there can be jitteriness and sleep disturbances. A well-designed double-blind study by Silverman et al.[11] examined the withdrawal syndrome following discontinuation of caffeine consumption in 62 adults who were low to moderate caffeine consumers. Results indicated increased symptoms of

TABLE 3-8 Neuropathies by Pattern of Involvement[7]

Focal	Multifocal
Entrapment	Diabetes mellitus
Common sites of compression	Vasculitis
Myxedema	Polyarteritis nodosa
Rheumatoid arthritis	Systemic lupus erythematosus
Amyloidosis	Sjögren's syndrome
Acromegaly	Sarcoidosis
Compressive neuropathies	Leprosy
Trauma	HIV/AIDS
Ischemic lesions	Multifocal variant of chronic inflammatory
Diabetes mellitus	demyelinating polyneuropathy (CIDP)
Vasculitis	Hereditary predisposition to
Leprosy	pressure palsies
Sarcoidosis	
Neoplastic infiltration	
or compression	

TABLE 3-9 Medications that May Cause Neuropathies

Axonal	Demyelinating	Neuronopathy
Vincristine (Oncovin, Vincasar PFS)	Amiodarone (Cordarone)	Thalidomide (Synovir)
Paclitaxel (Taxol)	Chloroquine	Cisplatin (Platinol)
Nitrous oxide	Suramin (Fourneau 309, Bayer 205, Germanin)	Pyridoxine
Colchicine (Probenecid, Col-Probenecid)	Gold	
Isoniazid (Laniazid)		
Hydralazine (Apresoline)		
Metronidazole (Flagyl)		
Pyridoxine (Nestrex, Beesix)		
Didanosine (Videx)		
Lithium		
Alfa interferon (Roferon-A, Intron A, Alferon N)		
Dapsone		
Phenytoin (Dilantin)		
Cimetidine (Tagamet)		
Disulfiram (Antabuse)		
Chloroquine (Aralen)		
Ethambutol (Myambutol)		
Amitriptyline (Elavil, Endep)		

depression, anxiety, fatigue, and headache after caffeine cessation. In addition, motor performance was disrupted and subjects provided qualitative comments that caffeine withdrawal was disruptive to their normal activities.

Frequency and Duration The frequency and duration of the patient's symptoms can help the clinician to classify the injury according to its stage of healing: acute (inflammatory), subacute (migratory and proliferative), and chronic (remodeling) (Table 3-11) (see *Orthopaedic Examination, Evaluation, and Intervention*, pp 101–109).

TABLE 3-10 The Identification of Drug Class by Suffix

Suffix	Drug class	Example
Cillin	Antibacterials	Amoxicillin
Micin		
Mycin		
Epam	Benzodiazepines	Diazepam
Olam		
Olol	Beta blockers	Atenolol
Pril	ACE inhibitors	Enalapril
Ipine	Ca++ Channel blockers	Nifedipine
Barbital	Barbiturates	Phenobarbital
Statin	Antihyperlipidemic	Lovastatin
Erol	Bronchodilators	Albuterol
Phylline		
Caine	Local anesthetic	Lidocaine
Amide	Oral hypoglycemics	Acetohexamide
Idine	H_2 blockers	Cimetidine

TABLE 3-11 Stages of Healing

Stage	General characteristics
Acute or inflammatory	The area is red, warm, swollen, and painful The pain is present without any motion of the involved area Usually lasts for 48–72 hours, but can be as long as 7–10 days
Subacute or tissue formation (neovascularization)	The pain usually occurs with the activity or motion of the involved area Usually lasts for 10 days to 6 weeks
Chronic or remodeling	The pain usually occurs after the activity Usually lasts from 6 weeks to 12 months

Aggravating and Easing Factors Of particular importance are the patient's chief complaint and the relationship of that complaint to specific aggravating activities or postures. Questions must be asked to determine whether the pain is sufficient to prevent sleep or to wake the patient at night, and the effect that activities of daily living (ADL), work, sex, and so forth have on the pain. Musculoskeletal conditions are typically influenced with movements or positions (Tables 3-12 and 3-13). Symptoms that are aggravated with movement and alleviated with rest indicate a mechanical source. Chemical or inflammatory pain is more constant and is less affected by movements or positions. Intermittent pain is usually caused by prolonged postures, by a loose intra-articular body, or by an impingement of a musculoskeletal structure. If no activities or postures are reported to aggravate the symptoms, the clinician needs to probe for more information.

Location The clinician should determine the location of the symptoms, as this can indicate which areas need to be included in the physical examination. Information about how the location of the symptoms has changed since the onset can indicate whether a condition is worsening or improving. In general, as a condition worsens, the pain distribution becomes more widespread and distal (peripheralizes). As the condition improves, the symptoms tend to become more localized (centralized). A body chart may be used to record the location of symptoms (Table 3-14).

TABLE 3-12 Differentiation between Musculoskeletal and Systemic Pain

Musculoskeletal pain	Systemic pain
Usually decreases with cessation of activity	Reduced by pressure
Generally lessens at night	Disturbs sleep
Is aggravated with mechanical stress	Is not aggravated by mechanical stress
Usually continuous or intermittent	Usually constant or in waves

Source: Meadows J: Orthopedic Differential Diagnosis in Physical Therapy. New York, McGraw-Hill, 1999.

TABLE 3-13 Differentiation of Systemic and Musculoskeletal Pain

Systemic	Musculoskeletal
Disturbs sleep	Generally lessens at night
Deep aching or throbbing	Sharp or superficial ache
Reduced by pressure	Usually decreases with cessation of activity
Constant, or waves of pain and spasm	
Is not aggravated by mechanical stress	Usually continuous or intermittent
Associated with:	Is aggravated by mechanical stress
Jaundice	Usually associated with nothing specific
Migratory arthralgias	
Skin rash	
Fatigue	
Weight loss	
Low grade fever	
Generalized weakness	
Cyclic and progressive symptoms	
History of infection	

Sources: Meadows J: Orthopedic Differential Diagnosis in Physical Therapy. New York, McGraw-Hill, 1999.
Magee DJ (ed): Orthopedic Physical Assessment. Philadelphia, PA, WB Saunders, 2002.

TABLE 3-14 Patient Pain Evaluation From

Name: _____

Date: _____ **Signature:** _____

Please use the diagram below to indicate where you feel symptoms right now. Use the following key to indicate different types of symptoms.

KEY: Pins and Needles = 000000   Stabbing = ///////   Burning = XXXXX   Deep Ache = ZZZZZZ

Please use the three scales below to rate your pain over the past 24 hours. Use the upper line to describe your pain level right now. Use the other scales to rate your pain at its worst and best over the past 24 hours.

RATE YOUR PAIN: 0 = NO PAIN, 10 = EXTREMELY INTENSE

1. Right now	0	1	2	3	4	5	6	7	8	9	10
2. At its worst	0	1	2	3	4	5	6	7	8	9	10
3. At its best	0	1	2	3	4	5	6	7	8	9	10

The term *referred pain* is used to describe those symptoms that have their origin at a site other than where the patient feels the pain. If the extremity appears to be the source of the symptoms, the clinician should attempt to reproduce the symptoms by loading the peripheral tissues. If this proves unsuccessful, a full investigation of the spinal structures must ensue.

Behavior of Symptoms Whether the pain is worsening, improving, or unchanging provides the clinician with valuable information. For example, a gradual increase in the intensity of symptoms over time may indicate to the clinician that the condition is worsening, or that the condition is nonmusculoskeletal in nature.[2,4]

The Nature of the Symptoms The clinician must determine whether pain is the only symptom, or whether there are other symptoms that accompany the pain, such as dizziness, bowel and bladder changes, radicular pain/numbness (Table 3-15), paresthesia, weakness, and increased sweating. Causes of generalized weakness include motor neuron disease, disorders of the neuromuscular junction, and myopathy.

Past History of Current Condition

It is important for the clinician to determine whether the patient has had successive onsets of similar symptoms in the past, as recurrent injury tends to have a detrimental affect on the potential for recovery. If it is a recurrent injury, the clinician should note how often, and how easily, the injury has recurred, and the success, or failure of previous interventions.

TABLE 3-15 Common Radicular Syndromes

Disk level	Nerve root	Motor deficit	Sensory deficit	Reflex compromise
Lumbar				
L3-4	L4	Quadriceps	Anterolateral thigh Anterior knee Medial leg and foot	Knee
L4-5	L5	Extensor hallucis longus	Lateral thigh Anterolateral leg Mid-dorsal foot	Medial hamstrings
L5-S1	S1	Ankle plantar flexors	Posterior leg Lateral foot	Ankle
Cervical				
C4-5	C5	Deltoid biceps	Anterolateral Shoulder and arm	Biceps
C5-6	C6	Wrist extensors biceps	Lateral forearm and hand Thumb	Brachioradialis Pronator teres
C6-7	C7	Wrist flexors Triceps Finger extensors	Middle finger	Triceps
C7-T1	C8	Finger flexors Hand intrinsics	Medial forearm and hand, ring and little fingers	None
T1-2	T1	Hand intrinsics	Medial forearm	None

Source: Magee DJ (ed): Orthopedic Physical Assessment. Philadelphia, PA, WB Saunders, 2002.

Past Medical and Surgical History

The patient's past medical history (PMH) can be obtained through a questionnaire (see *Orthopaedic Examination, Evaluation, and Intervention*, p 155). The PMH can provide information with regard to allergies, childhood illnesses, and previous trauma. In addition, information on any health conditions such as a cardiac problems, high blood pressure, or diabetes, should be elicited as these may impact exercise tolerance (cardiac problems, high blood pressure) and speed of healing (diabetes).

If the surgical history is related to the current problem, the clinician should obtain as much detail about the surgery as possible from the surgical report, including any complications, precautions, or postsurgical protocols.

Family History and General Health Status

The general health status refers to a review of the patient's health perception, physical and psychologic function, as well as any specific questions related to a particular body region, or complaint.[1] Certain diseases, such as rheumatoid arthritis, diabetes, cardiovascular disease, and cancer have familial tendencies.

Tests and Measures

The tests and measures (Table 3-16) component of the examination (see Figure 3-1), which serves as an adjunct to the history and systems review (see Chapter 4), involves the physical examination of the patient. The information from the history and the systems review serves as a guide for the clinician in determining which structures and systems require further investigation. The physical examination may also be modified based on the history—the examination of an acutely injured patient differs greatly from that of a patient in less discomfort or distress. In addition, the examination of a child differs in some respects to that of an adult. There are times when a complete examination

---

TABLE 3-16 Tests and Measures Related to the Neuromusculoskeletal Patterns

Aerobic capacity and endurance
Anthropometric characteristics
Circulation
Cranial and peripheral nerve integrity
Environmental, home, and work barriers
Ergonomics and body mechanics
Gait, locomotion, and balance
Integumentary integrity
Joint integrity and mobility
Motor function
Muscle performance (including strength, power, and endurance)
Orthotic, protective, and supportive devices
Pain
Posture
Range of motion
Reflex integrity
Sensory integrity
Work, community, and leisure integration

cannot be performed. For example, if the joint to be examined is too acutely inflamed, the clinician may defer some of the examination to the subsequent visit.

The decision about which tests to use should be based on the best available research evidence. A good test must distinguish between the other disorders that the target disorder might otherwise be confused with.[12]

Before proceeding with the tests and measures, a full explanation must be provided to the patient as to what procedures are to be performed and the reasons for these. A logical sequence must be followed (see Figure 3-1) so as to provide the clinician with relevant information.

Range of Motion

A normal joint has an available range of active, or physiological, motion, which is limited by a physiologic barrier (Figure 3-2) as tension develops within the surrounding tissues. At the physiologic barrier, there is an additional amount of passive range of motion (see Figure 3-2). Beyond the available passive range of motion, the anatomic barrier (see Figure 3-2) is found. This barrier cannot be exceeded without disruption to the integrity of the joint.

The range of motion examination should determine the exact directions of motion that elicit the symptoms. The diagnosis of restricted movement in the extremities can usually be simplified by comparing both sides, provided that at least one side is uninvolved.

Active Range of Motion

Active range of motion testing gives the clinician information about:

- The quantity of available physiologic motion (see Figure 3-2)
- The presence of muscle substitutions
- The willingness of the patient to move
- The integrity of the contractile and inert tissues
- The quality of motion
- Symptom reproduction
- The pattern of motion restriction

Active range of motion testing may be deferred if small and unguarded motions provoke intense pain, as this may indicate a high degree of joint irritability. The normal active range of motion for each of the joints is depicted in Table 3-17.

Full and pain-free active range of motion suggests normalcy for that movement, although it is important to remember that normal *range* of motion is not synonymous with normal motion.[13] Normal motion implies that the control of motion must also be present.

Single motions in the cardinal planes are usually tested first (see Figure 3-3). Dynamic and static testing in the cardinal planes follows if the single motions do not provoke symptoms. Dynamic testing involves repeated movements in specific directions. Repeated movements can give the clinician some valuable insight into the patient's condition:[14]

- Internal derangements tend to worsen with repeated motions
- The symptoms of a postural dysfunction remain unchanged with repeated motions

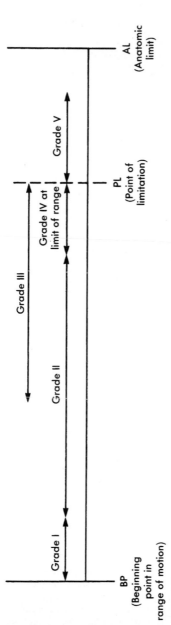

FIG. 3-2 Available joint range of motion. (*Reproduced with permission from Dutton M: Manual Therapy of the Spine, Fig. 3-3, p 44. New York, McGraw-Hill, 2001.*)

TABLE 3-17 Active Ranges of Joint Motions

Joint	Action	Degrees of motion
Shoulder	Flexion	0–180
	Extension	0–40
	Abduction	0–180
	Internal rotation	0–80
	External rotation	0–90
Elbow	Flexion	0–150
Forearm	Pronation	0–80
	Supination	0–80
Wrist	Flexion	0–60
	Extension	0–60
	Radial deviation	0–20
	Ulnar deviation	0–30
Hip	Flexion	0–100
	Extension	0–30
	Abduction	0–40
	Adduction	0–20
	Internal rotation	0–40
	External rotation	0–50
Knee	Flexion	0–150
Ankle	Plantar flexion	0–40
	Dorsiflexion	0–20
Foot	Inversion	0–30
	Eversion	0–20

- Pain from a dysfunction syndrome is increased with tissue loading, but ceases at rest
- Repeated motions can indicate the irritability of the condition
- Repeated motions can indicate to the clinician the direction of motion to be used as part of the intervention. If pain increases during repeated motion in a particular direction, exercising in that direction is not indicated. If pain only worsens in part of the range, repeated motion exercises can be used for that part of the range that is pain-free, or which does not worsen the symptoms.
- Pain that is increased after the repeated motions may indicate a retriggering of the inflammatory response, and repeated motions in the opposite direction should be explored.
- Static testing involves sustaining a position. Sustained static positions may be used to help detect postural syndromes.[15]

Combined motion testing (see Figure 3-3) may be used when the symptoms are not reproduced with the cardinal plane motion tests. Combined motions, as their name suggests use single plane motions with other motions superimposed. For example, at the elbow the single plane motion of elbow flexion is tested together with forearm supination and then forearm pronation. As with the single plane tests, the combined motions are testing statically and then dynamically in an effort to reproduce the patient's symptoms.

Compression and distraction may also be added to all of the active motion tests in an attempt to reproduce the symptoms.

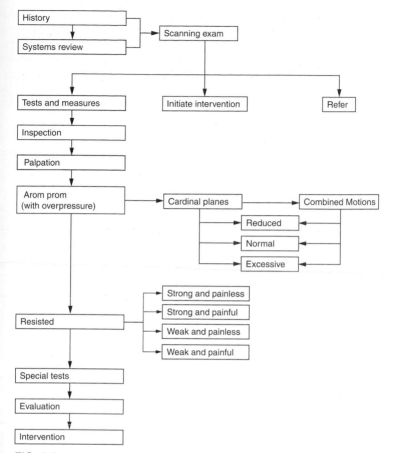

FIG. 3-3 Examination algorithm.

The active range of motion will be found to be either abnormal or normal. Abnormal motion is typically described as being reduced (Figure 3-4). It must be remembered though, that abnormal motion may also be excessive. Excessive motion is often missed and is erroneously classified as normal motion. To help determine whether the motion is normal or excessive, passive range of motion, in the form of passive overpressure, and the end-feel are assessed (see Figure 3-4).

Passive Range of Motion

If the active motions do not reproduce the patient's symptoms, or the active range of motion appears incomplete, it is important to perform gentle passive range of motion and over pressure, at the end of the active range in order to fully test the motion (see Figure 3-4). The passive overpressure should be

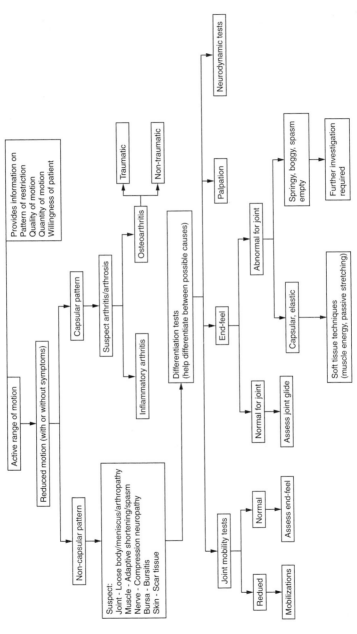

FIG. 3-4 Algorithm used for findings of apparent normal range of motion.

applied carefully in the presence of pain. The barrier to active motion should occur earlier in the range than the barrier to passive motion. Pain that occurs at the end-range of active and passive movement is suggestive of hypermobility or instability, a capsular contraction, or scar tissue that has not been adequately remodeled.[14]

Passive range of motion testing gives the clinician information about the integrity of the contractile and inert tissues, and the *end-feel*. Cyriax[16] introduced the concept of the end-feel, which is the quality of resistance at end range. The end-feel can indicate to the clinician the cause of the motion restriction (Tables 3-18 and 3-19).

The type of end-feel can help the clinician determine the presence of dysfunction (see Figure 3-4). For example, a hard, capsular end-feel indicates a pericapsular hypomobility, while a jammed or pathomechanic end-feel indicates a pathomechanic hypomobility. A normal end-feel would indicate normal range, whereas an abnormal end-feel would suggest abnormal range, either hypomobile, or hypermobile. An association between an increase in pain and abnormal-pathologic end-feels compared to normal end-feels has been demonstrated.[17]

The planned intervention, and its intensity, is based on the type of tissue resistance to movement demonstrated by the end-feel, and the acuteness of the condition (Table 3-20).[16] This information may indicate whether the resistance is caused by pain, muscle, capsule ligament, disturbed mechanics of the joint, or a combination.

Flexibility

The examination of flexibility is performed to determine if a particular structure, or group of structures, has sufficient extensibility to perform a desired activity. The extensibility and habitual length of connective tissue is a factor of the demands placed on it. A decrease in the length of the soft tissue structures, or adaptive shortening is very common in postural dysfunctions. Adaptive shortening can also be produced by:

- Restricted mobility
- Tissue damage—secondary to trauma
- Prolonged immobilization
- Disease
- *Hypertonia*. Hypertonic muscles can be identified through observation and palpation. Observation will reveal the muscle to be raised, and light palpation will provide information about tension, as the muscle will feel hard and may stand out from those around it.

Capsular and Noncapsular Patterns of Restriction

Cyriax[16] gave us the terms *capsular* and *noncapsular* pattern of restriction, which link impairment to pathology (Table 3-21). A capsular pattern of restriction is a limitation of pain and movement in a joint specific ratio, which is usually present with arthritis, or following prolonged immobilization (see Figure 3-4).[16]

A noncapsular pattern of restriction is a limitation in a joint in any pattern other than a capsular one, and may indicate the presence of either a derangement, a restriction of one part of the joint capsule, or an extra-articular lesion, that obstructs joint motion (see Figure 3-4).[16]

TABLE 3-18 Normal End-Feels

Type	Cause	Characteristics and examples
Bony	Produced by bone to bone approximation	Abrupt and unyielding with the impression that further forcing will break something. Examples: Normal: Elbow extension. Abnormal: Cervical rotation (may indicate osteophyte)
Elastic	Produced by the muscle-tendon unit. May occur with adaptive shortening.	Stretch with elastic recoil and exhibits constant-length phenomenon. Further forcing feels as if it will snap something. Examples: Normal: Wrist flexion with finger flexion, the straight leg raise, and ankle dorsiflexion with the knee extended. Abnormal: Decreased dorsiflexion of the ankle with the knee flexed.
Soft tissue approxi-mation	Produced by the contact of two muscle bulks on either side of a flexing joint where the joint range exceeds other restraints.	A very forgiving end-feel that gives the impression that further normal motion is possible if enough force could be applied. Examples: Normal: Knee flexion, elbow flexion in extremely muscular subjects. Abnormal: Elbow flexion with the obese subject.
Capsular	Produced by capsule or ligaments	• Various degrees of stretch without elasticity. Stretch ability is dependent on thickness of the tissue. • Strong capsular or extra-capsular ligaments produce a hard capsular end-feel while a thin capsule produces a softer one. • The impression given to the clinician is, if further force is applied something will tear. Examples: Normal: Wrist flexion (soft), elbow flexion in supination (medium), and knee extension (hard) Abnormal: Inappropriate stretch ability for a specific joint. If too hard, may indicate a hypomobility as a result of arthrosis; if too soft, a hypermobility.

TABLE 3-19 Abnormal End-Feels

Type	Causes	Characteristics and examples
Springy	Produced by the articular surface rebounding from an intra-articular meniscus or disk. The impression is that if forced further, something will collapse.	A rebound sensation as if pushing off from a sorbo rubber pad. Examples: Normal: Axial compression of the cervical spine. Abnormal: Knee flexion or extension with a displaced meniscus.
Boggy	Produced by viscous fluid (blood) within a joint.	A "squishy" sensation as the joint is moved toward its end range. Further forcing feels as if it will burst the joint. Examples: Normal: None Abnormal: Hemarthrosis at the knee
Spasm	Produced by reflex and reactive muscle contraction in response to irritation of the nociceptor predominantly in articular structures and muscle. Forcing it further feels as if nothing will give.	An abrupt and "twangy" end to movement that is unyielding while the structure is being threatened, but disappears when the threat is removed (kicks back). With joint inflammation, it occurs early in the range especially toward the close pack position to prevent further stress. With an irritable joint hypermobility, it occurs at the end of what should be normal range as it prevents excessive motion from further stimulating the nociceptor. Spasm in grade II muscle tears becomes apparent as the muscle is passively lengthened and is accompanied by a painful weakness of that muscle. Note: Muscle guarding is not a true end-feel as it involves a co-contraction Examples: Normal: None Abnormal: Significant traumatic arthritis, recent traumatic hypermobility, grade II muscle tears.
Empty	Produced solely by pain. Frequently caused by serious and severe pathologic changes that do not affect the joint or muscle and so do not produce spasm. Demonstration of this end-feel is, with the exception of acute sub-deltoid bursitis, de facto evidence of serious pathology. Further forcing simply increases the pain to unacceptable levels.	The limitation of motion has no tissue resistance component and the resistance is from the patient being unable to tolerate further motion due to severe pain. It is not the same feeling as voluntary guarding but rather it feels as if the patient is both resisting and trying to allow the movement simultaneously. Examples: Normal: None Abnormal: Acute subdeltoid bursitis, sign of the buttock
Facilitation	Not truly an end-feel as facilitated hypertonicity does not restrict motion. It can, however, be perceived near the end range.	A light resistance as from a constant light muscle contraction throughout the latter half of the range that does not prevent the end of range being reached. The resistance is unaffected by the rate of movement. Examples: Normal: None Abnormal: Spinal facilitation at any level

TABLE 3-20 Abnormal Barriers to Motion and Recommended Manual Techniques[16]

Barrier	End-feel	Technique
Pain	Empty	None
Pain	Spasm	None
Pain	Capsular	Oscillations (I, IV)
Joint adhesions	Early capsular	Passive articular motion stretch (I-V)
Muscle adhesions	Early elastic	Passive physiologic motion stretch
Hypertonicity	Facilitation	Hold/relax
Bone	Bony	None

TABLE 3-21 Capsular Patterns of Restriction[16]

Joint	Limitation of motion (passive angular motion)
Glenohumeral	External rotation > abduction > internal rotation (3:2:1)
Acromioclavicular	No true capsular pattern. Possible loss of horizontal adduction, pain (and sometimes slight loss of end range) with each motion
Sternoclavicular	See above: acromioclavicular joint
Humeroulnar	Flexion > Extension (±4:1)
Humeroradial	No true capsular pattern. Possible equal limitation of pronation and supination
Superior radioulnar	No true capsular pattern. Possible equal limitation of pronation and supination with pain at end ranges
Inferior radioulnar	No true capsular pattern. Possible equal limitation of pronation and supination with pain at end ranges
Wrist (carpus)	Flexion = Extension
Radiocarpal	See above (carpus)
Carpometacarpal	See above (carpus)
Midcarpal	See above (carpus)
1st carpometacarpal	Retroposition
Carpometacarpal 2-5	Fan > Fold
Metacarpophalangeal 2-5	Flexion > Extension (±2:1)
Interphalangeal	
Proximal (PIP)	Flexion > Extension (±2:1)
Distal (DIP)	
Hip	Internal rotation > Flexion > Abduction = Extension > other motions
Tibiofemoral	Flexion > Extension (±5:1)
Superior tibiofibular	No capsular pattern: pain at end range of translatory movements
Talocrural	Plantar flexion > Dorsiflexion
Talocalcaneal (subtalar)	Varus > Valgus
Midtarsal	
Talonavicular calcaneocuboid	Inversion (plantar flexion, adduction, supination) > dorsiflexion
1st metatarsophalangeal	Extension > Flexion (±2:1)
Metatarsophalangeal 2-5	Flexion >/= Extension
Interphalangeal 2-5	
Proximal	Flexion >/= Extension
Distal	Flexion >/= Extension

Joint Integrity and Mobility

The small motion, which is available at the joint surfaces, is referred to as *accessory* motion. This motion can only occur when resistance to active motion is applied, or when the patient's muscles are completely relaxed.[18]

A variety of different measurement scales have been proposed for judging the amount of accessory joint motion present between two joint surfaces, most of which are based on a comparison with a comparable contralateral joint using manually applied forces in a logical and precise manner (refer to Passive Accessory Mobility tests next).[19] Using these techniques to assess the joint glide, joint motion is described as hypomobile, normal, or hypermobile.[4,20,21]

Passive Accessory Mobility Tests

The passive articular mobility (PAM) tests involve the clinician assessing the arthrokinematic or accessory motions of a joint. In the spine these tests are referred to as passive physiologic accessory intervertebral motion (PPAIVM) testing.

The joint glides are tested in the loose pack position of a peripheral joint and, at the end of available range, in the spinal joints to avoid soft tissue tension affecting the results. By performing a joint glide, information about the integrity of the inert structures will be given (see Figure 3-4). There are two scenarios:

1. The joint glide is unrestricted. An unrestricted joint glide indicates two differing conclusions:

   a. The integrity of both the joint surface and the periarticular tissue is good. If this is the case, the patient's loss of motion must be due to a contractile tissue. With this scenario, the intervention should emphasize soft tissue mobilization techniques designed to change the length of a contractile tissue.

   b. The joint glide is unrestricted but excessive. Stress tests (see *Special Tests*) are then used to assess the integrity of the inert tissues, particularly the ligaments, and to determine whether instability exists at the joint. Instability at a joint may occur if the joint has undergone significant degenerative changes or trauma. The intervention for excessive motion that is impeding function focuses on stabilizing techniques designed to give secondary support to the joint through muscle action.

2. The joint glide is restricted. If the joint glide is restricted, the joint surface and periarticular tissues are implicated as the cause for the patient's loss of motion, although, as mentioned above, the contractile tissues cannot definitively be ruled out. The intervention for this type of finding initially involves a specific joint mobilization to restore the glide. Once the joint glide is restored following these mobilizations, the osteokinematic motion can be assessed again. If it is still reduced, the surrounding tissues have likely adaptively shortened. Distraction and compression can be used to help differentiate the cause of the restriction.

   a. *Distraction.* Traction is a force imparted passively by the clinician that results in a distraction of the joint surfaces.
      • If the distraction is limited, a contracture of connective tissue should be suspected.

- If the distraction increases the pain, it may indicate a tear of connective tissue, and may be associated with increased range.
- If the distraction eases the pain, it may indicate an involvement of the joint surface.

b. *Compression.* Compression is the opposite force to distraction, and involves an approximation of joint surfaces.

- If the compression increases the pain, a loose body or internal derangement of the joint may be present.
- If the compression decreases the pain, it may implicate the joint capsule.

Thus, by assessing joint motions in this manner, the clinician can determine:[18]

a. The cause of a limitation in a joint's physiologic range of motion[22]
b. The end-feel response of the tissues[16]
c. The stage of healing[23]
d. The integrity of the ligaments at a joint (for example, the Lachman test)

Based on the information gleaned from the joint glide assessment, the clinician makes clinical decisions as to which intervention to use (see Figures 3-4 and 3-5). If the joint play is felt to be restricted, and there is no indication of a bony end-feel, or severe irritability, joint mobilization techniques are used, with the grade determined by the stage of healing. If the joint play is found to be unrestricted, the clinician may decide to employ a technique that increases the extensibility of the surrounding connective tissues, as abnormal shortness of these connective tissues, including the ligaments, the joint capsule, and the periarticular tissues, can restrict joint mobility.

Muscle Performance—Strength, Power, and Endurance

Strength measures the ability with which musculotendinous units act across a bone-joint lever-arm system to actively generate motion, or passively resist movement against gravity and variable resistance.[24]

By definition, a contractile tissue is a tissue involved with a muscle contraction, and one that can be tested using an isolated muscle contraction. However, contractile tissues, such as tendons, which have no ability to contract, could be classified as inert, as while they are strongly affected by the contraction of their respective muscle bellies, they are also affected if passively stretched (see Chapter 1). Conversely, inert tissues, which also have no ability to contract, can be compressed, and therefore affected, during a contraction. Inert tissues are mainly tested with passive movement and ligament stress tests.

According to Cyriax, pain with a muscle contraction generally indicates an injury to the muscle or a capsular structure (Tables 3-22 and 3-23).[16] This can be confirmed by combining the findings from the isometric test with the findings of the passive motion and the joint distraction and compression. In addition to examining the integrity of the contractile and inert structures, strength testing may be used to examine the integrity of the myotomes. A myotome is defined as a muscle or group of muscles served by a single nerve root. *Key muscle* is a better, more accurate term, as the muscles tested are the most representative of the supply from a particular segment. Voluntary muscle strength testing remains somewhat subjective until a precise way of measuring muscle contraction is generally available.[24] Cyriax reasoned that if you isolate, and then apply tension to a structure, you could make a conclusion as to the integrity of that structure.[16] His work also introduced the concept of tissue

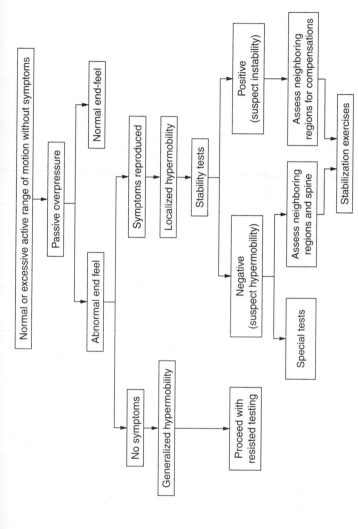

FIG. 3-5   Algorithm used for findings of abnormal range of motion.

TABLE 3-22 Differential Diagnosis of Muscle and Ligament Tissue Pathology

	Muscle	Ligament
Mechanism of injury	Overstretching Direct trauma	Overstretching
Contributing factors	Fatigue Muscle imbalance Inflexibility Inadequate warm-up	Fatigue Hypermobility/instability Decreased articular stability
Active movement	Pain on contraction or stretch (Grade I or II) No pain on contraction (Grade III) Weakness on contraction (Grades I–III)	Pain on stretch or distraction (Grade I or II) No pain on stretch (Grade III) Decreased range of motion
Passive movement	Pain on stretch Pain on compression	Pain on stretch (Grades I, II) No pain on stretch (Grade III) Decreased range of motion
Resisted isometric movement	Pain on contraction (Grade I or II) No pain on contraction (Grade III) Weakness on contraction (Grades I–III)	No pain (Grades I–III)
Special tests	If test isolates muscles, weakness and pain on contraction (Grade I or II) or weakness and no pain on contraction (Grade III)	Stress tests positive
Reflexes	Normal unless Grade III	Normal
Cutaneous distribution	Normal	Normal
Joint play/glide	Normal	Increased
Palpation of structure	Point tenderness Swelling (blood) Spasm	Point tenderness Swelling (blood/synovial fluid)
Diagnostic imaging	Positive MRI, arthrogram, and CT scan	Positive MRI, arthrogram, and CT scan Stress radiograph shows increased range of motion (ROM)

Source: Magee DJ (ed): Orthopedic Physical Assessment. Philadelphia, PA, WB Saunders, 2002.

TABLE 3-23 Differential Diagnosis of Contractile, Inert, and Nervous Tissue

	Contractile tissue	Inert tissue	Neural tissue
Pain	Cramping, dull, ache	Dull-sharp	Burning, lancinating
Paresthesia	No	No	Yes
Duration	Intermittent	Intermittent	Intermittent-constant
Dermatomal distribution	No	No	Yes
Peripheral nerve sensory distribution	No	No	Yes (if peripheral nerve involved)
End-feel	Muscle spasm	Boggy, hard capsular	Stretch

reactivity. Tissue reactivity is the manner in which different stresses and movements can alter the clinical signs and symptoms. This knowledge can be used to gauge any subtle changes to the patient's condition.[25]

Pain that occurs consistently with resistance, at whatever the length of the muscle, may indicate a tear of the muscle belly. Pain with muscle testing may indicate a muscle injury, a joint injury, or a combination of both (see Figure 3-3). Table 3-24 outlines four scenarios of muscle testing based on the work of Cyriax.[16,26]

Pain that does not occur during the test, but occurs upon the release of the contraction, is thought to have an articular source, produced by the joint glide that occurs following the release of tension.

The degree of significance with the findings in resisted testing depends on the position of the muscle, and the force applied (Table 3-25). For example, pain reproduced with a minimal contraction in the rest position for the muscle is more strongly suggestive of a contractile lesion than pain reproduced with a maximal contraction in the lengthened position for the muscle.

Whenever possible, the same muscle is tested on the opposite side, using the same testing procedure, and a comparison is made.

A number of scales have been devised to assess muscle strength (Tables 3-26 and 3-27).[27,28]

To be a valid test, strength testing must elicit a maximum contraction of the muscle being tested. Four strategies ensure this:

- *Placing the muscle to be tested in a shortened position.* This puts the muscle in an ineffective physiologic position, and has the effect of increasing motor neuron activity.
- *Having the patient perform an eccentric muscle contraction by using the command "Don't let me move you."* As the tension at each cross-bridge and the number of active cross-bridges is greater during an eccentric contraction, the maximum eccentric muscle tension developed is greater with an eccentric contraction than a concentric one (see Chapter 1).
- *Breaking the contraction.* It is important to break the patient's muscle contraction in order to ensure that the patient is making a maximal effort and that the full power of the muscle is being tested.
- *Holding the contraction for at least 5 seconds.* Weakness caused by nerve palsy has a distinct fatigability. The muscle demonstrates poor endurance as it is usually only able to sustain a maximum muscle contraction for about 2 to 3 seconds before complete failure occurs. This is based on the theories

TABLE 3-24 Findings from Muscle Testing

Finding	Possible explanation
Strong and painless contraction	Normal finding
Strong and painful contraction	Grade I contractile lesion
Weak and painless contraction	• Palsy • Complete rupture of the muscle-tendon unit
Weak and painful contraction	Serious pathology such as a significant muscle tear, fracture, tumor, etc.

TABLE 3-25 Strength Testing Related to Joint Position and Muscle Length

Muscle length	Rationale/purpose
Fully lengthened	• Muscle in position of passive insufficiency • Tightens the inert component of the muscle • Tests for muscle tears (tendoperiosteal tears) while using minimal force
Midrange	• Muscle in strongest position • Tests overall power of muscle
Fully shortened	• Muscle in its weakest position • Used for the detection of palsies especially if coupled with an eccentric contraction

TABLE 3-26 Muscle Grading

Grade	Value	Movement
5	Normal (100%)	Complete range of motion against gravity with maximal resistance
4	Good (75%)	Complete range of motion against gravity with some (moderate) resistance
3+	Fair+	Complete range of motion against gravity with minimal resistance
3	Fair (50%)	Complete range of motion against gravity
3−	Fair−	Some but not complete range of motion against gravity
2+	Poor+	Initiates motion against gravity
2	Poor (25%)	Complete range of motion with gravity eliminated
2−	Poor−	Initiates motion if gravity eliminated
1	Trace	Evidence of slight contractility but no joint motion
0	Zero	No contraction palpated

Source: Sapega AA: Muscle performance evaluation in orthopedic practice. J Bone Joint Surg 1990;72A:1562–1574.

TABLE 3-27 Muscle Grading According to Janda[28]

Grade	Interpretation
Grade 5: N (normal)	A normal, very strong muscle with a full range of movement and able to overcome considerable resistance. This does not mean that the muscle is normal in all circumstances (for example, when at the onset of fatigue or in a state of exhaustion).
Grade 4: G (good)	A muscle with good strength and a full range of movement, and able to overcome moderate resistance
Grade 3: F (fair)	A muscle with a complete range of movement against gravity only when resistance is not applied
Grade 2: P (poor)	A very weak muscle with a complete range of motion only when gravity is eliminated by careful positioning of the patient
Grade 1: T (trace)	A muscle with evidence of slight contractility but no effective movement
Grade 0	A muscle with no evidence of contractility

behind muscle recruitment wherein a normal muscle while performing a maximum contraction uses only a portion of its motor units, keeping the remainder in reserve to help maintain the contraction. A palsied muscle with its fewer functioning motor units, has very few, if any, in reserve. If a muscle appears to be weaker than normal, further investigation is required:

a. The test is repeated three times. Muscle weakness, resulting from disuse will be consistently weak and should not get weaker with several repeated contractions.

b. Another muscle that shares the same innervation (spinal nerve or peripheral nerve) is tested. Knowledge of both spinal nerve and peripheral nerve innervation will aid the clinician in determining which muscle to select.

Substitutions by other muscle groups during testing, indicates the presence of weakness. It does not, however, tell the clinician the cause of the weakness. The standard manual muscle testing positions as described by Kendall are depicted in Figures 3-6 through 3-40.

As always, these tests cannot be evaluated in isolation, but have to be integrated into a total clinical profile, before drawing any conclusion about the patient's condition.

Neurologic Testing

The evaluation of the transmission capability of the nervous system is performed to detect the presence of either an upper motor neuron (UMN) lesion or a lower motor neuron (LMN) lesion (refer to Chapter 4). In addition, the neurologic examination can often determine the exact site of the lesion.

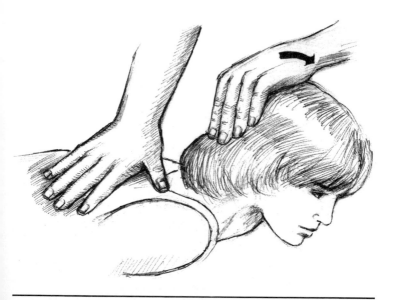

FIG. 3-6   Manual muscle testing position for the posterolateral head and neck extensors.

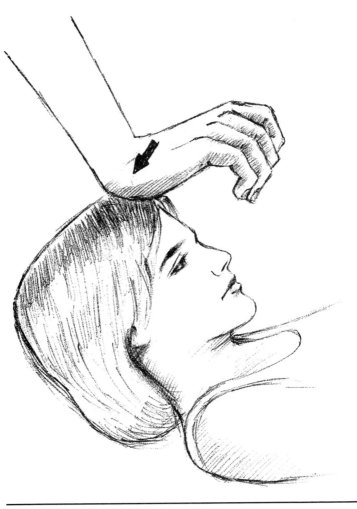

FIG. 3-7   Manual muscle testing position for the anterior head and neck flexors.

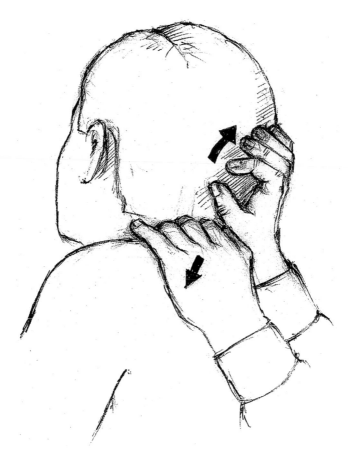

FIG. 3-8 Manual muscle testing position for the upper trapezius.

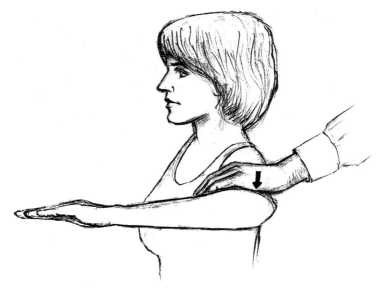

FIG. 3-9   Manual muscle testing position for the supraspinatus and middle deltoid.

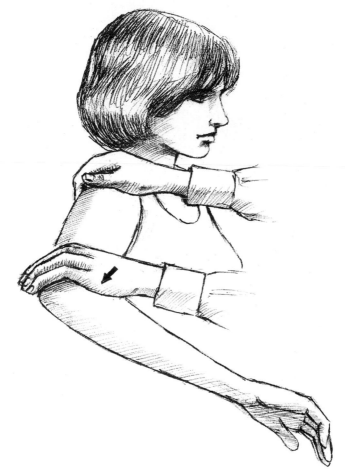

FIG. 3-10   Manual muscle testing position for the posterior deltoid.

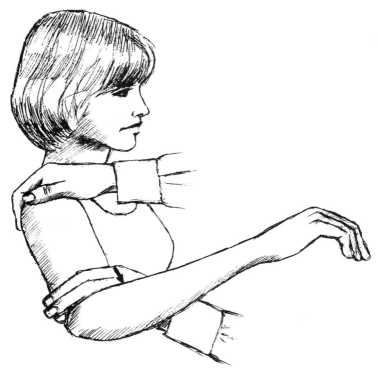

FIG. 3-11 Manual muscle testing position for the anterior deltoid.

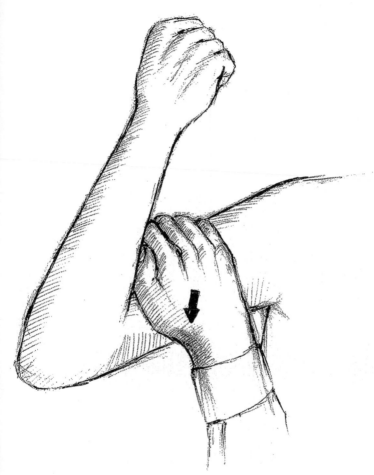

FIG. 3-12   Manual muscle testing position for the coracobrachialis.

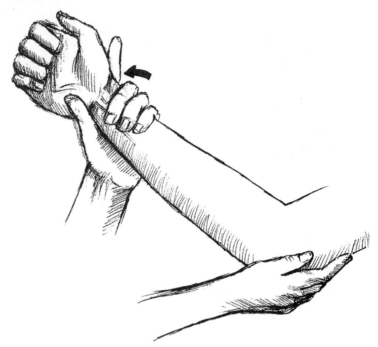

FIG. 3-13 Manual muscle testing position for the brachioradialis.

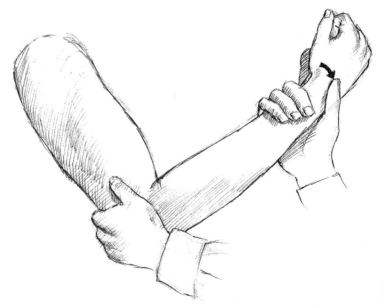

FIG. 3-14 Manual muscle testing position for the biceps.

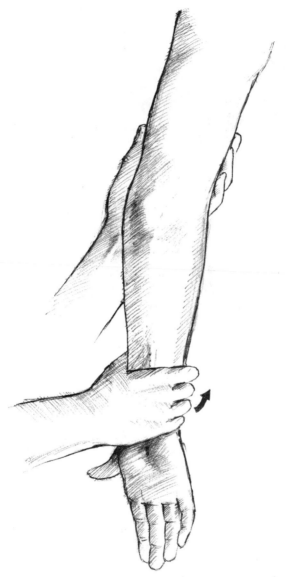

FIG. 3-15 Manual muscle testing position for the triceps brachii and anconeus.

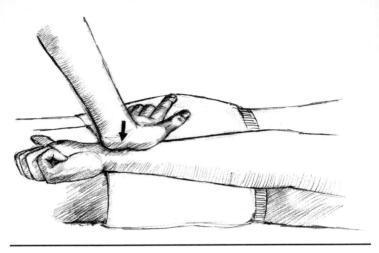

FIG. 3-16   Manual muscle testing position for the latissimus dorsi.

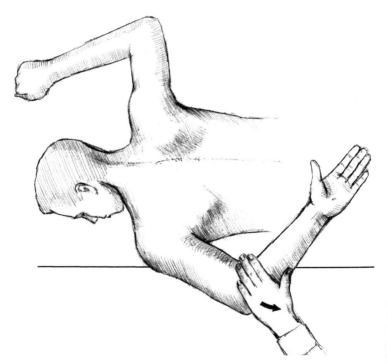

FIG. 3-17   Manual muscle testing position for the teres major.

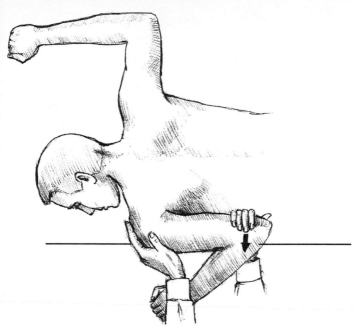

FIG. 3-18 Manual muscle testing position for the rhomboids and levator scapulae.

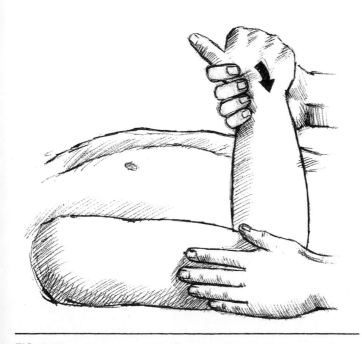

FIG. 3-19 Manual muscle testing position for the shoulder internal rotators.

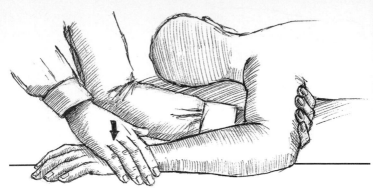

FIG. 3-20　Manual muscle testing position for the shoulder external rotators.

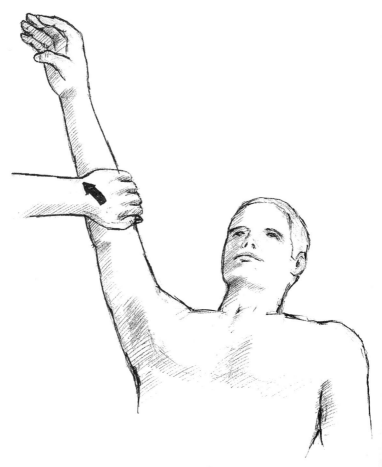

FIG. 3-21　Manual muscle testing position for the pectoralis major (lower fibers).

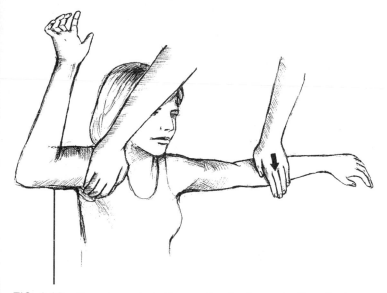

FIG. 3-22   Manual muscle testing position for the pectoralis major (upper fibers).

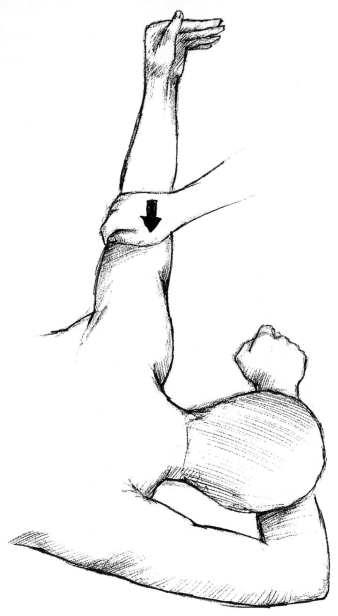

FIG. 3-23   Manual muscle testing position for the middle trapezius.

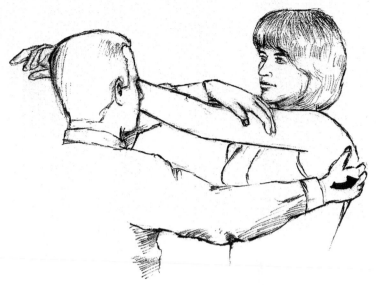

FIG. 3-24   Manual muscle testing position for the serratus anterior.

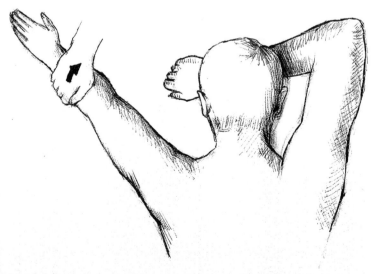

FIG. 3-25   Manual muscle testing position for the lower trapezius.

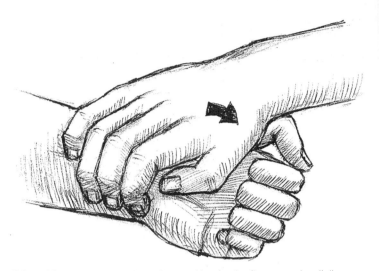

FIG. 3-26   Manual muscle testing position for the flexor carpi radialis.

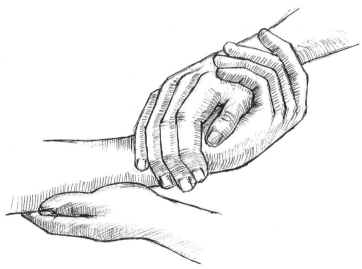

FIG. 3-27   Manual muscle testing position for the flexor carpi ulnaris.

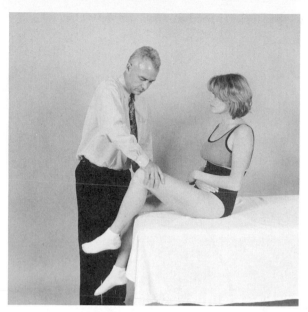

FIG. 3-28 Manual muscle testing position for the hip flexors. (*Reproduced with permission from Dutton M: Orthopaedic Examination, Evaluation, and Intervention, p 1182 (Fig. 25–28). New York, McGraw-Hill.*)

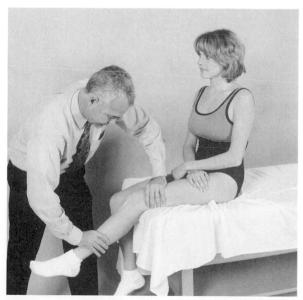

FIG. 3-29 Manual muscle testing position for the quadriceps femoris. (*Reproduced with permission from Dutton M: Orthopaedic Examination, Evaluation, and Intervention, p 1183 (Fig. 25–29). New York, McGraw-Hill.*)

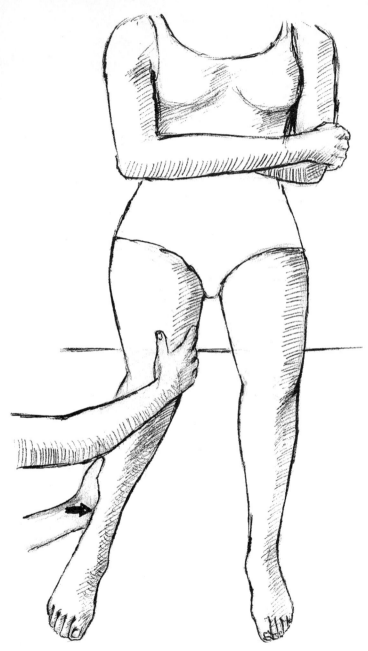

FIG. 3-30 Manual muscle testing position for the internal rotators of the hip.

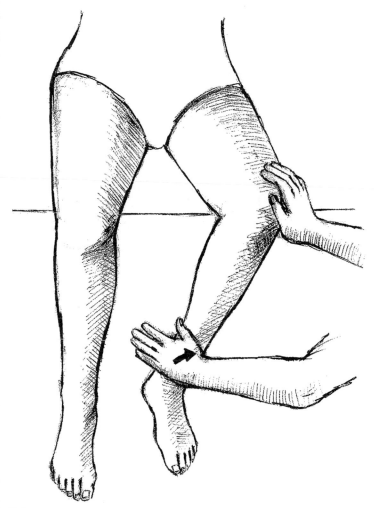

FIG. 3-31   Manual muscle testing position for the external rotators of the hip.

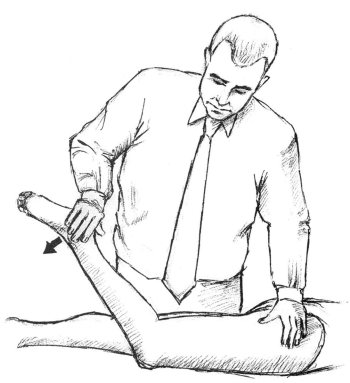

FIG. 3-32 Manual muscle testing position for the medial hamstrings.

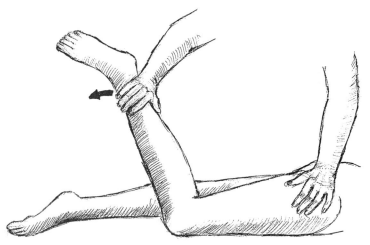

FIG. 3-33 Manual muscle testing position for the lateral hamstrings.

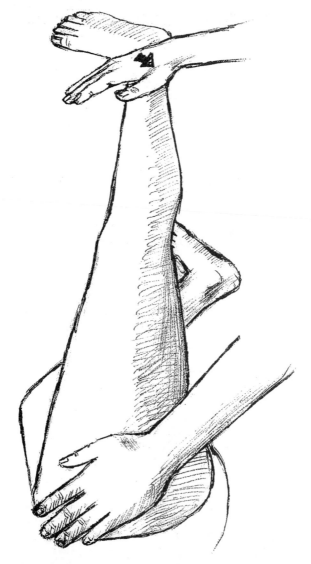

FIG. 3-34   Manual muscle testing position for the gluteus medius.

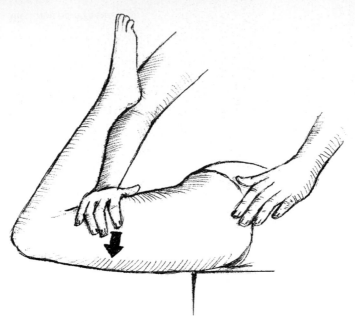

FIG. 3-35   Manual muscle testing position for the gluteus maximus.

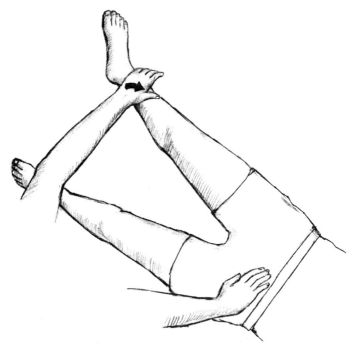

FIG. 3-36   Manual muscle testing position for the iliopsoas.

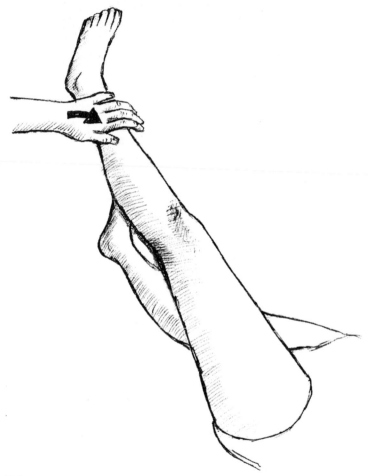

FIG. 3-37   Manual muscle testing position for the tensor of the fascia latae.

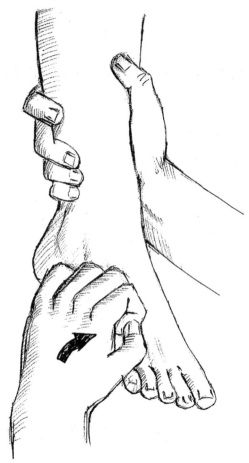

FIG. 3-38   Manual muscle testing position for the fibularis (peroneus) tertius.

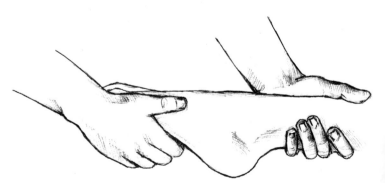

FIG. 3-39   Manual muscle testing position for the tibialis posterior.

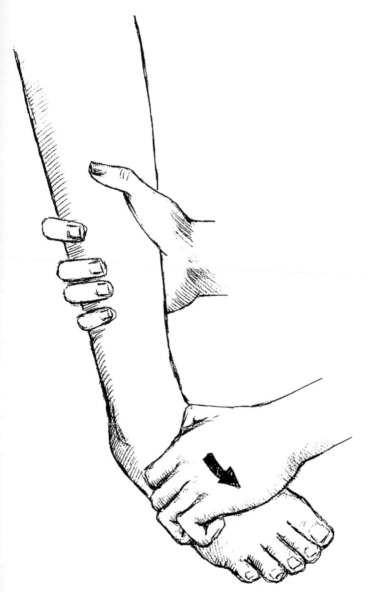

FIG. 3-40 Manual muscle testing position for the tibialis anterior.

Upper Motor Neuron Lesion

The UMN is located in the white columns of the spinal cord and the cerebral hemispheres. A UMN lesion is also known as a central palsy. It is characterized by spastic paralysis or paresis, little or no muscle atrophy, hyperreflexive DTRs in a nonsegmental distribution, and the presence of pathologic signs and reflexes (Table 3-28).

Lower Motor Neuron Lesion

An LMN lesion is also known as a peripheral palsy. These lesions can be caused by direct trauma, toxins, infections, ischemia, and compression. The characteristics of an LMN include muscle atrophy and hypotonus, a diminished or absent DTR of the areas served by a spinal nerve root, or a peripheral nerve and an absence of pathologic signs or reflexes.

The differing symptoms between a UMN and an LMN are the result of injuries to different parts of the nervous system. LMN impairment involves damage to a neurologic structure distal to the anterior horn cell, whereas the UMN impairment involves damage to a neurologic structure—proximal to the anterior horn cell—namely the spinal cord or central nervous system or both.

TABLE 3-28 Pathologic Reflexes

Reflex	Elicitation	Positive response	Pathology
Babinski's	Stroking of lateral aspect of side of foot	Extension of big toe and fanning of four small toes Normal reaction in newborns	Pyramidal tract lesion Organic hemiplegia
Chaddock's	Stroking of lateral side of foot beneath lateral malleolus	Same response as above	Pyramidal tract lesion
Oppenheim's	Stroking of anteromedial tibial surface	Same response as above	Pyramidal tract lesion
Gordon's	Squeezing of calf muscles firmly	Same response as above	Pyramidal tract lesion
Brudzinski's	Passive flexion of one lower limb	Similar movement occurs in opposite limb	Meningitis
Hoffmann's	"Flicking" of terminal phalanx of index, middle, or ring finger	Reflex flexion of distal phalanx of thumb and of distal phalanx of index or middle finger, whichever one was not "flicked"	Increased irritability of sensory nerves in tetany Pyramidal tract lesion
Lhermitte's	Neck flexion	An electric shock-like sensation that radiates down the spinal column into the upper or lower limbs	Abnormalities (demyelination) in the posterior part of the cervical spinal cord

Source: Magee DJ (ed): Orthopedic Physical Assessment. Philadelphia, PA, WB Saunders, 2002.

Spinal Reflexes

A reflex is a programmed unit of behavior in which a certain type of stimulus from a receptor automatically leads to the response of an effector. The assessment of reflexes is extremely important in the diagnosis and localization of neurologic lesions.[29] Reflex integrity is defined as the intactness of the neural path involved in a reflex.[1] Spinal or supraspinal (brain stem) pathways control reflexes using a hierarchy of control mechanisms. Of these control mechanisms, the spinal reflexes are the simplest (e.g., stretch reflex, withdrawal reflex) and are entirely contained in the spinal cord. The stretch reflex (myotactic) is an example of the spinal reflex.

Myotactic Reflex   The myotatic or DTR tests are used to determine the state of both the afferent and efferent peripheral nervous systems, and the ability of the CNS to inhibit the reflex.

Any muscle that possesses a tendon is capable of producing a DTR. Five of these are regularly tested: the biceps (C5), brachioradialis (C6), and triceps (C7) in the upper extremity, and the quadriceps (L4) and Achilles (S1) in the lower extremities (Table 3-29).

Deep tendon reflexes are graded as follows:

0	Absent (areflexia)
1+	Decreased (hyporeflexia)
2+	Normal
3+	Hyperactive (brisk)
4+	Hyperactive with clonus (hyperreflexive)

TABLE 3-29 Common Deep Tendon Reflexes

Reflex	Site of stimulus	Normal response	Pertinent central nervous system segment
Jaw	Mandible	Mouth closes	Cranial nerve V
Biceps	Biceps tendon	Biceps contraction	C5-6
Brachioradialis	Brachioradialis tendon or just distal to the musculotendinous junction	Flexion of elbow or pronation of forearm or both	C5-6
Triceps	Distal triceps tendon above the olecranon process	Elbow extension	C7-8
Patella	Patellar tendon	Leg extension	L3-4
Medial hamstrings	Semimembranosus tendon	Knee flexion	L5, S1
Lateral hamstrings	Biceps femoris tendon	Knee flexion	S1-2
Tibialis posterior	Tibialis posterior tendon behind medial malleolus	Plantar flexion of foot with inversion	L4-5
Achilles	Achilles tendon	Plantar flexion of foot	S1-2

Each of these categories can occur as a generalized, or local, phenomenon. The absence of a reflex signifies an interruption of the reflex arc. A hyperactive reflex denotes a release from cortical inhibitory influences. Reflex asymmetry has more pathologic significance than the absolute activity of the reflex. For example, a bilateral patella reflex of 3+ is less significant than a 3+ on the left and a 2+ on the right.

The causes of generalized hyporeflexia run the gamut from neurologic disease, chromosomal metabolic conditions, and hypothyroidism to schizophrenia and anxiety.[30] Hyporeflexia, if not generalized to the whole body, indicates an LMN or sensory paresis, which may be segmental (root), multisegmental (cauda equina), or nonsegmental (peripheral nerve).

True neurologic hyperreflexia contains a clonic component, and is suggestive of CNS (upper motor neuron) impairment such as a brainstem or cerebral impairment, spinal cord compression, or a neurologic disease. A brisk reflex is a normal finding, provided that it is not masking a hyperreflexia due to an incorrect testing technique. Unlike hyperreflexia, a brisk reflex does not have a clonic component.

As with hyporeflexia, the clinician should assess more than one reflex before coming to a conclusion about a hyperreflexia, and can confirm the presence of a UMN with the presence of the pathologic reflexes (see below).

Pathologic Reflexes

Individuals normally integrate pathologic reflexes as they develop, unless an injury or disease process results in a loss of this normal suppression by the cerebrum on the segmental level of the brainstem or spinal cord, resulting in a release of the primitive reflex.[31] Thus, the presence of pathologic reflexes is suggestive of CNS (upper motor neuron) impairment, and requires an appropriate referral (see Table 3-28).

Babinski In this test, the clinician applies noxious stimuli to sole of the patient's foot by running a pointed object along the plantar aspect.[32] A positive test, demonstrated by extension of the big toe and a splaying (abduction) of the other toes, is indicative of an injury to the corticospinal tract. The pyramidal tracts are not well developed in infants, and these signs, which are abnormal past the age of 3 years, are usually present.

Oppenheim The clinician applies noxious stimuli to the crest of the patient's tibia by running a fingernail along the crest. A positive test, demonstrated by the Babinski sign, is indicative of a UMN impairment.

Clonus The clinician passively applies a sudden dorsiflexion of the patient's ankle and the stretch is maintained during the test. The clinician notes a gradual increase in tone and then the transient occurrence of ankle clonus. In some patients, there is a more sustained clonus, and in others there is only a very short-lived finding. During the testing, the patient should not flex their neck as this can often increase the number of beats. A positive test, demonstrated by four or five reflex twitches of the plantar flexors (two to three twitches are considered normal), is indicative of UMN impairment.

Superficial Skin Reflexes The abdominal and cremaster reflexes are decreased or absent on the side, affected by a corticospinal tract lesion and thus, serve as adjuncts to the muscle stretch and plantar reflexes (Table 3-30).[33]

TABLE 3-30 Superficial Reflexes

Reflex	Normal response	Pertinent central nervous system segment
Upper abdominal	Umbilicus moves up and toward area being stroked	T7-9
Lower abdominal	Umbilicus moves down and toward area being stroked	T11-12
Cremasteric	Scrotum elevates	T12, L1
Plantar	Flexion of toes	S1-2
Gluteal	Skin tenses in gluteal area	L4-5, S1-3
Anal	Contraction of anal sphincter muscles	S2-4

Hoffmann's Sign   Hoffmann's sign is the upper limb equivalent of the Babinski. However, unlike the Babinski, some normal individuals can exhibit a present Hoffmann's sign.[33]

The clinician holds the patient's middle finger and briskly pinches the distal phalanx thereby applying a noxious stimulus to the nail bed of the middle finger.[33] Denno and Meadows[34] devised a dynamic version of the Hoffman's sign, which involves the patient performing repeated flexion and extension of the head before being tested for the Hoffmann's sign. A positive response for this test is the presence of the Hoffman's sign (Table 3-28).

Supraspinal Reflexes

The supraspinal reflexes produce movement patterns, which can be modulated by descending pathways and the cortex. A number of processes involved in locomotor function are oriented around these reflexes and are referred to as postural reflexes. Postural reflexes are those that help maintain postural equilibrium and stability during head, trunk, and extremity motions, as well as those that react in situations that have the potential to cause serious injury.

Cervicoocular and Vestibuloocular Reflexes   The cervicoocular reflexes (COR) and vestibuloocular reflexes (VOR) work together to maintain the position and *visual fixation* of the eyes during movements of the head and neck. The ability to track and focus on a moving target that is moving across a visual field is termed *smooth pursuit*, and requires a greater degree of voluntary control than the COR and VOR can provide. The area in the brain stem where this integration of horizontal eye movements takes place is the paramedian pontine reticular formation (PPRF).

Separate tests exist for visual fixation, VOR, and smooth pursuit (see *Orthopaedic Examination, Evaluation, and Intervention*, pp 66–68).

Sensory Testing

The dorsal roots of the spinal nerves are represented by a series of restricted peripheral sensory regions called dermatomes (see Chapter 2, Figure 2-2).

The peripheral sensory nerves are represented by a number of more distinct and circumscribed areas (see Chapter 2, Figure 2-2). Sensory testing is performed throughout the dermatomal areas. The segmental innervation of the skin has a high degree of overlap, especially in the thoracic spine, necessitating the clinician to test the full area of the dermatome. This is done in order to seek out the area of sensitivity, or autogenous area, which is a small region of the dermatome with no overlap, and the only area within a dermatome that is supplied exclusively by a single segmental level.[35] It is important to start with an area of normal sensation before moving toward an area of altered sensation to provide the patient with an appropriate reference point.

Pain sensation is generally tested with a pin or needle, and soft touch is adequately tested with a wisp of cotton. Mapping the area of involvement helps to categorize the abnormality into a specifically defined syndrome (i.e., dermatomal, nerve, nerve root, or glove and stocking pattern), a spinal cord lesion, or a peripheral nerve abnormality.[8] The proximal sensory examination should be compared with the distal examination, paying special attention to areas of numbness. Symmetric distal sensory loss is compatible with a polyneuropathy.

Vibration sense is tested by placing the stem of a 128- or 256-cps (cycles per second) tuning fork against several bony prominences, beginning at the most distal points. Loss of vibratory sensation occurs relatively early in a peripheral neuropathy such as those related to diabetes, alcoholism, vitamin B_{12} deficiency or dorsal column disease.[8] If the patient does not respond in the distal joints, the more proximal joints should be checked. The clinician should make sure the patient is responding to the vibration and not the pressure of the instrument by occasionally dampening the vibration and eliciting a response.[8]

Proprioception is tested by grasping the sides of the finger or toe being tested and asking the patient, whose eyes should be closed, to indicate whether the digit is moved into an up or a down position. A loss of position sense is associated with a nerve root lesion, a peripheral nerve abnormality or dorsal column disease.

Thermal sensation is tested with test tubes filled with water of various temperatures. Patients with normal thermal sensation should be able to distinguish between stimuli differing by a few degrees.[8] Unfortunately, this test relies on a subjective patient response, which is dependent on the patient's level of motivation and cognition.

Cranial Nerve Examination

With practice, the entire cranial nerve examination (refer to larger text) can be performed in approximately 5 minutes (Table 3-31).[36] The following may be used to help remember the order and tests for the cranial nerve examination:[37]

- Smell and see
- And look around,
- Pupils large and smaller.
- Smile, hear!
- Then say ah …
- And see if you can swallow.
- If you're left in any doubt,
- Shrug and stick your tongue right out.

TABLE 3-31 Cranial Nerves and Methods of Testing

Nerve	Afferent (sensory)	Efferent (motor)	Test
I. Olfactory	Smell	—	Identify familiar odors (e.g., chocolate, coffee)
II. Optic	Sight	—	Test visual fields
III. Oculomotor	—	Voluntary motor: levator of eyelid; superior, medial, and inferior recti; inferior oblique muscle of eyeball Autonomic: smooth muscle of eyeball	Upward, downward, and medial gaze Reaction to light
IV. Trochlear	—	Voluntary motor: superior oblique muscle of eyeball	Downward and lateral gaze
V. Trigeminal	Touch, pain: skin of face, mucous membranes of nose, sinuses, mouth, anterior tongue	Voluntary motor: muscles of mastication	Corneal reflex Face sensation Clench teeth: push down on chin to separate jaws
VI. Abducens	—	Voluntary motor: lateral rectus muscle of eyeball	Lateral gaze
VII. Facial	Taste: anterior tongue	Voluntary motor: facial muscles Autonomic: lacrimal, submandibular, and sublingual glands	Close eyes tight Smile and show teeth Whistle and puff cheeks Identify familiar tastes (e.g., sweet, sour)
VIII. Vestibulocochlear (acoustic nerve)	Hearing: ear Balance: ear	—	Hear watch ticking Hearing tests Balance and coordination test

(Continued)

TABLE 3-31 Cranial Nerves and Methods of Testing (*Continued*)

Nerve	Afferent (sensory)	Efferent (motor)	Test
IX. Glossopharyngeal	Touch, pain: posterior tongue, pharynx Taste: posterior tongue	Voluntary motor: unimportant muscle of pharynx Autonomic: parotid gland	Gag reflex Ability to swallow
X. Vagus	Touch, pain: pharynx, larynx, bronchi Taste: tongue, epiglottis	Voluntary motor: muscles of palate, pharynx, and larynx Autonomic: thoracic and abdominal viscera	Gag reflex Ability to swallow Say "Ahhh"
XI. Accessory	—	Voluntary motor: sternocleidomastoid and trapezius muscle	Resisted shoulder shrug
XII. Hypoglossal	—	Voluntary motor: muscles of tongue	Tongue protrusion (if injured, tongue deviates toward injured side)

Source: Hollinshead WH, Jenkins DB: Functional Anatomy of the Limbs and Back. Philadelphia, PA, WB Saunders, 1981.

Neurodynamic Mobility Tests

Neurodynamic mobility testing is designed to examine the neurologic structures for adaptive shortening and inflammation of the neural structures both centrally and peripherally (see *Orthopaedic Examination, Evaluation, and Intervention*, Chapter 12). These tests are used if a dural adhesion or irritation is suspected. The tests employ a sequential and progressive stretch to the dura until the patient's symptoms are reproduced.[38] Theoretically, if the dura is scarred, or inflamed, a lack of extensibility with stretching occurs. Because the sinuvertebral nerve innervates the dural sleeve, the pain caused by an inflamed dura, is felt by the patient at multisegmental levels, and is described as having an ache-like quality. If the patient experiences sharp or stabbing pain during the test, a more serious underlying condition should be suspected.

Tests for the lumbosacral plexus stress the sciatic nerve and include the slump test and the straight leg raise (SLR). The prone knee bend stresses the femoral nerve (see *Orthopaedic Examination, Evaluation, and Intervention*, Chapter 12).

Tests for the brachial plexus, the so-called upper limb tension tests (ULTT), include tests for the median, radial, and ulnar nerve (see *Orthopaedic Examination, Evaluation, and Intervention*, Chapter 12). Tests have also been designed to assess the neurodynamic mobility of the musculocutaneous, axillary, and suprascapular nerve (see *Orthopaedic Examination, Evaluation, and Intervention*, pp 368–369).

Palpation

Palpation can play a central role in the diagnosis.[39] Palpation should be performed at three levels of manual pressure: first with light pressure for conformity and temperature (tactile gnosis), second palpation for tissue induration and effusion, and finally palpation for tenderness.[40] By gradually increasing the manual pressure, the clinician will gain the confidence of the patient. The purpose of the palpatory examination is to:[41,42]

- Check for any vasomotor changes such as an increase in skin temperature that might suggest an inflammatory process.
- Localize specific sites of swelling.
- Identify specific anatomic structures and their relationship to one another (Table 3-32).
- Identify sites of point tenderness. Hyperalgic skin zones (HAZ) can be detected using skin drag, which consists of moving the pads of the fingertips over the surface of the skin, and attempting to sense resistance or drag.
- Identify soft tissue texture changes or myofascial restriction. Normal tissue is soft and mobile, and moves equally in all directions. Abnormal tissue may feel hard, sensitive, or somewhat crunchy or stringy.[43]
- Locate changes in muscle tone resulting from, trigger points, muscle spasm, hypertonicity, or hypotonicity.
- Determine circulatory status by checking distal pulses.
- Detect changes in the moisture of the skin.

TABLE 3-32 Palpation Points of Common Muscle Attachments

Landmark	Muscle/tendon attachment
Greater tuberosity of humerus	Supraspinatus
	Infraspinatus
	Teres minor
	Pectoralis major
Lesser tuberosity of humerus	Teres major
	Subscapularis
Medial epicondyle of humerus	Origin of common flexor tendon
Lateral epicondyle	Origin of common extensor tendon
Ulna tuberosity	Brachialis
Radial tuberosity	Biceps brachii
Anterior superior iliac spine	Rectus femoris
	Sartorius
Greater trochanter	Gluteus minimus
	Gluteus medius
	Vastus lateralis
	Piriformis
	Obturator internus
	Inferior gemelli
Lesser trochanter	Psoas major
Ischial tuberosity	Semitendinosus
	Semimembranosus
	Biceps femoris
	Adductor magnus

Aerobic Capacity and Endurance

Aerobic capacity endurance is the ability to perform work or participate in activity over time using the body's oxygen uptake, delivery, and energy release mechanisms.[1] Clinical indications for the use of the tests and measures for this category are based on the findings of the history and systems review.

The aerobic capacity and endurance of a patient can be measured using standardized exercise test protocols (e.g., ergometry, step tests, time/distance walk/run tests, treadmill tests), and the patient's response to such tests.[1]

Anthropometric Characteristics

Anthropometric characteristics are those traits that describe body dimensions, such as height, weight, girth, and body fat composition.[1] The use of an anthropometric examination and the subsequent measurements vary. Clearly, if there is a noticeable amount of effusion or swelling present, these measurements serve as an important baseline from which to judge the effectiveness of the intervention.

Swelling or edema may be localized at the site of the injury or diffused over a larger area. In general, the amount of swelling is related to the severity of the injury. However, there are cases in which serious injuries produce very limited swelling and minor injuries that cause significant swelling. These changes occur as a result of changes in the local circulation and an inability of the lymphatic system to maintain equilibrium.

A report of rapid swelling (within 2-4 hours) following a traumatic event may indicate bleeding into the joint. Swelling that is more gradual, occurring 8–24 hours following the trauma is likely caused by an inflammatory process or synovial swelling.

An edematous limb indicates poor venous return. Pitting edema is characterized by an indentation of the skin after the pressure has been removed.

The more serious reasons for swelling include fracture, tumor, congestive heart failure, and deep vein thrombosis (DVT).

Gait, Locomotion, and Balance

Gait analysis is an important component of the examination process, and should not just be reserved for those patients with lower extremity dysfunction (see *Orthopaedic Examination, Evaluation, and Intervention*, Chapter 13). Gait, like posture, varies between individuals, and a gait that differs from normal is not necessarily pathologic. The examination of gait is performed to highlight any breakdown within these reflexes, including imbalances of flexibility and/or strength, or compensatory motions (Tables 3-33 through 3-36).[44]

Special Tests

Special tests for each area are dependent on the special needs and structure of each joint. Numerous tests exist for each joint. These tests are usually performed only if there is some indication that they would be helpful in arriving at a diagnosis. The tests help confirm or implicate a particular structure and may also provide information as to the degree of tissue damage.

The interpretation of the findings from a special test depends on the skill and experience of the clinician, the specificity of the test, and the degree of familiarity with the test.

Imaging Studies

Although the ordering of imaging studies is not within the scope of physical therapy practice, clinicians frequently receive imaging study reports (see *Orthopaedic Examination, Evaluation, and Intervention*, pp 193–196). Thus, it is important for the clinician to know what relevance to attach to these reports, and the strengths and weaknesses of the various imaging techniques (Table 3-37). In general, imaging tests have a high sensitivity (few false negatives), but low specificity (high false-positive rate).

TABLE 3-33 Joint Motions and Muscle Activity at the Hip and Knee, and Joint Positions and Motions of the Tibia, Foot, and Ankle during Gait

Phase	Hip	Knee	Tibia	Ankle	Foot
• Heel strike	• Gluteus maximus and hamstrings work eccentrically to resist flexion moment at the hip. • Erector spinae working eccentrically to control trunk flexion • The hip begins to extend from a position of 20–40° of flexion • Reaction force anterior to the hip joint creating a flexion moment • Hip positioned in slight adduction and external rotation	• Positioned in full extension before heel contact, but flexing as heel makes contact • Reaction force behind knee causing flexion moment • Quadriceps femoris contracting eccentrically to control knee flexion	• Slight external rotation	• Moving into plantar flexion	• Supination
• Foot Flat	• Gluteus maximus and hamstrings contract concentrically to move hip toward extension • Hip moving into extension, adduction, and internal rotation	• In 20° of knee flexion, moving toward extension • Flexion moment • After foot is flat, quadriceps femoris activity becoming concentric to bring femur over tibia	• Internal rotation	• Plantar flexion to dorsiflexion over a fixed foot	• Pronation, adapting to support surface

Phase	Hip	Knee	Rotation	Ankle	Foot
• Midstance	• Hip moves through neutral position • Pelvis rotates posteriorly • Reaction force now posterior to hip joint creating an extension moment • Iliopsoas contracting eccentrically to resist hip extension • Gluteus medius creating reverse action to stabilize opposite pelvis	• In 15° of flexion, moving toward extension • Maximum flexion moment • Quadriceps femoris activity decreasing	• Neutral rotation	• 3° of dorsiflexion	• Neutral
• Heel off	• Hip positioned in 10°–15° of hip extension, abduction, and external rotation • Iliopsoas activity continuing • Extension moment decreases after double-limb support begins	• In 4° of flexion, moving toward extension • Maximum flexion moment • Quadriceps femoris activity decreasing	• External rotation	• 15° dorsiflexion toward plantar flexion • Maximum dorsiflexion moment	• Supination as foot becomes rigid for push-off
• Toe off	• Hip moving toward 10° of extension, abduction, and external rotation • Continued decrease of extension moment • Iliopsoas activity continuing • Adductor magnus working eccentrically to control pelvis	• Moving from near full extension to 40° of flexion • Reaction forces moving posterior to knee as knee flexes • Flexion moment • Quadriceps femoris contracting eccentrically	• External rotation	• 20° of plantar flexion • Dorsiflexion moment	• Supination

TABLE 3-34 Muscle Functions of the Lower Leg during the Stance Phase of Gait

Muscle	Action
Heel strike to weight acceptance	Eccentric—control pronation of subtalar joint
Anterior tibialis	Eccentric—decelerate plantar flexion and posterior shear of tibia on talus
Extensor hallucis longus	
Extensor digitorum	Eccentric—decelerate pronation of subtalar joint and internal rotation of the tibia
Posterior tibialis	
Soleus	
Gastrocnemius	
Midstance	
Posterior tibialis	Eccentric—decelerate forward movement of tibia
Soleus	
Flexor hallucis longus	Concentric—supinate subtalar and midtarsal joints
Flexor digitorum longus	
Posterior tibialis	
Soleus	
Gastrocnemius	
Push-off and Propulsion	
Fibularis (Peroneus) longus	Concentric—plantar flexion of first ray
Abductor hallucis	
Fibularis (Peroneus) brevis	Antagonist to supinators of subtalar and midtarsal joints
Flexor digitorum longus	Concentric—stabilize toes against ground
Extensor hallucis longus and brevis	Concentric—stabilize first metatarsophalangeal joint
Abductor hallucis	Concentric—stabilize midtarsal and forefoot, raise medial arch of foot in push-off
Abductor digit quinti	
Flexor hallucis brevis	
Flexor digitorum brevis	
Extensor digitorum brevis	
Interossei, lumbricals	

Source: Donatelli RA: Normal anatomy and biomechanics. In Donatelli RA (ed): Biomechanics of the Foot and Ankle, pp 3–31. Philadelphia, PA, WB Saunders, 1990.

TABLE 3-35 Some Causes of Antalgic Gait[37]

Bone disease	Fracture
	Infection
	Tumor
	Avascular necrosis (Legg-Calvé-Perthes disease. Osgood Schlatter's disease, Köhler's disease)
Muscle disorder	Traumatic rupture, contusion
	Cramp secondary to fatigue, strain, malposition, or claudication
	Inflammatory myositis
Joint disease	Traumatic arthritis
	Infectious arthritis
	Rheumatoid arthritis
	Crystalline arthritis (gout, pseudogout)
	Hemarthrosis
	Bursitis
Neurologic disease	Lumbar spine disease with nerve root irritation or compression
Other	Hip, knee, or foot trauma
	Corns, bunions, blisters, ingrown toenails

TABLE 3-36 Some Gait Deviations and Their Causes

Gait deviations	Reasons
Slower cadence than expected for person's age	Generalized weakness Pain Joint motion restrictions Poor voluntary motor control
Shorter stance phase on the involved side and a decreased swing phase on the uninvolved side • Shorter stride length on the uninvolved side • Decrease lateral sway over the involved stance limb • Decrease in cadence • Decrease in velocity • Use of an assistive device	Antalgic gait, resulting from a painful injury to the lower limb and pelvic region
Stance phase longer on one side	Pain Lack of trunk and pelvic rotation Weakness of lower limb muscles Restrictions in lower limb joints Poor muscle control Increased muscle tone
Lateral trunk lean (The purpose is to bring the center of gravity of the trunk nearer to the hip joint.)	Ipsilateral lean—hip abductor weakness (gluteus medius/trendelenburg gait) Contralateral lean—decreased hip flexion in swing limb Painful hip Abnormal hip joint (congenital dysplasia, coxa vara, etc.) Wide walking base Unequal leg length
Anterior trunk leaning (Occurs at initial contact to move the line of gravity in front of the axis of the knee)	Weak or paralyzed knee extensors, or gluteus maximus Decreased ankle dorsiflexion Hip flexion contracture
Posterior trunk leaning (Occurs at initial contact to bring the line of the external force behind the axis of the hip)	Weak or paralyzed hip extensors, especially the gluteus maximus (gluteus maximus gait) Hip pain Hip flexion contracture Inadequate hip flexion in swing Decreased knee range of motion
Increased lumbar lordosis (Occurs at the end of the stance period)	Inability to extend the hip, usually due to a flexion contracture or ankylosis
Pelvic drop during stance	Contralateral gluteus medius weakness Adaptive shortening of quadratus lumborum on the swing side Contralateral hip adductor spasticity
Excessive pelvic rotation	Adaptively shortened/spasticity of hip flexors on same side Limited hip joint flexion

(Continued)

TABLE 3-36 Some Gait Deviations and Their Causes (*Continued*)

Gait deviations	Reasons
Circumducted hip (Ground contact by the swinging leg can be avoided if it is swung outward [in order for natural walking to occur, the leg that is in its stance phase needs to be longer than the leg that is in its swing phase in order to allow toe clearance of the swing foot].)	Functional leg length discrepancy Arthrogenic stiff hip or knee
Hip hiking (The pelvis is lifted on the side of the swinging leg, by contraction of the spinal muscles and the lateral abdominal wall.)	Functional leg length discrepancy Inadequate hip flexion, knee flexion, or ankle dorsiflexion Hamstring weakness Quadratus lumborum shortening
Vaulting (The ground clearance of the swinging leg will be increased if the subject goes up on the toes of the stance period leg.)	Functional leg length discrepancy Vaulting occurs on the shorter limb side
Abnormal internal hip rotation (Produces a "toe in" gait)	Adaptive shortening of the iliotibial band Weakness of the hip external rotators Femoral anteversion Adaptive shortening of the hip internal rotators
Abnormal external hip rotation (Produces a "toe out" gait)	Adaptive shortening of the hip external rotators Femoral retroversion Weakness of the hip internal rotators
Increased hip adduction (scissor gait) (Results in excessive hip adduction during swing [scissoring], decreased base of support, and decreased progression of opposite foot)	Spasticity or contracture of ipsilateral hip adductors Ipsilateral hip adductor weakness Coxa vara
Inadequate hip extension/excessive hip flexion (Results in loss of hip extension in midstance [forward leaning of trunk, increased lordosis, and increased knee flexion and ankle dorsiflexion] and late stance [anterior pelvic tilt], and increased hip flexion in swing)	Hip flexion contracture Iliotibial band contracture Hip flexor spasticity Pain Arthrodesis (surgical or spontaneous ankylosis) Loss of ankle dorsiflexion
Inadequate hip flexion (Results in decreased limb advancement in swing, posterior pelvic tilt, circumduction, and excessive knee flexion to clear foot)	Hip flexor weakness Hip joint arthrodesis

(*Continued*)

TABLE 3-36 Some Gait Deviations and Their Causes (*Continued*)

Gait deviations	Reasons
Decreased hip swing through (psoatic limp) (Manifested by exaggerated movements at the pelvis and trunk to assist the hip to move into flexion)	Legg-Calvé-Perthes disease Weakness or reflex inhibition of the psoas major muscle
Excessive knee extension/ Inadequate knee flexion (Results in decreased knee flexion at initial contact and loading response, increased knee extension during stance, and decreased knee flexion during swing)	Pain Anterior trunk deviation/bending Weakness of the quadriceps. The hyperextension is a compensation and places the body weight vector anterior to the knee Spasticity of the quadriceps. This is noted more during the loading response and during the initial swing intervals Joint deformity
Excessive knee flexion/Inadequate knee extension (At initial contact or around midstance. Results in increased knee flexion in early stance, decreased knee extension in midstance and terminal stance, and decreased knee extension during swing)	Knee flexion contracture resulting in decreased step length, and decreased knee extension instance Increased tone/spasticity of hamstrings or hip flexors Decreased range of motion of ankle dorsiflexion in swing period Weakness of plantar flexors resulting in increased dorsiflexion in stance Lengthened limb
Inadequate dorsiflexion control ("foot slap") during initial contact to midstance	Weak or paralyzed dorsiflexors Lack of lower limb proprioception
Steppage gait during the acceleration through deceleration of the swing phase Exaggerated knee and hip flexion are used to lift the foot higher than usual, for increased ground clearance resulting from a foot drop.	Weak or paralyzed dorsiflexor muscles Functional leg length discrepancy
Increased walking base (>20 cm)	Deformity such as hip abductor muscle contracture Genu valgus Fear of losing balance Leg length discrepancy
Decreased walking base (<10 cm)	Hip adductor muscle contracture Genu varum
Excessive eversion of calcaneus during initial contact through midstance	Excessive tibia vara (refers to the frontal plane position of the distal 1/3 of the leg as it relates to the supporting surface) Forefoot varus Weakness of tibialis posterior Excessive lower extremity internal rotation (due to muscle imbalances, femoral anteversion)

(*Continued*)

TABLE 3-36 Some Gait Deviations and Their Causes (*Continued*)

Gait deviations	Reasons
Excessive pronation during mid-stance through terminal stance	Insufficient ankle dorsiflexion (less than 10°)
	Increased tibial varum
	Compensated forefoot or rearfoot varus deformity
	Uncompensated forefoot valgus deformity
	Pes planus
	Long limb
	Uncompensated medial rotation of tibia or femur
	Weak tibialis anterior
Excessive supination during initial contact through midstance	Limited calcaneal eversion
	Rigid forefoot valgus
	Pes cavus
	Uncompensated lateral rotation of the tibia or femur
	Short limb
	Plantar flexed 1st ray
	Upper motor neuron muscle imbalance
Excessive dorsiflexion	Compensation for knee flexion contracture
	Inadequate plantar flexor strength
	Adaptive shortening of dorsiflexors
	Increased muscle tone of dorsiflexors
	Pes calcaneus deformity
Excessive plantar flexion	Increased plantar flexor activity
	Plantar flexor contracture
Excessive varus	Contracture
	Overactivity of the muscles on the medial aspect of the foot
Excessive valgus	Weak invertors
	Foot hypermobility
Decreased or absence of propulsion (plantar flexor gait)	Inability of plantar flexors to perform function resulting in a shorter step length on the involved side.

Sources: Giallonardo LM: Clinical evaluation of foot and ankle dysfunction. Phys Ther 1988;68:1850–1856.
Epler M: Gait. In Richardson JK, Iglarsh ZA (eds): Clinical Orthopaedic Physical Therapy, pp 602–625. Philadelphia, PA, WB Saunders, 1994.
Hunt GC, Brocato RS: Gait and foot pathomechanics. In Hunt GC (ed): Physical Therapy of the Foot and Ankle. Edinburgh, Churchill Livingstone, 1988.
Krebs DE, et al: Hip biomechanics during gait. J Orthop Sports Phys Ther 1998;28(1):51–59.
Larish DD, Martin PE, Mungiole M: Characteristic patterns of gait in the healthy old. Ann N Y Acad Sci 1987;515:18–32.
Levine D, Whittle M: Gait analysis: The lower extremities. Orthopaedic Physical Therapy Home Study Course—The Lower Extremity, vol. 92–1. La Crosse, WI: Orthopaedic Section, APTA, 1992.
Perry J: Gait Analysis: Normal and Pathological Function. Thorofare, NJ, Slack Inc, 1992.
Song KM, Halliday SE, Little DG: The effect of limb-length discrepancy on gait. J Bone Joint Surg 1997;79A:1690–1698.

TABLE 3-37 Strengths and Weaknesses of Various Imaging Studies

Imaging study	Advantages	Disadvantages
Plain-film, or conventional radiograph	Helpful in detecting fractures and subluxations in patients with a history of trauma Highlight the presence of degenerative joint disease	Do not provide an image of soft tissue structures such as muscles, tendons, ligaments, and intervertebral disks
Stress radiograph	Helpful in assessing spinal mobility and stability in the spine	Patient may not tolerate stress position
Arthrogram	Outlines the soft tissue structures of a joint that would otherwise not be visible with a plain-film radiograph Good for detecting internal derangements	Mildly invasive May require imaging guidance to place the needle
Myelography	Provides image of the spinal cord, nerve roots, dura mater, and the spinal canal	Potential for a postmyelogram headache Potential for seizure (rare)
Computed tomography (CT)	Provides good visualization of the shape, symmetry, and position of structures by delineating specific areas Quicker scan than MRI Better detail of bone than MRI	Generally limited to axial plane Soft tissue contrast not as good as MRI
Magnetic resonance imaging (MRI)	Excellent tissue contrast No streak artifacts Ability to provide cross-sectional images Noninvasive nature Complete lack of ionizing radiation Can take images of any plane	Expensive Time consuming Poor visualization of cortical bone detail or calcifications Limited spatial resolution compared with CT
Diagnostic ultrasound	Readily available Noninvasive Much less expensive than CT or MRI Can be used in any plane (sagittal, coronal, axial, and at any obliquity) Can detect soft tissue injuries, tumors, bone infections, bone mineral density, and arthropathy	Not a sharp, clear image compared to images produced by other radiologic modalities Because of the degrees of obliquity, one cannot easily tell what one is looking at with knowledge of cross-sectional anatomy; sonographer identifies anatomic segment. Visualization of structures limited by bone and gas (lung, bowel)

REFERENCES

1. Guide to physical therapist practice. Phys Ther 2001;81:S13–S95.
2. Goodman CC, Snyder TEK: Differential Diagnosis in Physical Therapy. Philadelphia, PA, WB Saunders, 1990.
3. Goodman CC, Snyder TK: Introduction to the interviewing process. In Goodman CC, Snyder TK (eds): Differential Diagnosis in Physical Therapy, pp 7–42. Philadelphia, PA, WB Saunders, 1990.
4. Maitland G: Vertebral Manipulation. Sydney, Butterworth, 1986.
5. McKenzie R, May S: History. In McKenzie R, May S (eds): The Human Extremities: Mechanical Diagnosis and Therapy, pp 89–103. Waikanae, New Zealand, Spinal Publications, 2000.
6. Rowland LP: Diseases of the motor unit. In Kandel ER, Schwartz JH, Jessell TM (eds): Principles of Neural Science, pp 695–712. New York, McGraw-Hill, 2000.
7. McKnight JT, Adcock BB: Paresthesias: A practical diagnostic approach. Am Fam Physician 1997;56:2253–2260.
8. Poncelet AN: An algorithm for the evaluation of peripheral neuropathy. Am Fam Physician 1998;57:755–764.
9. Boissonnault WG: Examination in Physical Therapy Practice: Screening for Medical Disease. New York, Churchill Livingstone, 1991.
10. Magarey ME: Examination of the cervical and thoracic spine. In Grant R (ed): Physical Therapy of the Cervical and Thoracic Spine, pp 109–144. New York, Churchill Livingstone, 1994.
11. Silverman K, et al.: Withdrawal syndrome after the double-blind cessation of caffeine consumption. N Engl J Med 1992;327:1109–1114.
12. Jaeschke R, Guyatt G, Sackett DL: Users guides to the medical literature: III. How to use an article about a diagnostic test. B. What are the results and will they help me in caring for my patients? JAMA 1994;27:703–707.
13. Farfan HF: The scientific basis of manipulative procedures. Clin Rheum Dis 1980;6:159–177.
14. McKenzie R, May S: Physical examination. In McKenzie R, May S (eds): The Human Extremities: Mechanical Diagnosis and Therapy, pp 105–121. Waikanae, New Zealand, Spinal Publications, 2000.
15. McKenzie RA: The Lumbar Spine: Mechanical Diagnosis and Therapy. Waikanae, New Zealand, Spinal Publication, 1981.
16. Cyriax J: Textbook of Orthopaedic Medicine, Diagnosis of Soft Tissue Lesions, 8th ed. London, Bailliere Tindall, 1982.
17. Petersen CM, Hayes KW: Construct validity of Cyriax's selective tension examination: Association of end-feels with pain at the knee and shoulder. J Orthop Sports Phys Ther 2000;30:512–527.
18. Williams PL, et al: Gray's Anatomy. London, Churchill Livingstone, 1989.
19. Riddle DL: Measurement of accessory motion: Critical issues and related concepts. Phys Ther 1992;72:865–874.
20. Maitland G: Peripheral Manipulation, 3rd ed. London, Butterworth, 1991.
21. Kaltenborn FM: Manual Mobilization of the Extremity Joints: Basic Examination and Treatment Techniques, 4th ed. Oslo, Norway, Olaf Norlis Bokhandel, Universitetsgaten, 1989.
22. Maitland GD: Passive movement techniques for intra-articular and periarticular disorders. Aust J Physiother 1985;31:3–8.
23. Grieve GP: Common Vertebral Joint Problems. New York, Churchill Livingstone, 1981.
24. Cocchiarella L, Andersson GBJ (eds): American Medical Association, Guides to the Evaluation of Permanent Impairment, 5th ed. Chicago, American Medical Association, 2001.
25. Tovin BJ, Greenfield BH: Impairment-based diagnosis for the shoulder girdle. In Evaluation and Treatment of the Shoulder: An Integration of the Guide to Physical Therapist Practice, pp 55–74. Philadelphia, PA, FA Davis, 2001.

26. Cyriax JH, Cyriax PJ: Illustrated Manual of Orthopaedic Medicine. London, Butterworth, 1983.
27. Sapega A.: Muscle performance evaluation in orthopedic practice. J Bone Joint Surg 1990;72A:1562–1574.
28. Janda V: Muscle Function Testing, pp 163–167. London, Butterworth, 1983.
29. Waxman SG: Correlative Neuroanatomy, 24th ed. New York, McGraw-Hill, 1996.
30. Adams RD, Victor M: Principles of Neurology, 5th ed. New York, McGraw-Hill, 1993.
31. Halle JS: Neuromusculoskeletal scan examination with selected related topics. In Flynn TW (ed): The Thoracic Spine and Rib Cage: Musculoskeletal Evaluation and Treatment, pp 121–146. Boston, Butterworth-Heinemann, 1996.
32. Dommisse GF, Grobler L: Arteries and veins of the lumbar nerve roots and cauda equina. Clin Orthop 1976;115:22–29.
33. Gilman S: The physical and neurologic examination. In Gilman S (ed): Clinical Examination of the Nervous System, pp 1–34. New York, McGraw-Hill, 2000.
34. Denno JJ, Meadows GR: Early diagnosis of cervical spondylotic myelopathy: A useful clinical sign. Spine 1991;16:1353–1355.
35. Dutton M: Manual Therapy of the Spine: An Integrated Approach. New York, McGraw-Hill, 2002.
36. Goldberg S: The Four Minute Neurological Examination. Miami, Medmaster, 1992.
37. Judge RD, Zuidema GD, Fitzgerald FT: Head. In Judge RD, Zuidema GD, Fitzgerald FT (eds): Clinical Diagnosis, pp 123–151. Boston, Little, Brown, 1982.
38. Butler DS: Mobilization of the Nervous System. New York, Churchill Livingstone, 1992.
39. Farrell JP: Cervical passive mobilization techniques: The Australian approach. Am J Phys Med Rehabil: State-of-the-Art Reviews 1990;4:309–334.
40. Feagin JA Jr: The office diagnosis and documentation of common knee problems. Clin Sports Med 1989;8:453–459.
41. Dyson M, et al.: The stimulation of tissue regeneration by means of ultrasound. Clin Sci 1968;35:273–285.
42. Dyson M, Suckling J: Stimulation of tissue repair by ultrasound: A survey of the mechanisms involved. Physiotherapy 1978;64:105–108.
43. Ramsey SM: Holistic manual therapy techniques. Prim Care 1997;24:759–785.
44. Ayub E: Posture and the upper quarter. In Donatelli RA (ed): Physical Therapy of the Shoulder, pp 81–90. New York, Churchill Livingstone, 1991.

4 | Systems Review

OVERVIEW

With the advent of Direct Access, it has become increasingly critical that clinicians construct a screening tool that incorporates a review of systems (ROS) and becomes an integral part of the examination process. The ROS (Table 4-1) is the part of history taking that identifies possible health problems that require consultation with, or referral to, another health care provider. The ROS can either be used to assess the general health of a patient or can be used to assess a specific system (Table 4-2). As with other testing procedures, the depth of the screen is based on the clinical findings.

In the arena of physician referrals, the ideal role of the physical therapist is to serve as a second pair of eyes for the busy physician. The purpose of the ROS for the physical therapist differs from that of the medical profession. While the physician uses the information from the ROS to rule in or out the contribution of the organ systems to the client's chief complaint, the physical therapist conducts an ROS to confirm that the patient's signs and symptoms are neuromusculoskeletal in nature and not referred from viscera (Table 4-3), and to ensure that the presence of serious pathology does not pass undetected.

Although most serious pathologies may have characteristic findings that alert the clinician (Table 4-4), some serious and chronic pathologies can masquerade as benign conditions. It was Grieve[1] who coined the term *masqueraders* to indicate those conditions which mimic a musculoskeletal state, but whose cause may be more insidious requiring skilled intervention elsewhere. The clinical findings outlined in Table 4-5 should always alert the clinician to the presence of serious pathology.[2]

MEDICAL HISTORY TAKING

The medical history portions of the ROS that deserve special attention include past and current illnesses and surgeries that may impact the choice of examination and intervention, and past episodes of similar signs and symptoms. Family history of medical conditions such as diabetes, heart disease, cancer, and the current health status of family members must also be included.

The medical history can also provide the clinician with information about current medications the patient is taking. These include prescription drugs and over-the-counter medications. Depending on the type of medication, the clinician may need to determine the reasons the patient was prescribed the medications and the frequency and amounts of the dosages being taken.

REVIEW OF SPECIFIC SYSTEMS

The components and tests used to assess the specific systems are outlined in Table 4-2.

124

TABLE 4-1 Components of the ROS (Review of Systems)

- Musculoskeletal: gross range of motion, functional strength, and symmetry
- Neuromuscular: general movement patterns
- Integumentary: skin integrity, color, scar, temperature, patient's height, and weight
- Communication or Learning Ability: ability of a patient to make needs known, consciousness, orientation, expected emotional or behavioral responses, patient learning preferences.

TABLE 4-2 Assessment of Specific Systems in the ROS

System	Test
Cardiovascular or pulmonary	*Pulse.* The normal resting pulse is between 60 and 100 beats per minute. Lower rates (bradycardia) indicate athletic conditioning. Higher rates (tachycardia) may indicate an anxious patient, recent exertion, or underlying pathology. There is normally a transient increase in pulse rate with inspiration, followed by a slowing with expiration.[a]
	Respiratory Rate. Normal respiratory rate is between 8 and 14 per minute in adults, and slightly quicker in children. A number of breathing patterns are characteristic of disease[a]
	Cheyne-Stokes respiration, characterized by a periodic, regular, sequentially increasing depth of respiration, occurs with serious cardiopulmonary or cerebral disorders.
	Biot's respiration, characterized by irregular spasmodic breathing and periods of apnea is almost associated with hypoventilation caused by central nervous system disease.
	Kussmaul's respiration, characterized by deep, slow breathing, indicates acidosis as the body attempts to blow off carbon dioxide.
	Blood Pressure. The normal adult blood pressure can vary over a wide range. The normal systolic range varies from 95 to 140 mm Hg, generally increasing with age. The normal diastolic range is 60 to 90 mm Hg. The pressure should be determined in both arms.
	Temperature. "Normal" body temperature of the adult is 98.4°F (37°C). However, a temperature in the range of 96.5°F and 99.4°F are not at all uncommon. Fever is a temperature exceeding 100°F.[a] The temperature is generally taken by placing the bulb of a thermometer under the patient's tongue for 1–3 minutes depending on the device. In most individuals, there is a diurnal (occurring everyday) variation in body temperature of 0.5°F to 2°F. The lowest ebb is reached during sleep. Menstruating women have a well-known temperature pattern that reflects the effects of ovulation, with the temperature dropping slightly before menstruation, and then dropping further 24–36 hours prior to ovulation.[a] Coincident with ovulation, the temperature rises and remains at a somewhat higher level until just before the next menses.

(Continued)

TABLE 4-2 Assessment of Specific Systems in the ROS (*Continued*)

System	Test
Integumentary	• The intactness of the skin, including the ability of the skin to serve as a barrier to environmental threats (e.g., bacteria, parasites).[b] • Edema • Skin changes. These include but are not limited to rashes, blemishes, scarring, color, and pliability.
Musculoskeletal	The clinician observes and notes any impairments in gross symmetry, gross range of motion, or gross strength (see scanning examination).
Neuromuscular	The clinician observes and notes any impairment of gait, locomotion, balance, coordination, motor control, and motor learning (see scanning examination). In addition, the clinician observes for peripheral and cranial nerve integrity, and notes any indication of neurologic compromise such as tremors, or facial tics.

[a]Judge RD, Zuidema GD, Fitzgerald FT: Vital signs. In Judge RD, Zuidema GD, Fitzgerald FT (eds): Clinical Diagnosis, pp 49–58. Boston, Little, Brown, 1982.
[b]Guide to physical therapist practice. Phys Ther 2001;81:S13–S95.

TABLE 4-3 Potential Areas of Cutaneous Referral from Various Viscera

Visceral organ	Pain referral
Heart (T1-5) Bronchi and lung (T2-4)	Under the sternum, base of the neck, over the shoulders, over the pectorals and down one or both arms L > R
Esophagus (T5-6)	Pharynx, lower neck, arms, midline chest from the upper to the lower sternum
Gastric (T6-10)	Lower thoracic to upper abdomen
Gall bladder (T7-9)	Upper abdomen, lower scapular and thoracolumbar
Pancreas	Upper lumbar or upper abdomen
Kidneys (T10-L1)	Upper lumbar, occasionally anterior abdomen about 2 inches lateral to the umbilicus
Urinary bladder (T11-12)	Lower abdomen or low lumbar
Uterus	Lower abdomen or low lumbar

Source: Head H: Studies in Neurology, p 653. London, Oxford Medical, 1920.

TABLE 4-4 Signs and Symptoms of Serious Pathology

Sign or symptom	Possible cause
Fevers, chills, or night sweats	Systemic problem (infection, cancer, disease). Increased sweating can have a myriad of causes ranging from increased body temperature because of exertion, fever, apprehension, and compromise to the autonomic system. Night sweats are of particular concern as they can often indicate the presence of a systemic problem.[1]

(*Continued*)

TABLE 4-4 Signs and Symptoms of Serious Pathology (*Continued*)

Sign or symptom	Possible cause
Recent unexplained weight changes	An unexplained weight gain could be a result of congestive heart failure, hypothyroidism, or cancer.[2]
	An unexplained weight loss could result from a gastrointestinal disorder, hyperthyroidism, cancer, or diabetes.[2]
Malaise or fatigue	Systemic disease
	Thyroid disease
	Iron deficiency
Unexplained nausea or vomiting	Never a good sign
Dizziness	Although most causes of dizziness can be relatively benign, dizziness may signal a more serious problem, especially if the dizziness is associated with trauma to the neck or head, or with motions of cervical rotation and extension (vertebral artery compromise). The clinician must ascertain whether the symptoms result from vertigo, nausea, giddiness, unsteadiness, fainting, etc. Vertigo requires that the patient's physician be informed for further investigation. However, in of itself, it is not usually a contraindication to the continuation of the examination.
Unilateral, bilateral, or quadrilateral paresthesias.	The seriousness of the paresthesia depends on its distribution. Quadrilateral paresthesia always indicates the presence of central nervous system involvement.
Shortness of breath	With the exception of exertion as a cause, reports of shortness of breath should never be ignored. The most common nonbenign cause is a cardiovascular problem.
Bowel or bladder dysfunction	Bowel and bladder dysfunction may indicate involvement of the cauda equina
Night pain	Malignancy
Pain following eating	Gastrointestinal problems
Weakness	Any weakness should be investigated by the clinician to determine whether it is the result of spinal nerve root compression, a peripheral nerve lesion, disuse, inhibition due to pain or swelling, an injury to the contractile or inert tissues (muscle, tendon, bursa, etc.), or a more serious pathology such as a fracture.
A gradual increase in the intensity of the pain	Radiating pain refers to an increase in pain intensity and distribution. Radiating pain typically travels distal from the site of the injury.
Radicular pain	Nerve root irritation
Numbness	Numbness that is a dermatomal pattern indicates spinal nerve root compression.

Sources: D'Ambrosia R: Musculoskeletal Disorders: Regional Examination and Differential Diagnosis, 2nd ed. Philadelphia, PA, JB Lippincott, 1986. Goodman CC, Snyder TEK: Differential Diagnosis in Physical Therapy. Philadelphia, PA, WB Saunders, 1990.

TABLE 4-5 Examination Findings and the Possible Conditions Causing Them[5]

Findings	Possible condition
Dizziness	Upper cervical impairment, vertebrobasilar ischemia, craniovertebral ligament tear. May also be relatively benign.
Quadrilateral paresthesia	Spinal cord compression, vertebrobasilar ischemia
Bilateral upper limb paresthesia	Spinal cord compression, vertebrobasilar ischemia
Hyperreflexia	Spinal cord compression, vertebrobasilar ischemia
Babinski or clonus sign	Spinal cord compression, vertebrobasilar ischemia
Consistent swallow on transverse ligament stress tests	Craniovertebral joint instability, retro pharyngeal hematoma, rheumatoid arthritis
Nontraumatic capsular pattern	Rheumatoid arthritis, ankylosing spondylitis, neoplasm
Arm pain lasting >6–9 months	Neoplasm
Persistent root pain <30 years	Neoplasm
Radicular pain with coughing	Neoplasm
Pain worsening after 1 month	Neoplasm
More than one level involved (cervical region)	Neoplasm
Paralysis	Neoplasm or neurologic disease
Trunk and limb paresthesia	Neoplasm
Bilateral root signs and symptoms	Neoplasm
Nontraumatic strong spasm	Neoplasm
Nontraumatic strong pain in the elderly patient	Neoplasm
Signs worse than symptoms	Neoplasm
Radial deviator weakness	Neoplasm
Thumb flexor weakness	Neoplasm
Hand intrinsic weakness and/or atrophy	Neoplasm, thoracic outlet syndrome, carpal tunnel syndrome
Horner's syndrome	Superior sulcus tumor, breast cancer, cervical ganglion damage, brainstem damage
Empty end-feel	Neoplasm
Severe posttraumatic capsular pattern	Fracture
Severe posttraumatic spasm	Fracture
Loss of ROM posttrauma	Fracture
Posttraumatic painful weakness	Fracture

THE SCANNING EXAMINATION

Other tests that may be incorporated as part of the ROS include the scanning examination (Tables 4-6, 4-7).[3] Designed by Cyriax,[4] the scanning examination is based on sound anatomic and pathologic principles and follows a logical sequence (Figure 4-1).

TABLE 4-6 Typical Sequence of the Upper or Lower Quarter
Scanning Examinations

<table>
<tr><td align="center">Initial observation</td></tr>
</table>

This involves everything from the initial entry of the patient including his or her gait, demeanor, standing and sitting postures, obvious deformities and postural defects, scars, radiation burns, creases, and birthmarks.

Patient history

Scanning examination

Active range of motion

Passive overpressure

Resistive tests

Deep tendon reflexes

Sensation testing

Special tests

The Cyriax scanning (screening) examination traditionally follows the history and is often incorporated as part of the systems review. The purpose of the scanning examination is to help rule out the possibility of symptom referral from other areas, and to ensure that all possible causes of the symptoms are examined (Table 4-8). The scanning examination is used when there is no history to explain the signs and/or symptoms, or when the signs and/or symptoms are unexplainable.

The scanning examination is divided into two examinations: one for the lower quarter/quadrant and the other for the upper quarter/quadrant. The tests that comprise the scanning examination are designed to detect neurologic weakness (Tables 4-9, 4-10), the patient's ability to perceive sensations, and the inhibition of the deep tendon reflexes (DTR) and other reflexes by the central nervous system.

TABLE 4-7 Components of the Scanning Examination and the
Structures Tested

Active ROM	Willingness to move, ROM, integrity of contractile and inert tissues, pattern of restriction (capsular, or noncapsular), quality of motion, and symptom reproduction
Passive ROM	Integrity of inert and contractile tissues, ROM, end-feel, and sensitivity
Resisted	Integrity of contractile tissues (strength, sensitivity)
Stress	Integrity of inert tissues (ligamentous or disc stability)
Dural	Dural mobility
Neurologic	Nerve conduction
Dermatome	Afferent (sensation)
Myotome	Efferent (strength, fatigability)
Reflexes	Afferent-efferent and central nervous systems

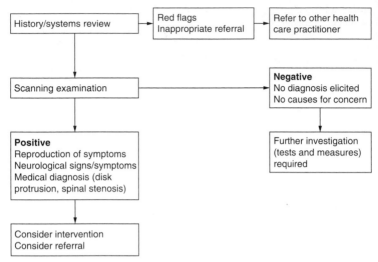

FIG. 4-1 Schematic representation of the scanning examination sequence.

The entire scanning examination should take no more than few minutes to complete and is routinely carried out unless there is some good reason for postponing it, such as recent trauma when a modified differential diagnostic examination is used.[5] The scanning examination should be carried out until the clinician is confident that there is no serious pathology present. For example,

TABLE 4-8 Signs and Symptoms Requiring Neurologic Assessment

1. Headaches that are sudden, severe, and diffuse
2. Headaches that awaken one from sleep
3. Headaches associated with projectile vomiting, but no nausea
4. Unilateral pulsating pain in synchrony with the heartbeat
5. Headaches that worsen with activity or exertion
6. Headaches that begin or worsen with recumbency
7. Focal tenderness over the temporal artery in someone over the age of 60
8. Sudden, intense, and sharp pain of short duration that is either spontaneous or triggered by a mild stimulus
9. Severe pain around the sinuses or teeth
10. Headaches associated with other symptoms
11. Cognitive impairment
12. Visual disturbances (i.e., blindness, diplopia, distortions, spots, or loss of vision on one side)
13. Numbness or altered sensation
14. Loss of strength or coordination
15. Loss or alteration of smell, taste, or hearing
16. Fever or associated systemic illness
17. Difficulty swallowing
18. Loss or impairment of voice, chronic cough

Source: Isaacs E, Bookout M: Screening for pathological origins of head and facial pain. In Boissonnault WG (ed): Examination in Physical Therapy Practice: Screening for Medical Disease, pp 175–189. Philadelphia, PA, WB Saunders, 1995.

TABLE 4-9 Lower Quarter Scanning Motor Examination

Muscle action	Muscle tested	Root level	Peripheral nerve
Hip flexion	Iliopsoas	L1-2	Femoral n. to iliacus and lumbar plexus to psoas
Knee extension	Quadriceps	L2-4	Femoral
Hamstrings	Biceps femoris, semimembranosus, and semitendinosus	L4-S3	Sciatic
Dorsiflexion with inversion	Tibialis anterior	Primarily L4	Deep peroneal
Great toe extension	Extensor hallucis longus	Primarily L5	Deep peroneal
Ankle eversion	Peroneus longus and brevis	Primarily S1	Superficial peroneal nerve
Ankle plantarflexion	Gastrocnemius and soleus	Primarily S1	Tibial
Hip extension	Gluteus maximus	L5-S2	Inferior gluteal nerve

the patient history may indicate to the clinician that the patient's condition is in the acute stage of healing. In these situations, most if not all of the joint motions may produce symptoms. While deeming the patient's condition as acute is not a diagnosis in the true sense, it can be used for the purpose of planning the intervention. (Refer to Chapter 5.)

Often the scanning examination does not generate enough signs and symptoms to formulate a working hypothesis or a diagnosis. In which case, further testing with the tests and measures is required in order to proceed (Figure 4-1).

TABLE 4-10 Upper Quarter Scanning Motor Examination

Resisted action	Muscle tested	Root level	Peripheral nerve
Shoulder abduction	Deltoid	Primarily C5	Axillary
Elbow flexion	Biceps brachii	Primarily C6	Musculocutaneous
Elbow extension	Triceps brachii	Primarily C7	Radial
Wrist extension	Extensor carpi radialis longus, brevis, and extensor carpi ulnaris	Primarily C6	Radial
Wrist flexion	Flexor carpi radialis and flexor carpi ulnaris	Primarily C7	Median n. for radialis and ulnar n. for ulnaris
Finger flexion	Flexor digitorum superficialis, flexor digitorum profundus, and lumbricales	Primarily C8	Median n. superficialis, both median and ulnar n. for profundus and lumbricales
Finger abduction	Dorsal interossei	Primarily T1	Ulnar

REFERENCES

1. Grieve GP: The Masqueraders. In Boyling JD, Palastanga N (eds): Grieve's Modern Manual Therapy, pp 841–856. Edinburgh, Churchill Livingstone, 1994.
2. Stetts DM: Patient Examination. In Wadsworth C (ed): Current Concepts of Orthopaedic Physical Therapy—Home Study Course 11.2.2. La Crosse, WI, Orthopaedic Section, APTA, 2001.
3. Guide to physical therapist practice. Phys Ther 2001;81:S13–S95.
4. Cyriax J: Textbook of Orthopaedic Medicine, Diagnosis of Soft Tissue Lesions, 8th ed. London, Bailliere Tindall, 1982.
5. Meadows J: Orthopedic Differential Diagnosis in Physical Therapy. New York, McGraw-Hill, 1999.

5 | The Evaluation

Once the history, review of systems (ROS), and the tests and measures are completed, an evaluation is made based on the information gathered by adding and subtracting the various findings (Figure 5-1).[1] According to Grieve,[2] an evaluation is the level of judgment necessary to make sense of the findings in order to identify a relationship between the symptoms reported and the signs of disturbed function. One of the challenges for the clinician is how to attach relevance to all the information gleaned from the examination. This judgment process can be viewed as a continuum, which is often based on experience. At one end of the continuum is the novice who uses very clear-cut signposts, while at the other end there is the experienced clinician who has a vast bank of clinical experiences from which to draw.[3] The clinician's knowledge base is therefore critical in the evaluation process.[4]

CLINICAL DECISION MAKING

Decision making in clinical practice should be based on the best available evidence. When integrating evidence into clinical decision-making, an understanding of how to appraise the quality of the evidence offered by the clinical tests is important (see *Orthopaedic Examination, Evaluation, and Intervention*, pp 197–202). One of the major problems in evaluating studies in the literature is that of deciding whether the results are definite enough to indicate an effect other than chance. Judging the strength of the evidence becomes an important part of the decision-making process. The standard for the assessment of the efficacy and value of a test or intervention is the clinical trial, that is, a prospective study assessing the effect and value of a test or intervention against a control in human subjects.[5] Unfortunately, many of the experimental studies that deal with physical therapy topics are not clinical trials, as there is no control to judge the efficacy of the test or intervention and there are no tests or interventions from which to draw comparisons.[6] The ideal clinical trial includes a blinded, randomized design and a control group (Table 5-1). The control can be a current standard practice, a placebo, or no active intervention.[5] Clinicians must constantly remind themselves that without information gathered from controlled clinical trials, they have limited scientific basis for their tests or interventions.[7]

PHYSICAL THERAPY DIAGNOSIS

The diagnostic process is essentially an exercise in probability revision,[8,9] with the creation of a diagnosis involving a combination of hypothesis testing and pattern recognition.[1] The best indicator for the correctness of a diagnosis is the quality of the hypothesis considered, for if the appropriate diagnosis is not considered from the start, any subsequent inquiries will be misdirected.[4]

Concepts of what constitutes a diagnosis have a long history in medicine. The concept used in the medical profession is based on a system in which a particular organism is identified as responsible for a cluster of signs and symptoms, giving rise to an etiologic-based diagnosis and classification system. One of the disadvantages of the medical system is that multiple categorizations are used for the same clinical problem and therefore diagnosis. In an ideal classification system, component categories are mutually exclusive and jointly exhaustive.[10] The other problem with using a medical model is that physicians diagnose conditions that

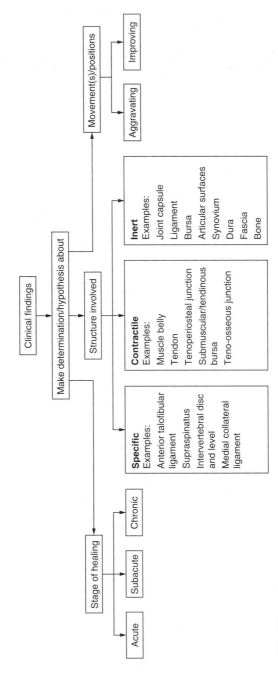

FIG. 5-1   The evaluation.

TABLE 5-1 A Hierarchy of Evidence Grading

	Level of evidence grading				
	A	B	C	D	E
Type of study			Nonrandomized trial with concurrent or historical controls Case study	Cross sectional study Case series Case report	Expert consensus Clinical experience
	Randomized clinical trials	Cohort study	Study of sensitivity and specificity of a diagnostic test Population based descriptive study		

are out of the scope of physical therapy. To address this issue, separate classification systems have evolved within the field of physical therapy. One such system is outlined in the *Guide to Physical Therapist Practice*.[11] This system focuses on the consequences of a disease, disorder, or injury versus the causes, and uses a model of disablement versus the traditional medical model.[12] In this diagnostic classification system, a patient is placed in categories called "preferred practice patterns," according to an identification of the patient's primary impairments and certain associated conditions.[13] One of the disadvantages of this system is that the potential for a classification problem occurs when the defining characteristics and intervention of one pattern are essentially the same as those of another pattern.[12,13] Other models developed within physical therapy use movement impairment syndromes[14] and treatment-based classification[15] systems to avoid this classification problem.[13] It is critical that the classification of musculoskeletal pain disorders be contingent on understanding and identifying the factors underlying a disorder, while understanding the healing stage of the disorder and the potential contribution of both organic and nonorganic factors that relate to it.[16]

Once the diagnosis has been determined, one of two scenarios generally exist:

1. The clinical findings warrant a referral to another health care practitioner. A complete and accurate evaluation can only be made when all potential causes for the symptoms have been ruled out. The clinician should resist the urge to categorize a condition based on a small number of findings. In such cases, knowledge of differential diagnosis is essential (see *Orthopaedic Examination, Evaluation, and Intervention*, pp 210–284), so that the clinician can systematically rule out all the causes for the pain. Patients may be referred to physical therapy with a nonspecific diagnosis, an incorrect diagnosis, or no diagnosis at all.[17] Physical therapists are responsible for thoroughly examining each patient and then either treating the patient according to established guidelines or referring the patient elsewhere.[18]

2. The data from the clinical findings is organized into clusters, syndromes, or categories called preferred practice patterns (Table 5-2), and an intervention can be commenced (refer to Chapter 6). With the implementation of the

TABLE 5-2 Preferred Practice Patterns[11]

Musculoskeletal practice pattern	Impairments
Pattern 4A	Primary prevention/risk factor reduction for skeletal demineralization
Pattern 4B	*Impaired posture*
	This pattern is often the result of a combination of other practice patterns including practice patterns C, E, F, and G, and includes impairments of motor function, muscle performance, joint mobility, localized inflammation, and range of motion.
	The pathologies associated with this pattern include vertebral pathology, neural compression syndromes, entrapment syndromes, myofascial syndromes, impingement syndromes, and referred pain.
	Clinical findings can include pain with sustained positions, limited range of motion in a noncapsular pattern of restriction, altered kinematics, positive impingement tests, neurologic findings (thoracic outlet, limb tension tests), trigger points, and palpable tenderness of specific muscles.
Pattern 4C	*Impaired muscle performance*
	This pattern is associated with a combination of other practice patterns including practice patterns D through J, and thus includes impairments of motor function, muscle performance, joint mobility, localized inflammation, and range of motion.
	The *pathologies* and *clinical findings* associated with this pattern include those that the pattern is associated with (practice patterns D through J).
Pattern 4D	*Impaired joint mobility, motor function, muscle performance, and range of motion associated with connective tissue dysfunction*
	Pattern D refers to an increased laxity or instability of the joint or hypomobility caused by capsular restriction. The *primary impairments* in pattern D include decreased motor control and muscle performance.
	Characteristic of this pattern is the complaint of the joint "slipping" or "popping out" during activities of extreme motion.
	The *pathologies* associated with this pattern include osteoarthritis, rheumatoid arthropathy, adhesive capsulitis, tendinitis, capsulitis, bursitis, synovitis, and ligament pathology.
	Clinical findings associated with this pattern can include pain, altered kinematics, crepitus, and positive apprehension.
Pattern 4E	*Impaired joint mobility, motor function, muscle performance, and range of motion associated with localized inflammation*
	In addition to those conditions producing impaired range of motion, motor function, and muscle performance attributed to inflammation, practice pattern E includes conditions that cause pain and muscle guarding without the presence of structural changes.

(Continued)

TABLE 5-2 Preferred Practice Patterns[11] (*Continued*)

Musculoskeletal practice pattern	Impairments
	The *pathologies* include: sprains and strains of the joints, internal derangements of the joint, including muscle tears, and periarticular syndromes—tendinitis, bursitis, capsulitis, and tenosynovitis. The *clinical findings* include pain with active and resisted motions, tenderness to palpation, localized edema, redness, and increased skin temperature.
Pattern 4F	*Impaired joint mobility, motor function, muscle performance, and range of motion, or reflex integrity secondary to spinal disorders* This pattern involves impaired motor function, muscle performance, range of motion, and joint mobility. The *pathologies* associated with this pattern include adverse neural tension and nerve root irritation. The clinical findings associated with this pattern can include positive limb tension tests, signs and symptoms of nerve, and nerve root compression.
Pattern 4G	*Impaired joint mobility, motor function, muscle performance, and range of motion associated with fracture* The treatment of most fractures is beyond the scope of practice for a physical therapist.
Patterns 4H and 4I	*Impaired joint mobility, motor function, muscle performance, and range of motion associated with joint arthroplasty, or with bony or soft tissue surgical procedures* Pattern H is associated with impaired joint mobility, muscle performance, and range of motion due to joint arthroplasty. Pattern I involves impaired joint mobility, motor function, muscle performance, and range of motion associated with bony or soft tissue surgical procedures. The clinical findings and treatment following a surgical procedure will vary according to each individual and the procedure performed.
Pattern 4J	*Impaired gait, locomotion, and balance and impaired motor function, secondary to lower extremity amputation*
Pattern 5F	*Impaired peripheral nerve integrity and muscle performance associated with peripheral nerve injury* This pattern involves decreased muscle strength, impaired proprioception, impaired sensory integrity, and difficulty with manipulation skills. The *pathologies* include carpal tunnel syndrome, cubital tunnel syndrome, radial tunnel syndrome, tarsal tunnel syndrome, and paroxysmal positional vertigo. The clinical findings can include diminished deep tendon reflexes, positive limb tension tests, and signs and symptoms of peripheral nerve compression

Guide to Physical Therapist Practice, the focus of the examination process has changed to one where an accurate diagnosis is made within appropriate practice patterns. However, it is worth noting that most of the time, these patterns do not occur in isolation. Patients often present with a mixture of signs and symptoms that indicate one or more possible problem areas.

For example, patterns such as impaired posture (practice pattern B), impaired muscle performance (practice pattern C), and impairment caused by localized inflammation (practice pattern F), can occur concurrently with each other. Once these impairments have been highlighted, a determination can be made as to the reason for those impairments, the relationship between the impairments, and the patient's functional limitations or disabilities.

PROGNOSIS

The prognosis is the predicted level of function that the patient will attain within a certain time frame. This prediction helps guide the intensity, duration, and frequency of the intervention, and aids in justifying the intervention. Knowledge of the severity of an injury, the age and physical status of a patient, and the healing processes of the various tissues involved, are among the factors used in determining the prognosis. In addition, as the clinician cannot be with the patient at all times, patient education and patient responsibility become extremely important in determining the prognosis.

REFERENCES

1. Cwynar DA, McNerney T: A primer on physical therapy. Lippincotts Prim Care Pract 1999;3:451–459.
2. Grieve GP: Common Vertebral Joint Problems. New York, Churchill Livingstone, 1981.
3. Coutts F: Changes in the musculoskeletal system. In Atkinson K, Coutts F, Hassenkamp A (eds): Physiotherapy in Orthopedics, pp 19–43. New York, Churchill Livingstone, 1999.
4. Jones MA: Clinical reasoning in manual therapy. Phys Ther 1992;72:875–884.
5. Friedman LM, Furberg CD, DeMets DL: Fundamentals of Clinical Trials, pp 2, 51, 71. Chicago, Mosby-Year Book, 1985.
6. Bloch R: Methodology in clinical back pain trials. Spine 1987;12:430–432.
7. Schiffman EL: The role of the randomized clinical trial in evaluating management strategies for temporomandibular disorders. In Fricton JR, Dubner R (eds): Orofacial Pain and Temporomandibular Disorders. Advances in Pain Research and Therapy, vol 21, pp 415–463. New York, Raven Press, 1995.
8. Sox HC Jr: Probability theory in the use of diagnostic tests: an introduction to critical study of the literature. Ann Intern Med 1986;104:60–66.
9. Fritz JM, Wainner RS: Examining diagnostic tests: an evidence-based perspective. Phys Ther 2001;81:1546–1564.
10. Kendell RE: Clinical validity. Psychol Med 1989;19:45–55.
11. Guide to physical therapist practice. Phys Ther 2001;81:S13–S95.
12. Jette AM: Diagnosis and classification by physical therapists: a special communication. Phys Ther 1989;69:967.
13. Zimny NJ: Clinical Commentary: Diagnostic classification and orthopaedic physical therapy practice: what we can learn from medicine. J Orthop Sports Phys Ther 2004;34:105–115.
14. Sahrmann SA: Diagnosis and Treatment of Movement Impairment Syndromes. St Louis, MO, Mosby, 2001.
15. Delitto A, Erhard RE, Bowling RW: A treatment-based classification approach to low back syndrome: identifying and staging patients for conservative management. Phys Ther 1995;75:470–489.
16. Elvey R, O'Sullivan PB: A contemporary approach to manual therapy. In Jull G, Boyling JD (eds): Modern Manual Therapy. Philadelphia, PA, WB Saunders, 2004.
17. Clawson AL, Domholdt E: Content of physician referrals to physical therapists at clinical education sites in Indiana. Phys Ther 1994;74:356–360.
18. Leerar PJ: Differential diagnosis of tarsal coalition versus cuboid syndrome in an adolescent athlete. J Orthop Sports Phys Ther 2001;31:702–707.

6 | The Intervention

According to the "*Guide to Physical Therapist Practice*," an intervention is "the purposeful and skilled interaction of the physical therapist and the patient/client and, when appropriate, with other individuals involved in the patient/client care, using various physical therapy procedures and techniques to produce changes in the condition consistent with the diagnosis and prognosis."[1] The physical therapy intervention comprises three components (Table 6-1): coordination, communication, and documentation; patient/client related instruction; and direct interventions (Table 6-2).[1]

A physical therapy intervention is most effectively addressed from a problem-oriented approach, based on the evaluation, the patient's functional needs, and on mutually agreed-on goals.[1] The most successful intervention programs are those that are custom designed from a blend of clinical experience and scientific data, with the level of improvement achieved related to goal setting and the attainment of those goals (Table 6-3).

INTERVENTION PRINCIPLES

A number of principles should guide the intervention through the various stages of healing. These include:

- Control pain, inflammation, and swelling (edema)
- Promote and progress healing
- As appropriate, instruct the patient on a therapeutic exercise program that:
  - Corrects any imbalances between strength and flexibility
  - Addresses postural and movement dysfunctions
  - Integrates the open and closed kinetic chains
  - Incorporates neuromuscular reeducation
  - Maintains or improves the overall strength and fitness
  - Improves the functional outcome of the patient

Control Pain and Inflammation

The clinician has a number of tools at his or her disposal to help control pain, inflammation, and swelling (edema). These include the application of electrotherapeutic and physical modalities, gentle range of motion exercises, and graded manual techniques. During the acute stage of healing, the principles of PRICEMEM (**P**rotection, **R**est, **I**ce, **C**ompression, **E**levation, **M**anual therapy, **E**arly motion, and **M**edications) are recommended. The modalities used during the acute phase involve the application of cryotherapy, electrical stimulation, pulsed ultrasound, and iontophoresis. Modalities used during the later stages of healing include thermotherapy, phonophoresis, electrical stimulation, ultrasound (US), iontophoresis, and diathermy (Tables 6-4, 6-5). The applications of cold and heat are taught to the patient at the earliest opportunity.

Gentle manual techniques (Grade I or II joint mobilizations) may also be used to help with pain. As the patient progresses, gentle passive muscle stretching may be introduced. Self-stretching and self-mobilization techniques are taught to the patient at the earliest and the most appropriate opportunity.

TABLE 6-1　Components of an Intervention

Coordination, Communication, and Documentation

These interventions may include case management, communication with other health care providers or insurers, and the coordination of care with the patient/client or significant others involved in the care of the patient/client. This is to ensure a continuum of care among health care providers. Other interventions may include documentation of care, discharge planning, education plans, patient care conferences, record reviews, and referrals to other professionals or resources.

Patient Related Instruction

Patient education can include, but is not limited to verbal, written, or pictorial instructions, which may be part of a home program. Computer assisted instruction and demonstrations by the patient/client or caregivers are also examples of instructions that may be given. Audiovisual aides and demonstrations of exercises or functional activities may be used. This enables the patient/client to continue with his or her program when out of the clinic, either independently or with assistance.

Direct Interventions

Direct interventions are selected based on the findings in the evaluation and examination of the patient/client, diagnosis, prognosis, and anticipated outcomes and goals for the individual. Direct interventions are performed with or on the patient. This section encompasses the largest component of patient care. Examples of direct interventions include but are not limited to: therapeutic exercise, aerobic exercise, functional training, manual therapy, and use of assistive devices, and modalities.

Source: Cwynar DA, McNerney T: A primer on physical therapy. Lippincotts Prim Care Pract 1999;3:451–459.

TABLE 6-2　Direct Interventions

- Therapeutic exercise (including aerobic conditioning)
- Functional training in self-care and home management [activities of daily living (ADL)]
- Functional training in community and work integration and reintegration [instrumental activities of daily living (IADL)]
- Manual therapy
- Prescription, application, and fabrication of devices and equipment
- Airway clearance techniques
- Wound management
- Electrotherapeutic modalities
- Physical agents and mechanical modalities

TABLE 6-3　Key Questions for Intervention Planning

- What is the stage of healing: acute, subacute, or chronic?
- How long do you have to treat the patient?
- What does patient do for activities?
- How compliant is the patient?
- How much skilled physical therapy is needed?
- What needs to be taught to prevent recurrence?
- Are there any referrals needed?
- What has worked for other patients with similar problems?
- Are there any precautions?
- What is your skill level?

Source: Guide to physical therapist practice. Phys Ther 2001;81:S13–S95.

TABLE 6-4 Indications and Contraindications for the Use of
Therapeutic Modalities

Therapeutic modality	Physiologic responses (indications for use)	Contraindications and precautions
Electrical stimulating currents—high voltage	Pain modulation Muscle reeducation Muscle pumping contractions Retard atrophy Muscle strengthening Increase range of motion Fracture healing Acute injury	Pacemakers Thrombophlebitis Superficial skin lesions
Electrical stimulating currents—low voltage	Wound healing Fracture healing Iontophoresis	Malignancy Skin hypersensitivities Allergies to certain drugs
Electrical stimulating currents— interferential	Pain modulation Muscle reeducation Muscle pumping contractions Fracture healing Increase range of motion	Same as high voltage
Electrical stimulating currents—Russian	Muscle strengthening	Pacemakers
Electrical stimulating currents—MENS	Fracture healing Wound healing	Malignancy Infections
Shortwave diathermy and microwave diathermy	Increase deep circulation Increase metabolic activity Reduce muscle guarding/spasm Reduce inflammation Facilitate wound healing Analgesia Increase tissue temperatures over a large area	Metal implants Pacemakers Malignancy Wet dressings Anesthetized areas Pregnancy Acute injury and inflammation Eyes Areas of reduce blood flow Anesthetized areas
Cryotherapy—cold packs, ice massage	Acute injury Vasoconstriction— decreased blood flow Analgesia Reduce inflammation Reduce muscle guarding/spasm	Allergy to cold Circulatory impairments Wound healing Hypertension

(Continued)

TABLE 6-4 Indications and Contraindications for the Use of Therapeutic Modalities (*Continued*)

Therapeutic modality	Physiologic responses (indications for use)	Contraindications and precautions
Thermotherapy—hot whirlpool, paraffin, hydrocollator, infrared lamps	Vasodilation—increased blood flow Analgesia Reduce muscle guarding/spasm Reduce inflammation Increase metabolic activity Facilitate tissue healing	Acute and postacute trauma Poor circulation Circulatory impairments Malignancy
Low-power laser	Pain modulation (trigger points) Facilitate wound healing	Pregnancy Eyes
Ultraviolet	Acne Aseptic wounds Folliculitis Pityriasis rosea Tinea Septic wounds Sinusitis Increase calcium metabolism	Psoriasis Eczema Herpes Diabetes Pellagra Lupus erythematosus Hyperthyroidism Renal and hepatic insufficiency Generalized dermatitis Advanced atherosclerosis
Ultrasound	Increase connective tissue extensibility Deep heat Increased circulation Treatment of most soft tissue injuries Reduce inflammation Reduce muscle spasm	Infection Acute and postacute injury Epiphyseal areas Pregnancy Thrombophlebitis Impaired sensation Eyes Malignancy
Intermittent compression	Decrease acute bleeding Decrease edema	Circulatory impairment

Source: Prentice WE: Using therapeutic modalities in rehabilitation. In Prentice WE, Voight ML (eds): Techniques in Musculoskeletal Rehabilitation, pp 289–303. New York, McGraw-Hill, 2001.

Promote and Progress Healing

The promotion and progression of tissue repair involves a delicate balance between protection and the application of controlled functional stresses to the damaged structure (Tables 6-6, 6-7). Tissue repair can be viewed as an adaptive life process in response to both intrinsic and extrinsic stimuli.[2] These stimuli can be in the form of normal movements, manual techniques, and therapeutic exercises, or any one of them. Although physical therapy cannot

TABLE 6-5 Clinical Decision-Making on the Use of Various Therapeutic Modalities during the Various Stages of Healing

Phase	Approximate time frame	Clinical picture	Possible modalities used	Rationale for use
Initial acute	Injury-Day 3	Swelling, pain to touch, pain on motion	CRYO ESC IC LPL Rest	↓ Swelling, ↓ Pain ↓ Pain ↓ Swelling ↓ Pain
Inflammatory response	Days 1–6	Swelling subsides, warm to touch, discoloration, pain to touch, pain on motion	CRYO ESC IC LPL Range of motion	↓ Swelling, ↓ Pain ↓ Pain ↓ Swelling ↓ Pain
Fibroblastic repair	Days 4–10	Pain to touch, pain on motion, swollen	THERMO ESC LPL IC Range of motion Strengthening	Mildly ↑ circulation ↓ Pain-muscle pumping ↓ Pain Facilitate lymphatic flow
Maturation-remodeling	Day 7– Recovery	Swollen, no more pain to touch, decreasing pain on motion	ULTRA ESC LPL SWD MWD Range of motion Strengthening Functional activities	Deep heating to ↑ circulation ↑ Range of motion, ↑ strength ↓ Pain ↓ Pain Deep heating to ↑ circulation Deep heating to ↑ circulation

CRYO = Cryotherapy; ESC = electrical stimulating currents; IC = intermittent compression; LPL = low-power laser; MWD = microwave diathermy; SWD = short-wave diathermy; THERMO = thermotherapy; ULTRA = ultrasound; ↓ decrease; ↑ increase.
Source: Prentice WE: Using therapeutic modalities in rehabilitation. In Prentice WE, Voight ML (eds): Techniques in Musculoskeletal Rehabilitation, pp 289–303. New York, McGraw-Hill, 2001.

accelerate the healing process, it can ensure that the healing process is not delayed or disrupted, and that it occurs in an optimal environment.[3] In addition to excess stress, detrimental environments such as prolonged immobilization must be avoided (Table 6-8). The rehabilitation procedures chosen to progress the patient will depend on the type of tissue involved, the extent of tissue damage, and the stage of healing (Table 6-9 to Table 6-11). The intervention must be related to the signs and symptoms present rather than the actual diagnosis.

TABLE 6-6 Ligament Injuries

Grade	Signs	Implications
First degree (mild)	Minimal loss of structural integrity No abnormal motion Little or no swelling Localized tenderness Minimal bruising	Minimal functional loss Early return to training—some protection may be necessary
Second degree (moderate)	Significant structural weakening Some abnormal motion Solid end-feel to stress More bruising and swelling Often associated hemarthrosis and effusion	Tendency to recurrence Need protection from risk of further injury May need modified immobilization May stretch out further with time
Third degree (complete)	Loss of structural integrity Marked abnormal motion Significant bruising Hemarthrosis	Needs prolonged protection Surgery may be considered Often permanent functional instability

TABLE 6-7 Classification of Muscle Injury

Type	Related factors
Exercise-induced muscle injury (delayed muscle soreness)	Increased activity Unaccustomed activity Excessive eccentric work Viral infections Secondary to muscle cell damage Onset at 24–48 hours after exercise
Strains First degree (mild): minimal structural damage, minimal hemorrhage, early resolution Second degree (moderate): partial tear, large spectrum of injury, significant early functional loss Third degree (severe): complete tear, may require aspiration, may require surgery	Sudden overstretch Sudden contraction Decelerating limb Insufficient warm-up Lack of flexibility Increasing severity of strain associated with greater muscle fiber death, more hemorrhage, and more eventual scarring Steroid use or abuse Previous muscle injury Collagen disease
Contusions Mild, moderate, severe Intramuscular vs. intermuscular	Direct blow, associated with increasing muscle trauma and tearing of fiber proportionate to severity
Avulsions Bony	Specific sites vulnerable May be complication of stress fractures Osteoporosis
Apophyseal Muscle	Skeletally immature but well developed muscle strength Associated with steroid injection or generalized collagen disorders

Source: Reid DC: Sports Injury Assessment and Rehabilitation. New York, Churchill Livingstone, 1992.

TABLE 6-8 Structural Changes in the Types of Muscle Following Immobilization in a Shortened Position

Structural characteristics	Muscle fiber type and changes		
	Slow oxidative	Fast oxidative glycolytic	Fast glycolytic
Number of fibers	Moderate decrease	Minimal increase	Minimal increase
Diameter of fibers	Significant decrease	Moderate decrease	Moderate decrease
Fiber fragmentation	Minimal increase	Minimal increase	Significant increase
Myofibrils	Minimal decrease and disoriented	Degenerated and rounded	Wavy
Nuclei	Degenerated and rounded	Moderate decrease, degenerated	Degenerated and rounded
Mitochondria	Moderate decrease, degenerated,	Minimal decrease	Minimal decrease, degenerated, swollen
Sarcoplasmic reticulum	Minimal decrease, orderly arrangement	Moderate decrease	Minimal decrease
Myofilaments	Minimal decrease and disorganized		Minimal decrease and wavy
Z band	Moderate decrease		Faint or absent
Vesicles	Abnormal configuration		
Basement membrane	Minimal increase		
Register of sarcomeres	Irregular projections		
Fatty infiltration	Shifted with time		
Collagen	Minimal increase	Minimal increased invasion	Minimal increased invasion
Macrophages	Minimal increase between fibers		
Satellite cells	Minimal increased invasion		
Target cells	Minimal increase		

Source: Gossman MR, Sahrmann SA, Rose SJ: Review of length-associated changes in muscle. Phys Ther 1982;62:1799–1808.

TABLE 6-9 Stages of Healing

Stage	General characteristics
Acute or inflammatory	The area is red, warm, swollen, and painful
	The pain is present without any motion of the involved area
	Usually lasts for 48–72 hours, but can be as long as 7–10 days
Subacute or tissue formation (neovascularization)	The pain usually occurs with the activity or motion of the involved area
	Usually lasts for 10 days to 6 weeks
Chronic or remodeling	The pain usually occurs after the activity
	Usually lasts from 6 weeks to 12 months

TABLE 6-10 Prognostic Factors for Muscle Injury

Parameter	Prognostic factors	
	Positive	Negative
Site	Belly tears Intermuscular contusions	Musculotendinous junction tears Intramuscular contusions
Severity	Partial tears (1st degree and mild 2nd degree) First injury	Complete tears (severe 2nd degree and 3rd degree tears) Re-tear
Clinical signs	Minimal loss of range Minimal swelling Little pain	Significant loss of range Obvious tense swelling Extreme pain
Complications	Usually preserved function Compartment syndrome rare Myositis ossificans less likely Often complete resolution Early resolution expected	Loss of function Compartment syndromes a distinct range with large bleeds Myositis ossificans more prevalent Tendency for recurrent tears Prolonged disability possible

TABLE 6-11 Intervention of Tendinitis and Overuse Syndromes

Grade	Symptoms	Intervention
I	Pain only after activity Does not interfere with performance Often generalized tenderness Disappears before next exercise session	Modification of activity Assessment of training pattern Possibly NSAIDs
II	Minimal pain with activity Does not interfere with intensity or distance	Modification of activity Physical therapy, NSAIDs; consider orthotics
III	Usually localized tenderness Pain interferes with activity Usually disappears between sessions Definite local tenderness	Significant modification of activity Assess training schedule Physical therapy, NSAIDs, consider orthotics Usually need to temporarily discontinue aggravating motion
IV	Pain does not disappear between activity sessions Seriously interferes with ntensity of training Significant local sign of pain, tenderness, crepitus, swelling	Design alternate program May require splinting Physical therapy and NSAIDs
V	Pain interferes with sport and activities of daily living Symptoms often chronic or recurrent Signs of tissue changes and altered associated muscle function	Prolonged rest from activity NSAIDs plus other medical therapies Consider splint or cast Physical therapy May require surgery

Therapeutic Exercise

Therapeutic exercise is the foundation of physical therapy and a fundamental component of the vast majority of interventions. Prescribed accurately, therapeutic exercise can be used to restore, maintain, and improve a patient's functional status by increasing strength, endurance, and flexibility.

Initially, activity should be modified to prevent further injury. This is preferable to total rest, except in severe cases. Patients must be advised to let pain be their guide and that pain-free range of motion activities must be continued to prevent loss of function. The promotion and progression of tissue repair involves a delicate balance between protection and the application of controlled functional stresses to the damaged structure. The goal of the functional exercise progression is to identify the motion or motions that the patient is able to exercise into without eliciting symptoms other than postexercise soreness.[4]

A hierarchy for ROM and resistive exercises exists.[5] This hierarchy is based on patient tolerance and response to ensure that any progress made is done in a safe and controlled fashion. The hierarchy for the ROM exercises is depicted in Table 6-12.

A similar hierarchy exists for resisted exercises. The hierarchy for the progression of resistive exercises is depicted in Table 6-13.[5,6]

A number of principles can be used to guide the clinician in the progression of therapeutic exercise:[7]

* Exercise according to the stage of healing and degree of irritability. The degree of irritability of each condition can often indicate the stage of healing to the clinician. The degree of irritability can be determined by inquiring about the vigor, duration, and intensity of the pain. Greater irritability is associated with very acutely inflamed conditions. The characteristic sign for an acute inflammation is pain at rest, which is diffuse in its distribution and often referred from the site of the primary condition.[8] Chronic conditions usually have low irritability but have an associated loss of active and passive ROM. Therapeutic exercises should be introduced as per the exercise hierarchy described above. The degree of movement and the speed of progression are both guided by the signs and symptoms.
* Exercise initially in cardinal planes progressing as quickly as allowed to exercising in the functional planes.
* Initiate with exercises that utilize a short lever arm. These exercises serve to decrease the amount of torque at the joint. Extremity exercises can be adapted to include short levers by flexing the extremity or by exercising with the extremity closer to the body.
* Achieve the closed pack position at the earliest opportunity. The closed pack position of a joint is its position of maximum stability. It is also the position of maximum ligamentous and capsular tautness, so care needs to be taken in achieving this position.
* Reproduce the forces and loading rates that will approach the patient's functional demands, as the rehabilitation progresses.

TABLE 6-12 Hierarchy for the ROM Exercises

* Passive ROM
* Active assisted ROM
* Active ROM

TABLE 6-13 Hierarchy for the Progression of Resistive Exercises

- Single-angle submaximal isometrics performed in the neutral position
- Multiple-angle submaximal isometrics performed at various angles of the range
- Multiple-angle maximal isometrics
- Small arc submaximal isotonics
- Full ROM submaximal isotonics
- Functional ROM submaximal isotonics

Exercise progressions for all the joints are provided in the larger text. All exercise progressions should include:[9]

- *Variation.* Variation to the exercises can be provided by altering:
  - The plane of motion
  - The range of motion
  - The body position
  - The exercise duration
  - The exercise frequency
- *Safe progression.* A safe progression is ensured if the exercises are progressed from:
  - Slow to fast
  - Simple to complex
  - Stable to unstable
  - Low force to high force

INTERVENTION GOALS

Acute Phase

The goals of the acute phase should include:

- Maximizing patient comfort by decreasing pain and inflammation
- Protection of the injury site
- Restoration of pain-free range of motion throughout the entire kinetic chain
- Retardation of muscle atrophy
- Minimizing the detrimental effects of immobilization and activity restriction[10–15]
- Attainment of early neuromuscular control
- Improving soft tissue extensibility
- Increasing functional tolerance
- Maintaining general fitness
- Appropriate management of scar tissue
- Encouraging the patient toward independence with the home exercise program
- Progression of the patient to the functional stage

Functional Phase

The functional phase addresses any tissue overload problems and functional biomechanical deficits. The goals of the functional phase should address:

- Attainment of full range of pain-free motion
- Restoration of normal joint kinematics
- Improvement of muscle strength to within normal limits

- Improvement of neuromuscular control
- Restoration of normal muscle force couples
- Correction of any deficits in the whole kinetic chain that are involved in an activity to which the patient is planning to return.
- Performance of activity-specific progressions before full return to function.

The selection of intervention procedures, and the intervention progression, must be guided by continuous reexamination of the patient's response to a given procedure, making the reexamination of patient dysfunction before, during, and after each intervention, essential.[16] There are three possible scenarios following a reexamination:

1. The patient's function has improved. In this scenario, the intensity of the intervention may be incrementally increased.
2. The patient's function has diminished. In this scenario, the intensity and the focus of the intervention must be changed. Further review of the home exercise program may be needed. The patient may require further education on activity modification and the use of heat and ice at home. The working hypothesis used to formulate a diagnosis must be reviewed. Further investigation is needed.
3. There is no change in the patient's function. Depending on the elapse of time since the last visit, there may be a reason for the lack of change. This finding may indicate the need for a change in the intensity of the intervention. If the patient is in the acute or subacute stage of healing, a decrease in the intensity may be warranted, to allow the tissues more of an opportunity to heal. In the chronic stage, an increase in intensity may be warranted.

REFERENCES

1. Guide to physical therapist practice, Phys Ther 2001;81:S13–S95.
2. Dehne E, Tory R: Treatment of joint injuries by immediate mobilization based upon the spiral adaption concept. Clin Orthop 1971;77:218–232.
3. McKenzie R, May S: Introduction. In McKenzie R, May S (eds): The Human Extremities: Mechanical Diagnosis and Therapy, pp 1–5. Waikanae, New Zealand, Spinal Publications, 2000.
4. Hyman J, Liebenson C: Spinal stabilization exercise program. In Liebenson C (ed): Rehabilitation of the Spine: A Practitioner's Manual, pp 293–317. Baltimore, MD, Williams & Wilkins, 1996.
5. Ierna GF, Murphy DR: Management of acute soft tissue injuries of the cervical spine. In Murphy DR (ed): Conservative Management of Cervical Spine Disorders, pp 531–552. New York, McGraw-Hill, 2000.
6. Davies GJ: Compendium of isokinetics. In: Clinical Usage and Rehabilitation Techniques, 4th ed. Onalaska, WI, S & S, 1992.
7. Litchfield R, et al.: Rehabilitation of the overhead athlete. J Orthop Sports Phys Ther 1993;2:433–441.
8. Maitland G: Peripheral Manipulation, 3rd ed. London, Butterworth, 1991.
9. Cook G, Voight ML: Essentials of functional exercise: A four-step clinical model for therapeutic exercise prescription. In Prentice WE, Voight ML (eds): Techniques in Musculoskeletal Rehabilitation, pp 387–407. New York, McGraw-Hill, 2001.
10. Booth FW: Physiologic and biochemical effects of immobilization on muscle. Clin Orthop 1987;219:15–21.
11. Eiff MP, Smith AT, Smith GE: Early mobilization versus immobilization in the treatment of lateral ankle sprains. Am J Sports Med 1994;22:83–88.
12. Akeson WH, et al.: Collagen cross-linking alterations in the joint contractures: Changes in the reducible cross-links in periarticular connective tissue after 9 weeks immobilization. Connect Tissue Res 1977;5:15.

13. Akeson WH, et al.: Effects of immobilization on joints. Clin Orthop 1987;219:28–37.
14. Akeson WH, Amiel D, Woo SL-Y: Immobility effects on synovial joints: the pathomechanics of joint contracture. Biorheology 1980;17:95–110.
15. Woo SL-Y, et al.: Connective tissue response to immobility: a correlative study of biochemical and biomechanical measurements of normal and immobilized rabbit knee. Arthritis Rheum 1975;18:257–264.
16. Yoder E: Physical therapy management of nonsurgical hip problems in adults. In Echternach JL (ed): Physical Therapy of the Hip, pp 103–137. New York, Churchill Livingstone, 1990.

7 | The Shoulder Complex

OVERVIEW

The shoulder complex is composed of articulations between the humerus, glenoid, scapula, acromion, clavicle, and the surrounding soft tissue structures that connect them. This compound set of articulations can present a diagnostic challenge. The specific joints of the shoulder complex include the glenohumeral joint (G-H joint), the acromioclavicular joint (A-C joint), the sternoclavicular joint (S-C joint), and the scapulothoracic articulation (see *Orthopaedic Examination, Evaluation, and Intervention*, pp 406–417). In addition, if optimal shoulder function is to occur, motion also has to be available at the cervicothoracic junction and at the connections between the first three ribs and the sternum and spine.

The muscles of the shoulder complex can be divided into three anatomic groups: thoracoscapular (rhomboids, levator scapulae, serratus anterior, and the trapezius muscles), thoracohumeral (latissimus dorsi and pectoralis major) and the scapulohumeral (supraspinatus, infraspinatus, teres minor, and subscapularis [rotator cuff]), and deltoid.[1] Functionally, these muscles can be divided into four groups (see *Orthopaedic Examination, Evaluation, and Intervention*, pp 417–420):[2]

- *Scapular pivoters (trapezius, serratus anterior, rhomboids, and levator scapulae).* The primary function of the scapular pivoters is to support posture. In addition, the trapezius and the serratus anterior muscles help rotate the scapula upward, and the trapezius and the rhomboids aid scapular retraction.[3]
- *Humeral propellers (latissimus dorsi, pectoralis major, and pectoralis minor)*
- *Humeral positioners (deltoid)*
- *Shoulder protectors (rotator cuff, biceps brachii).* These muscles are referred to as the protectors of the shoulder since they fine-tune the humeral head position during arm elevation.[2]

The shoulder complex is endowed with a unique blend of mobility and stability:

- The degree of mobility is contingent on a healthy articular surface, intact muscle-tendon units (Table 7-1), and supple capsuloligamentous restraints (Table 7-2).
- The degree of stability is dependent on a combination of ligamentous and capsular restraints, surrounding musculature and the glenoid labrum (see *Orthopaedic Examination, Evaluation, and Intervention*, pp 423–427). Static joint stability is provided by the integrity of the osseous articular structures and the capsulolabral complex (Table 7-3), and dynamic stability by the rotator cuff muscles (Table 7-3) and the scapular pivoters (see Table 7-1).[4]

EXAMINATION

The overall success of the intervention for a dysfunctional shoulder complex depends almost exclusively on an accurate diagnosis. In the vast majority of cases, an accurate diagnosis can be established with a detailed history and a thorough physical examination supplemented on occasion with appropriate radiographic and laboratory examinations.[5,6]

TABLE 7-1 Muscles of the Shoulder Complex According to Their Actions on the Scapular and at the Glenohumeral Joint

Scapular abductors
Trapezius
Serratus anterior (upper fibers)

Scapular adductors
Levator scapulae
Rhomboids

Scapular flexors
Serratus anterior (lower fibers)

Scapular Extensor
Pectoralis minor

Scapular external rotators
Trapezius
Rhomboids

Shoulder flexors
Coracobrachialis
Short head biceps
Long head biceps
Pectoralis major
Anterior deltoid

Shoulder extensors
Triceps
Posterior deltoid
Teres minor
Teres major
Latissimus dorsi

Shoulder abductors
Supraspinatus
Deltoid

Shoulder adductors
Subscapularis
Pectoralis major
Latissimus dorsi
Teres major
Teres minor

Shoulder internal rotators
Pectoralis major
Serratus anterior
Subscapularis
Latissimus dorsi
Teres major

Shoulder external rotators
Infraspinatus
Supraspinatus
Deltoid
Teres minor

TABLE 7-2 Ligaments of the Shoulder

Ligament	Description	Function
Clavicular ligaments		
Coracoclavicular ligament	Comprised of the conoid and trapezoid ligaments	Reinforces the connection between the coracoid process Stabilizes the acromio-clavicular joint
Acromioclavicular ligament	Runs between the acromion process and the clavicle	Reinforces the connection between the acromion and the clavicle
Sternoclavicular ligaments		
Sternoclavicular ligament	Comprised of anterior and posterior ligaments	Reinforces the connection between the sternum and the clavicle
Interclavicular ligament	Connects the superior-medial sternal ends of each clavicle with the capsular ligaments and the upper sternum	Strengthens the articular capsule
Costoclavicular ligament	The strongest of the sternoclavicular ligaments	Reinforces the connection between the first rib and the clavicle and stabilizes the joint
Glenohumeral ligaments		
Glenohumeral ligaments	Distinct capsular thickenings limiting excessive rotation and translation of the humeral head by reinforcing the connection between the glenoid fossa and the humerus	
Inferior glenohumeral ligament	A complex—parts include the anterior band, axillary pouch, and the posterior band	Provides anterior stabilization, especially during abduction of the arm
Middle glenohumeral ligament	Strongest of the glenohumeral ligaments	Provides anterior stabilization during the combined motion of external rotation and 45° of abduction
Superior glenohumeral ligament	Runs from glenoid rim to anatomic neck	Works in conjunction with the coracohumeral ligament to provide inferior stabilization during adduction
Coracohumeral ligament	Runs from the lateral end of the coracoid process and inserts either side of the greater and lesser tuberosities	Provides anterior support by tightening with flexion
Transverse humeral ligament	Traverses the bicipital groove	Maintains the long head of the biceps muscle in the intertubercular groove

(*Continued*)

TABLE 7-2 Ligaments of the Shoulder (*Continued*)

Ligament	Description	Function
	Intrinsic ligaments of the scapula	
Superior transverse scapular ligament	Attached by one end to the base of the coracoid process, and by the other to the medial end of the scapular notch	Reinforces the connection between the coracoid process and the medial border of the scapular notch
Inferior transverse scapular ligament	An inconstant fibrous band that passes from the lateral border of the spine of the scapula to the posterior margin of the glenoid cavity	Reinforces the connection between the lateral aspect of the root of the spine of the scapula and the margin of the glenoid fossa
Coracoacromial ligament	Runs from the coracoid process to the anterior-inferior aspect of the acromion, with some of its fibers extending to the A-C joint.	Reinforces the connection between the coracoid process and the acromion, stabilizing the joint

TABLE 7-3 Restraints About the Glenohumeral Joint

Passive (static)	Active (dynamic)	
Capsule	Supraspinatus	
Labrum	Infraspinatus	
Coracohumeral ligament	Subscapularis	Humeral stabilizers
Superior glenohumeral ligament	Teres minor	
Middle glenohumeral ligament	Pectoralis major	
Inferior glenohumeral ligament	Latissimus dorsi	
Geometry of humeral articular surface	Biceps (long head)	
Geometry of glenoid articular surface	Triceps	Movers of glenohumeral joint
Coracoacromial ligament	Deltoid	
Articular cartilage compliance	Teres major	
Joint cohesion	Serratus anterior	
	Latissimus dorsi	
	Trapezius	
	Rhomboids	Movers of scapula
	Levator scapulae	
	Pectoralis minor	

Source: Magee DJ: Shoulder. In Orthopedic Physical Assessment, pp 90–142. Philadelphia, PA, WB Saunders, 1992.

History

Since shoulder pain has a broad spectrum of patterns and characteristics, a good history is the cornerstone of proper diagnosis (Table 7-4). Handedness and occupation are key elements to determine during the history.[7] Age can also be an important factor as it is well recognized that certain shoulder pathologies are related to age. For example degenerative rotator cuff tears tend to occur more often in the over 45-age group, whereas traumatic tears are more likely to occur in the younger population.

Determining the location of the pain can provide some clues as to the cause (Figure 7-1). Many shoulder pathologies have key findings that can help guide the examiner (Table 7-5).

Stiffness or loss of motion may be the major symptom in patients with adhesive capsulitis (frozen shoulder), dislocation, or G-H joint arthritis. Pain with throwing (such as pitching a baseball) suggests anterior glenohumeral instability. The shoulder pathologies that can present with specific subjective complaints are outlined in Table 7-6.

Once the location, quality, distribution, and aggravating and relieving factors of the shoulder symptoms have been established, the possibility of referred symptoms should be excluded (Table 7-7).[3] This includes questions about neck pain and previous neck injury and questions that attempt to establish a relationship between head and neck movements and symptom reproduction. Symptoms that originate from the neck and that radiate below the elbow are suggestive of a cervical spine disorder.[3]

Systems Review

The clinician should be able to determine the suitability of the patient for physical therapy. The differential diagnosis for shoulder pain is outlined in Table 7-8.[8] Table 7-9 can be used to help differentiate between the common causes of shoulder pain (see also Chapter 4). To aid further in the diagnosis, inquiries should be made for a history of rheumatoid arthritis, diabetes, neurofibromatosis, neoplasms, cardiac diseases, and gout as well as other systemic diseases.[7] For example, diaphragmatic irritation from a gallbladder or hepatic disorder will often yield shoulder pain, as can the Pancoast tumor with its coincident Horner's syndrome.[7] Pneumonia, cardiac ischemia, and peptic ulcer disease can also present with shoulder pain.[3] A history of malignancy raises the possibility of metastatic disease. If the clinician is concerned with any signs or symptoms of a visceral, vascular, neurogenic, psychogenic, spondylogenic, or systemic disorder that is out of the scope of physical therapy, the patient should be referred back to his or her physician or another appropriate health care provider.

TABLE 7-4 Important Factors in the Patient's History

All patients	Shoulder patients
Age	Overhead use—athletics/repetitive work
Hand dominance	Night pain
Occupation	Upper extremity symptoms
Onset	Neck pain
Mechanism?	Previous episodes?
Duration of symptoms	Previous rehabilitation?
	Surgical history

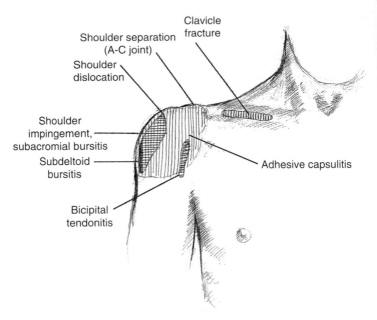

FIG. 7-1 Pain location and possible diagnoses.

The patient should be asked about paresthesias and muscle weakness. Brachial plexus lesions and cervical and upper thoracic spine disorders frequently cause shoulder symptoms. In addition to the cervical and upper thoracic joints, the related joints referring symptoms to the shoulder require clearing. These include the

TABLE 7-5 Key Findings in the History and Physical Examination and Their Probable Diagnosis

Finding	Probable diagnosis
Scapular winging, trauma, recent viral illness	Serratus anterior or trapezius dysfunction
Seizure and inability to passively or actively rotate affected arm externally	Posterior shoulder dislocation
Supraspinatus or infraspinatus wasting	Rotator cuff tear; suprascapular nerve entrapment
Pain radiating below elbow; decreased cervical range of motion	Cervical disk disease
Shoulder pain in throwing athletes; anterior glenohumeral joint pain and impingement	Glenohumeral joint instability
Pain or "clunking" sound with overhead motion	Labral disorder
Nighttime shoulder pain	Impingement
Generalized ligamentous laxity	Multidirectional instability

TABLE 7-6 Subjective Patient Complaints Related to Specific Diagnoses

Specific complaint	Pathology
Intermittent mild pain with overhead activities	Impingement (Stage I)
Mild to moderate pain with overhead or strenuous activities	Impingement (Stage II)
Pain at rest or with activities. Night pain may occur. Weakness is noted.	Impingement (Stage III)
Night pain. Weakness noted predominantly in abductors and external rotators. Loss of motion noted.	Rotator cuff tears (Full thickness). Night pain, with or without weakness could suggest malignancy
Inability to perform activities of daily living as a result of loss of motion. Loss of motion may be perceived as weakness.	Adhesive capsulitis (Frozen shoulder)
Apprehension to mechanical shifting limits activity. Slipping, popping, or sliding may present as subtle instability.	Anterior instability
Apprehension usually associated with horizontal abduction and external rotation. Anterior or posterior pain may be present.	Posterior instability
Slipping or popping of the humeral head posteriorly. This may be associated with forward flexion and internal rotation, while the shoulder is under a compressive load.	
Looseness of the shoulder in all directions. Pain may or may not be present.	Multidirectional instability
Localized pain, swelling, deformity, tenderness localized to A-C joint	Acromioclavicular (A-C) joint pathology

temporomandibular joint, costosternal joint, costovertebral and costotransverse joint, and the elbow and forearm.[9,10] The sympathetic dystrophies can also cause shoulder symptoms.[7,11] The Cyriax scanning examination can help highlight the presence or absence of the more insidious causes of shoulder symptoms and can also help the clinician whether a spinal nerve root or peripheral nerve palsy is present (Table 7-10) (see also Chapter 4). The patient should be asked about previous corticosteroid injections, particularly in the setting of osteopenia or rotator cuff tendon atrophy.[3]

Tests and Measures

The examination of the shoulder complex must be done in a systematic, thorough manner (see *Orthopaedic Examination, Evaluation, and Intervention*, pp 433–461). Table 7-11 demonstrates a stepwise approach for evaluating shoulder pain that begins at the neck, proceeds to the sternoclavicular, acromioclavicular, and scapulothoracic components of the shoulder joint, then focuses on particular anatomic sites, rotator cuff strength, and impingement signs, followed by glenohumeral tests (see Table 7-11).

TABLE 7-7 Peripheral Neuropathies About the Shoulder

Involved nerve root	Muscle weakness	Sensory alteration	Reflexes involved	Mechanism
Suprascapular nerve (C5-6)	Supraspinatus, infraspinatus (external rotation)	Superior aspect of shoulder from the clavicle to spine of scapula	None	Compression Traction (scapular protraction plus horizontal adduction) Direct blow Space occupying lesion
Axillary (circumflex) nerve (posterior cord; C5-6)	Deltoid, teres minor (abduction)	Pain in posterior aspect of shoulder radiating into arm Deltoid area Anterior shoulder pain	None	Anterior glenohumeral dislocation Fracture of surgical neck of humerus Forced abduction
Radial nerve (C5-8, T1)	Triceps, wrist extensors, finger extensors (shoulder, wrist, and hand extension)	Dorsum of hand	Triceps	Fracture humeral shaft Direct pressure (e.g., crutch palsy) Direct blow
Long thoracic nerve (C5-6, (C7))	Serratus anterior (scapular control)		None	Traction Compression against internal chest wall (backpack injury) Heavy effort above shoulder height Repetitive strain
Musculocutaneous nerve (C5-7)	Coracobrachialis, biceps, brachialis (elbow flexion)	Lateral aspect of forearm	Biceps	Compression Muscle hypertrophy Direct blow Fracture (clavicle and humerus) Dislocation (anterior) Shoulder surgery

Nerve	Muscles affected	Signs and symptoms		Cause of injury
Spinal accessory nerve (cranial nerve XI: C3-4)	Trapezius (shoulder elevation)	Brachial plexus symptoms possible because of drooping of shoulder Shoulder aching	None	Direct blow Traction (shoulder depression and neck rotation to opposite side)
Subscapular nerve (posterior cord; C5-6)	Subscapularis, teres major (internal rotation)	None	None	Direct blow Traction
Dorsal scapular nerve (C5)	Levator scapulae, rhomboid major, rhomboid minor (scapular retraction and elevation)	None	None	Direct blow Compression
Lateral pectoral nerve (C5-6)	Pectoralis major, pectoralis minor	None	None	Direct blow
Thoracodorsal nerve (C6-7, (C8))	Latissimus dorsi	None	None	Direct blow
Supraclavicular nerve		Mild clavicular pain Sensory loss over anterior shoulder	None	Compression

Source: Magee DJ: Shoulder. In Orthopedic Physical Assessment, pp 90–142. Philadelphia, PA, WB Saunders, 1992.

TABLE 7-8 Differential Diagnosis of Shoulder Pain

- Referred sources
- Neck
- Subdiaphragm
- Ribs
- Sternoclavicular joint
- Acromioclavicular joint
- Sprains (I–VI)
- Fractures distal clavicle (I–III)
- Instability—horizontal
- Degenerative
- Osteolysis
- Scapulothoracic bursitis
- Glenohumeral
- Rotator cuff
- Tear (complete vs. partial)
- Tendinitis
- Biceps tendinitis/tear
- Impingement
- Adhesive capsulitis—frozen shoulder
- Instability
- Unidirectional—anterior vs. posterior
- Multidirectional instability
- Labral tears—anterosuperior vs. Bankart

Source: Spindler K, Dovan T, McCarty E: Clinical cornerstone. Excerpta Med 2001;3:26–37.

TABLE 7-9 Differential Diagnosis of Common Causes of Shoulder Pain

Etiology	Physical examination	Laboratory findings	Radiographic findings
Autoimmune inflammatory disorders	Fluctuant sub-deltoid mass Erythema, tenderness	Elevated ESR Positive ANA, positive RF	Joint destruction
Septic/infectious causes	Fluctuant sub-deltoid mass Erythema, ten-derness	Aspirate Gram stain/culture	Bursal effusion (MRI, ultra-sound)
Crystal deposition	Anterolateral tenderness Positive impinge-ment signs	Aspiration: apatite crystals	Intrabursal rice bodies
Trauma (rotator cuff injury)	Anterior/lateral tenderness Positive impingement signs Supraspinatus challenge	None	Hooked acromion Tendon calcifi-cation Decreased acromio-humeral distance MRI: supraspinatus tendon tear

ESR = erythrocyte sedimentation rate; ANA = antinuclear antibody; RF = rheumatoid factor; NSAIDs = nonsteroidal anti-inflammatory drugs; MRI = magnetic resonance imaging.
Source: Salzman KL, Lillegard WA, Butcher JD: Upper extremity bursitis. Am Fam Phys 1997;56:1797–1806,1811–1812.

TABLE 7-10 Indications of Peripheral Nerve Damage at the Shoulder

Atrophied muscle	Peripheral nerve	Cause	Appearance
Deltoid	Axillary	Anterior dislocation	Squared appearance of the lateral shoulder[a]
Posterior deltoid	Axillary	Multidirectional instability[b]	
Infraspinatus or supraspinatus	Suprascapular	Rotator cuff tear[5] Nerve entrapment	Slight indent over fossae. Confirmed by pushing the examining finger into the respective muscle bellies
Trapezius	Spinal accessory		Appearance of a shoulder girdle that droops in association with a protracted inferior border of the scapula and an elevated acromion.[c,d]
Serratus anterior	Long thoracic		Prominent superior medial border of the scapula and a depressed acromion

[a]Hawkins RJ, Bokor DJ: Clinical evaluation of shoulder problems. In Rockwood CA Matsen FA (eds): The Shoulder. Philadelphia, PA, WB Saunders, 1990.
[b]Silliman FJ, Hawkins RJ: Clinical examination of the shoulder complex. In Andrews JR, Wilk KE (eds): The Athlete's Shoulder. New York, Churchill Livingstone, 1994.
[c]Barron OA, Levine WN, Bigliani LU, Surgical management of chronic trapezius dysfunction. In Warner JJP, Iannotti JP, Gerber C (eds): Complex and Revision Problems in Shoulder Surgery, pp 377–384. Philadelphia, PA, Lippincott-Raven, 1997.
[d]Kibler BW: The role of the scapula in athletic shoulder function. Am J Sports Med 1998;26(2):325–337.

A complete physical examination includes observation and palpation, assessment of range of motion and strength, and provocative shoulder testing for possible impingement syndrome and glenohumeral instability.[3] The neck and the elbow should also be examined to exclude the possibility that the shoulder pain is referred from a pathologic condition in either of these regions.

The closed and open packed positions and the capsular patterns for the joints of the shoulder complex are outlined in Table 7-12. The clinician should list all positive findings because multiple diagnoses are quite possible (Figure 7-2).

TABLE 7-11 Shoulder Examination Flow

Cervical Spine Examination	Result
Abnormal findings • Trapezius muscle spasm • Nerve root symptoms • Degenerative joint disease on examination or x-ray • Other	Continue assessment of cervical spine
Normal cervical spine findings	Proceed to shoulder assessment
Shoulder Range of Motion Abnormal active range of motion Normal passive range of motion	Causes include: • Pain • Rotator cuff tear • Nerve deficit
Restricted passive range of motion	Causes include: • Adhesive capsulitis (frozen shoulder), normal x-ray • Degenerative joint disease, abnormal x-ray • Pain due to impingement, A-C arthritis • Chronic dislocation
Normal active range of motion	Palpate for areas of tenderness to refine diagnosis • S-C joint • Sprain • Instability • DJD (degenerative joint disease) • A-C joint • Sprain • Instability • Osteolysis • Fracture • Biceps tendon • Impingement • Tendinitis • Adjacent labral injury

Evaluate Rotator Cuff Strength
Weakness
• Administer subacromial Xylocaine (Impingement test)
• Consider rotator cuff tear
• MRI may be warranted
• Neurologic injury
• Nerve root
• Burner
No weakness
Evaluate for subacromial impingement
Impingement signs
Positive
• Consider tendinitis or bursitis
• Possible rotator cuff tear—partial or complete
• Evaluate with MRI or arthroscopy
Negative
• Consider glenohumeral instability or glenoid labrum tear
• Glenohumeral instability/Labral tests

(Continued)

TABLE 7-11 Shoulder Examination Flow (*Continued*)

Instability

Anatomic lesion confirmed by physical exam, x-ray, MRI, examination under anesthesia, arthroscopy
- Anterior
- Posterior
- Inferior
- Multidirectional
- Functional instability
- Internal impingement
- Secondary impingement

Labral signs confirmed by physical examination, MRI, arthroscopy
- With instability
- Without instability
- No evidence of instability or labral pathology
- Training error
- Overuse
- Normal adaptation to increased loads

Observation

Observation of the shoulder complex can be divided into two static and dynamic factors. The static factors consider physiologic age and appearance, posture, generalized diseases such as rheumatoid arthritis, generalized distress, and distress related to the shoulder.[5] The dynamic factors consider generalized distress with movement, shoulder distress with movements, and the performance of simple functional tasks.[5]

TABLE 7-12 Close Packed, Open Packed, and Capsular Patterns of the Shoulder Complex

	Close packed	Open packed	Capsular pattern
Glenohumeral	90° of glenohumeral abduction and full external rotation; or full abduction and external rotation	55° abduction, 30° horizontal adduction	External rotation, abduction, internal rotation
Acromioclavicular	90° abduction	Arm resting by side	Pain at extremes of range, especially horizontal adduction and full elevation
Sternoclavicular	Full arm elevation and shoulder protraction	Arm resting by side	Pain at extremes of range, especially horizontal adduction and full elevation

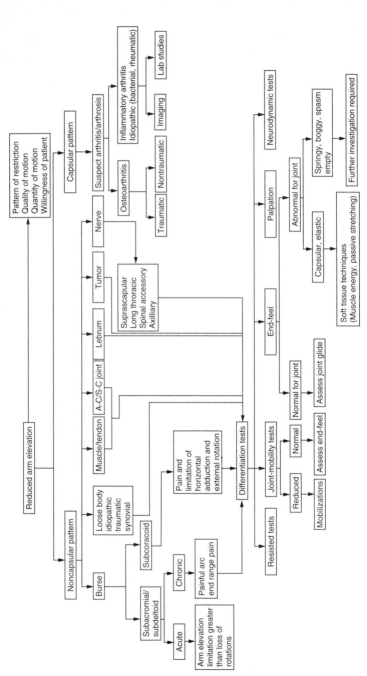

FIG. 7-2 Causes of painful arm elevation.

Static Observation Observation of the shoulder requires adequate visualization of the entire upper extremity, shoulder girdle, chest, and back. The examination is performed with the shirt off for male patients, and a sleeveless shirt for female patients. Both shoulders should be visible to allow comparative inspection and the observation should be from all views.[7] To ensure this, the observation should be systematically divided into anterior, lateral, posterior, and superior aspects.[5]

The clinician initially observes the attitude of the shoulder and notes the overall position of the upper extremity. Symmetry of right and left sides, or lack thereof, should also be noted. A painful shoulder is often held higher than the uninvolved side, or it may be held by the patient in a protective manner across the abdomen, often supported by the opposite extremity.[5]

The clinician should note muscle mass and tone, deformities, scars, masses, ecchymosis, discoloration, swelling, and any venous distention. Examples of possible deformities are listed in Table 7-13.

Discoloration from bruising may be present from a recent fracture, rotator cuff injury, or biceps rupture.[5] Specific atrophy can imply certain diagnoses. For example, muscle weakness or atrophy, especially post trauma, might indicate peripheral nerve damage (Tables 7-7, 7-10).[12]

The scapular position is initially examined with the arms by the side. The clinician notes any signs of winging (see Table 7-13), elevation, depression, adduction, abduction, and rotation. Winging of the scapula is usually evident at the inferior border, but can be found anywhere along the entire border.[5,9,12] A number of tests, outlined in Chapter 14 of the larger text, can be used to assess the position of the scapular relative to the uninvolved side.

Dynamic Observation Given the importance of the scapulothoracic joint to overall shoulder function, it is important to examine the scapulohumeral rhythm during humeral abduction. The ability of the patient to perform full abduction will vary according to the presenting pathology and pain. The first 20° to 30° of abduction do not normally require scapulothoracic motion. Frequently in the unstable shoulder, the scapula does not move with its normal rhythm.[5] After 90° of elevation, 60° of the motion has occurred at the G-H joint, with the remaining 30° consisting of scapular motion. After the first 90°, the rest of the elevation occurs at a 2:1 glenohumeral to scapula ratio, although this ratio is not consistent throughout the range of motion. By internally rotating the arm (palm down), further glenohumeral abduction may continue to 120°. Beyond 120°, full abduction is possible only when the humerus is externally rotated (palm up). Observation of the scapulohumeral rhythm should reveal that the scapula stops its rotation when the arm has been elevated to approximately 140°. On completion of the abduction, the inferior angle of the scapula should be in close proximity to the midline of the thorax, and the vertebral border of the scapula should be rotated 60°. Movement beyond these points may indicate excessive scapular abduction.[13] At the end of range the scapula should slightly depress, posteriorly tilt, and adduct.[13] Scapular control is provided primarily by the scapular pivoters (trapezius, serratus anterior, rhomboids, and levator scapulae). Thus, a dysfunctional scapulohumeral rhythm requires a thorough assessment of these muscles in terms of strength and length.

Palpation

Palpation must be systematic and focus on specific anatomic structures. The optimal methods of palpating the shoulder tendons occur in regions where there is the least amount of overlying soft tissue.[14] The shoulder girdle should

TABLE 7-13 Shoulder Deformities and Their Possible Reasons

Deformity present	Possible reason
Squaring off the shoulder with an anterior prominence of the humeral head	Anterior dislocation of the shoulder
Neck appears fuller, shorter on the affected side	Sprengel deformity (most common congenital deformity of the shoulder)
An elevated scapula	
Clavicle tilted superiorly about 25°	
An exaggeration of the A-C joint prominence	Third degree acromioclavicular separation
Excessive prominence of the spine of the scapula	Supraspinatus and infraspinatus wasting
"Popeye" appearance of the biceps muscle belly with elbow flexion	Rupture of the long head of the biceps
Scapular winging	Weakness of the serratus anterior
	Weakness of the trapezius
	Glenohumeral joint pathology

Sources: Yocum LA: Assessing the shoulder. History, physical examination, differential diagnosis, and special tests used. Clin Sports Med 1983;2:281–289.
Boublik M, Hawkins RJ: Clinical examination of the shoulder complex. J Orthop Sports Phys Ther 1993;18:379–385.
Alcheck DW, Dines DM: Shoulder injuries in the throwing athlete. J Am Acad Orthop Surgeons 1995;3:159–165.
Ayub E: Posture and the upper quarter. In Donatelli RA (ed): Physical Therapy of the Shoulder, pp 81–90. New York, Churchill Livingstone, 1991.
Barron OA, Levine WN, Bigliani LU: Surgical management of chronic trapezius dysfunction. In Warner JJP, Iannotti JP, Gerber C (eds): Complex and Revision Problems in Shoulder Surgery, pp 377–384. Philadelphia, PA, Lippincott-Raven, 1997.
Boerger TO, Limb D: Suprascapular nerve injury at the spinoglenoid notch after glenoid neck fracture. J Shoulder Elbow Surg 2000;9:236–237.
Bowling RW, Rockar PA, Erhard R: Examination of the shoulder complex. Phys Ther 1986;66:1886–1893.
Brody LT Shoulder. In Wadsworth C (ed): Current Concepts of Orthopedic Physical Therapy—Home Study Course. La Crosse, WI, Orthopaedic Section, APTA, 2001.
Butters KP: The scapula. In Rockwood CA, Matsen FA (eds): The Shoulder, pp 335–336. Philadelphia, PA, WB Saunders, 1990.
Cappel K, et al.: Clinical examination of the shoulder. In Tovin BJ, Greenfield B (eds): Evaluation and Treatment of the Shoulder—An Integration of The Guide to Physical Therapist Practice, pp 75–131. Philadelphia, PA, FA Davis, 2001.

be palpated for warmth, tenderness, deformity, and crepitus. Often, trigger points of pain from myofascial syndromes or isolated muscle spasm will be determined with selective palpation of the shoulder girdle structures.[7] Palpation should include examination of the acromioclavicular and sternoclavicular joints, medial scapula, posterior rotator cuff, anterior rotator cuff, deltoid, the cervical spinous processes and the biceps tendon (see *Orthopaedic Examination, Evaluation, and Intervention*, pp 436–437). Other structures to palpate include the spine of the scapula, the acromion, the subacromial bursa, the greater tuberosity, the coracoid process and the clavicle (Figure 7-3).[3]

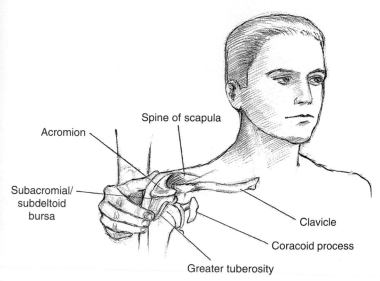

FIG. 7-3   Shoulder palpation.

Active and Passive Range of Motion

Owing to the complex nature of the arthrokinematics, osteokinematics, and myokinetics of this region, the actual clinical value of active movements are limited if used in isolation. Loss of motion at the shoulder complex is most commonly caused by pain (Table 7-14). It is important to determine the degree of pain as well as the arc of motion in which the pain occurs (Figure 7-4).[5,9,12]

TABLE 7-14 Diagnosing from the Point in the Range the Pain is Reproduced

AROM	AROM	AROM	PROM	PROM	PROM
Limited range and pain between 70° and 110° of elevation	Full range but pain between 70° and 110° of elevation	Full range but pain at 120°–160°/160°–180° range	Full and pain free	Restriction of all movements	Pain on adduction
• Rotator cuff impingement • Rotator cuff tear • Subacromial bursitis	• Subacromial bursitis	• A-C joint pathology	• Rotator cuff tear • Chronic instability	• Adhesive capsulitis	• A-C joint pathology

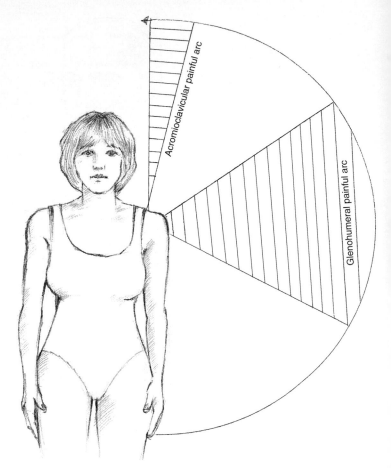

FIG. 7-4 Arm elevation.

Active motion is assessed first and the patient is asked to move the arm and shoulder actively through the available range of motion (Table 7-15). Ranges of motion that need to be documented are total elevation (forward elevation in the sagittal plane and abduction in the coronal plane), internal and external rotation with the arm by the side and in the 90° abducted position (if the patient is able to achieve) (Figure 7-5), horizontal adduction, and shrugging of the shoulders. Internal rotation can be tested further with the patient's arm at the side and the forearm behind his or her back (Figure 7-6). This measurement for internal rotation is assessed by the position reached with the extended thumb up the dorsal aspect of the spine using the spinous processes as landmarks. The interpretation of the active motion tests is outlined in Chapter 14 of *Orthopaedic Examination, Evaluation, and Intervention*. Passive

TABLE 7-15 Normal Ranges for Movements of the Shoulder Complex and Potential Causes of Pain

Motion	Range norms (degrees)	End-feel	Potential source of pain
Elevation— flexion	160–180	Tissue stretch	• Suprahumeral impingement • Stretching of glenohumeral, acromioclavicular, sternoclavicular joint capsule • Triceps tendon if elbow flexed
Extension	50–60	Tissue stretch	• Stretching of glenohumeral joint capsule • Severe suprahumeral impingement • Biceps tendon if elbow extended
Elevation— abduction	170–180	Tissue stretch	• Suprahumeral impingement • Acromioclavicular arthritis at terminal abduction
External rotation	80–90	Tissue stretch	• Anterior glenohumeral instability
Internal rotation	60–1000	Tissue stretch	• Suprahumeral impingement rotation • Posterior glenohumeral instability

Sources: Warner JJP, Caborn DNM, Berger RA et al.: Dynamic capsuloligamentous anatomy of the glenohumeral joint. J Shoulder Elbow Surg 1993;2:115–133.

Turkel SJ, Panio MW, Marshall JL et al.: Stabilizing mechanisms preventing anterior dislocation of the glenohumeral joint. J Bone Joint Surg [Am] 1981; 63:1208–1217.

Pagnani MJ, Warren RF. Stabilizers of the glenohumeral joint. J Shoulder Elbow Surg 1994; 3:173–190.

O'Connell PW, Nuber GW, Mileski RA et al.: The contribution of the glenohumeral ligaments to anterior stability of the shoulder joint. Am J Sports Med 1990;18:579–584.

Karduna AR, Williams GR, Williams JL et al.: Kinematics of the glenohumeral joint: Influences of muscle forces, ligamentous constraints, and articular geometry. J Orthop Res 1996;14:986–993.

Davies GJ, DeCarlo MS: Examination of the shoulder complex. In Bandy WD (ed): Current Concepts in the Rehabilitation of the Shoulder. Sports Physical Therapy Section—Home Study Course. LaCrosse, WI, Sports Physical therapy Section, APTA, 1995.

range of motion (PROM) testing follows the active range of motion testing, even if the active range of motion appears to be normal. The PROM tests take the form of passive overpressure superimposed on the active motion. PROM is performed to determine the end-feel.[15] Pain often occurs in the extremes of motion in the presence of joint instability. A patient with a loss of active motion but normal PROM is more likely to have muscle weakness than joint disease.

Given the importance of the scapulothoracic joint to overall shoulder function, it is important to examine the scapulothoracic joint arthrokinematics.[16]

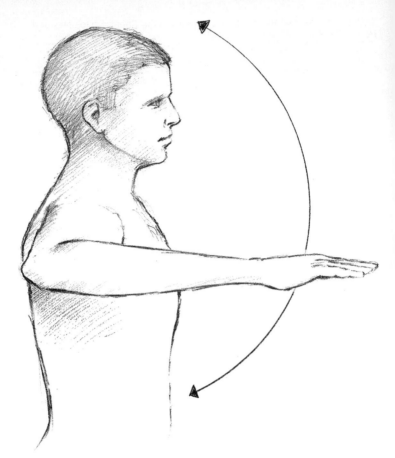

FIG. 7-5 Measuring internal rotation and external rotation.

Disorders of the glenohumeral articulation, such as osteoarthritis, adhesive capsulitis, can increase the relative contribution to motion by the scapulothoracic articulation.[5,9,12] Rotator cuff tears or labral lesions may cause catching pain and result in a hesitant scapulohumeral rhythm.[5,9,12]

Typically, 170° to 180° of elevation is possible in both flexion and abduction, with the upper portion of the arm able to be placed adjacent to the head. If pain occurs with glenohumeral elevation, the point in the range where the pain occurs can be diagnostic in implicating the cause (see Table 7-14; Figure 7-4).[17]

The patient then completes the motions of shoulder girdle elevation (shrug) and depression, and shoulder protraction and retraction. An inability to shrug the shoulder may indicate trapezius palsy.[18] Hiking of the shoulder and the scapula is often seen in patients with large rotator cuff tears.[19]

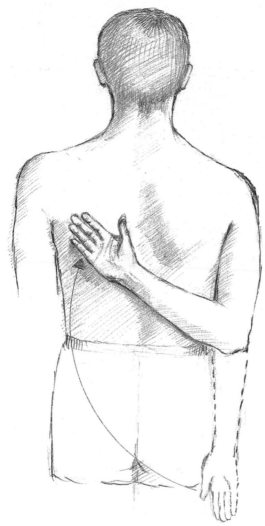

FIG. 7-6   Internal rotation of the shoulder.

A discrepancy between active and passive motion may indicate a painful periarticular condition.[19] Loss of active motion with preservation of passive motion is caused by rotator cuff tear[20] or, rarely, suprascapular nerve injury.[21,22] A severely restricted active abduction pattern with no pain is suggestive of a rupture of the supraspinatus or deltoid. Loss of both active and passive motion is usually caused by adhesive capsulitis.[23]

Resisted

In addition to pain, shoulder dysfunction is often caused or exacerbated by loss of motion or weakness (Table 7-16). The resistive tests assess the function and neurologic status of the important muscle groups of the upper kinetic chain (Table 7-17), including the cervical musculature. The comprehensiveness of the strength testing and neurologic examination of the shoulder complex is determined by the chief complaint and general status of the patient. Lesions such as brachial plexus or cervical root injuries may require extensive muscle, sensory, and reflex testing.[5] Weakness on isometric testing needs to be analyzed for the type (increasing weakness with repeated contractions of the same resistance indicating a palsy versus consistent weakness with repeated contractions, which could suggest a deconditioned muscle or a significant muscle tear), and the pattern of neurologic weakness (spinal nerve root, nerve trunk, or peripheral nerve) (Tables 7-18, 7-19). Localized, individual isometric muscle tests around the shoulder girdle can also give the clinician information about patterns of weakness other than from spinal nerve root or peripheral nerve palsies (e.g., instabilities, postural dysfunction), and also help to isolate the pain generators.

Given the importance of the scapulothoracic joint to overall shoulder function, it is important to examine the scapulothoracic muscles.[16] Increased activity of the upper trapezius muscle, or imbalances between the upper and lower trapezius muscle during shoulder elevation may have adverse effects on the kinematics of the scapula.[24-27] Routine strength testing should include the rotator cuff muscles, deltoid, and scapular pivoters.

The supraspinatus can be tested using the "empty can" test, having the patient abduct the shoulders to 90° in forward flexion with the thumbs pointing downward (Figure 7-7). The patient then attempts to elevate the arms against examiner resistance. The function of the infraspinatus and teres minor muscles are tested with the patient's arms at the sides, the patient flexes both elbows to 90°, while the examiner provides resistance against external rotation (Figure 7-8).

The function of the subscapularis is assessed with the Gerber "lift-off test." The patient rests the dorsum of the hand on the back in the lumbar area. Inability to move the hand off the back by further internal rotation of the arm suggests injury to the subscapularis muscle.[28] If the patient is unable to place the hand behind the back, a modified version of the lift-off test is used. In this version, the patient places the hand of the affected arm on the abdomen and resists the examiner's attempts to externally rotate the arm.

The deltoid is tested in forward flexion for the anterior third, straight abduction for the middle third, and in extension for the posterior third. The

TABLE 7-16 Common Muscle Imbalances of the Shoulder Complex

Muscles prone to tightness	Muscles prone to inactivity or lengthening
Upper trapezius	Middle and lower trapezius
Levator scapulae	Rhomboids
Pectoralis major and minor	Serratus anterior
Upper cervical extensors	Deep neck flexors
Sternocleidomastoid	Subscapularis
Scalenes	Supraspinatus
Teres major and minor	Infraspinatus

TABLE 7-17 Muscle Groups Tested in the Shoulder Examination[1]

Trunk flexors, extensors, and obliques
Scapulothoracic elevators
Scapulothoracic depressors
Scapulothoracic protractors
Scapulothoracic retractors
Scapulothoracic upward rotators
Scapulothoracic downward rotators
Glenohumeral flexors
Glenohumeral extensors
Glenohumeral abductors
Glenohumeral adductors
Glenohumeral internal rotators
Glenohumeral external rotators
Glenohumeral horizontal flexors
Glenohumeral horizontal extensors
Elbow flexors
Elbow extensors
Forearm supinators
Forearm pronators
Wrist flexors
Wrist extensors
Hand intrinsics

Source: Davies GJ, DeCarlo MS: Examination of the shoulder complex. In Bandy WD (ed): Current Concepts in the Rehabilitation of the Shoulder. Sports Physical Therapy Section—Home Study Course. LaCrosse, WI, Sports Physical Therapy Section, APTA, 1995.

TABLE 7-18 Shoulder Girdle Muscle Function and Innervation

Muscles	Peripheral nerve	Nerve root	Motions
Pectoralis major	Pectoral	C5-8	Adduction, horizontal adduction, and internal rotation Clavicular fibers—forward flexion Sternocostal fibers—extension
Latissimus dorsi	Thoracodorsal	C7(C6,8)	Adduction, extension, and internal rotation
Teres major	Subscapular	C5-8	Adduction, extension, horizontal abduction, and internal rotation
Teres minor	Axillary	C5(6)	Horizontal abduction (also a weak external rotator)
Deltoid	Axillary	C5(6)	Anterior—forward flexion, horizontal adduction Middle—abduction Posterior—extension, horizontal abduction
Supraspinatus	Suprascapular	C5(6)	Abduction
Subscapularis	Subscapular	C5-8	Adduction, and internal rotation
Infraspinatus	Suprascapular	C5(C6)	Abduction, horizontal abduction, and external rotation

TABLE 7-19 Peripheral Nerve Tests

Spinal accessory nerve	Inability to abduct the arm beyond 90°
	Pain in shoulder with abduction
Musculocutaneous nerve	Weak elbow flexion with forearm supinated
Long thoracic nerve	Pain on flexing fully extended arm
	Inability to flex fully extended arm
	Winging of scapula at 90° of forward flexion
Suprascapular nerve	Increased pain on forward shoulder flexion
	Pain increased with scapular abduction
	Pain increased with cervical rotation to opposite side
Axillary nerve	Inability to abduct arm with neutral rotation

serratus anterior is evaluated by having the patient push off a wall while standing. Winging of the scapula during this maneuver is classic when paralysis of the long thoracic nerve is involved.[25,29]

The serratus anterior muscle can also be tested using the full push-up to stress the serratus anterior muscle to demonstrate scapular winging.

A key finding, particularly with rotator cuff problems, is pain accompanied by weakness. True weakness should be distinguished from weakness that is caused by pain. A patient with subacromial bursitis with a tear of the rotator

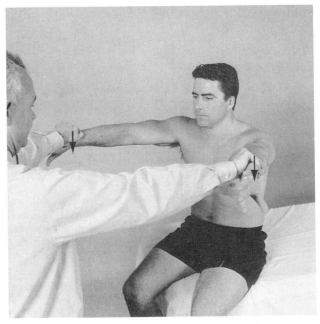

FIG. 7-7   Empty can test for supraspinatus.

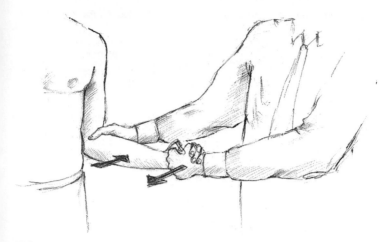

FIG. 7-8   Resisted test for infraspinatus and teres minor.

cuff often has objective rotator cuff weakness caused by pain when the arm is positioned in the arc of impingement. Conversely, the patient will have normal strength if the arm is not tested in abduction.[30]

Functional Testing

The assessment of shoulder function is an integral part of the examination of the shoulder complex. The term *shoulder function* can include tests for biomechanical dysfunction and tests assessing the patient's ability to perform the basic functions of activities of daily living.

Biomechanical Function   There are only two functional motions within the shoulder girdle: arm elevation using a combination of flexion and abduction, and arm extension with adduction. All other motions of the shoulder are parts or composites of these two basic functional sets.

Basic Function Testing   By referring to Table 7-20, the clinician is able to determine the functional status of the patient for basic functions simply by measuring the amount of available range of motion (see Table 7-15). For example, humeral motions necessary for eating and drinking have been reported at 5° to 45° of flexion, 5°–35° of abduction, and 5°–25° of internal rotation relative to the trunk.[31] Combing hair has been found to require 112° of arm elevation.[32]

Assessment tools such as those outlined in Tables 7-21 and 7-22 can be used as functional tests of the shoulder.

Examination of the Passive Restraint System and Neighboring Joints

If following the range of motion and the strength and functional movement tests, the clinician is unable to determine a working hypothesis from which to treat the patient, further examination is required. This more detailed examination

TABLE 7-20 Range of Motion Necessary at the Shoulder for Basic Functional Activities[1,2]

Activity	Necessary range of motion
Eating	70°–100° horizontal adduction
	45°–60° abduction
Combing hair	30°–70° horizontal adduction
	105°–120° abduction
	90° external rotation
Reach perineum	75°–90° horizontal adduction
	30°–45° abduction
	90° or greater internal rotation
Tuck in shirt	50°–60° horizontal adduction
	55°–65° abduction
	90° internal rotation
Position hand behind head	10°–15° horizontal adduction
	110°–125° forward flexion
	90° external rotation
Put an item on a shelf	70°–80° horizontal adduction
	70°–80° forward flexion
	45° external rotation
Wash opposite shoulder	60°–90° forward flexion
	60°–120° horizontal adduction

Sources: Matsen FH III, Lippitt SB, Sidles JA, et al.: Practical Evaluation of Management of the Shoulder, pp 19–150. Philadelphia, PA, WB Saunders, 1994.
Magee DJ: Shoulder. In Magee DJ (ed): Orthopedic Physical Assessment, p 196. Philadelphia, PA, WB Saunders, 1992.

involves the assessment of the mobility and stability of the passive restraint systems of the shoulder girdle.

Passive Accessory Motion Tests The passive accessory motion (PAM) tests are performed at the end of the patient's available range to determine if the joint itself is responsible for the loss of motion. A knowledge of the physiologic and accessory motions that accompany each motion is necessary (Table 7-23).

For all these tests, the patient is positioned in supine, with his or her head supported on a pillow, while the clinician is standing facing the patient.

- *Distraction or compression of the G-H joint.* The clinician stabilizes the shoulder girdle and the anterior thorax. With one hand, the clinician gently grasps the proximal one-third of the humerus. The clinician distracts/compresses (Figure 7-9) the G-H joint perpendicular to the plane of the glenoid fossa (30° off the sagittal plane). The quantity of motion is noted and compared with the other side.
- *Inferior glide of the G-H joint.* The clinician palpates and stabilizes the coracoid process of the scapula and the lateral clavicle. With the other hand, the clinician gently grasps proximal to the patient's shoulder. The humerus is glided inferiorly at the G-H joint, parallel to the superior-inferior plane of the glenoid fossa (Figure 7-10). The quantity of motion is noted and compared with the other side.

TABLE 7-21 Functional Testing of the Shoulder

Starting Position	Action	Functional test
Sitting, cuff weight attached to wrist	Forward flex arm to 90° elbow extended	Raise 4- to 5-pound weight: Functional Raise 1- to 3-pound weight: Functionally Fair Raise arm without weight: Functionally Poor Cannot raise arm: Nonfunctional
Sitting, cuff weight attached to wrist	Extend shoulder, elbow extended	Raise 4- to 5-pound weight: Functional Raise 3- to 4-pound weight: Functionally Fair Raise arm without weight: Functionally Poor Cannot extend arm: Nonfunctional
Sitting with hand behind low back	Shoulder internal rotation	Raise 5-pound weight: Functional Raise 1- to 3-pound weight: Functionally Fair Raise arm without weight: Functionally Poor Cannot raise arm: Nonfunctional
Side lying, cuff weight attached to wrist	Shoulder external rotation	Raise 5-pound weight: Functional Raise 3- to 4-pound weight: Functionally Fair Raise arm without weight: Functionally Poor Cannot Raise arm: Nonfunctional
Sitting, cuff weight attached to wrist	Shoulder abduction to 90°	Raise 5-pound weight: Functional Raise 3- to 4-pound weight: Functionally Fair Raise arm without weight: Functionally Poor Cannot raise arm: Nonfunctional

(Continued)

177

TABLE 7-21 Functional Testing of the Shoulder (*Continued*)

Starting Position	Action	Functional test
Sitting, arm abducted to 145°	Shoulder adduction	Pull 5-pound weight: Functional Pull 3- to 4-pound weight: Functionally Fair Pull 1- to 2-pound weight: Functionally Poor Cannot pull 1-pound weight: Nonfunctional
Sitting	Shoulder elevation (shoulder shrug)	Five Repetitions: Functional Three to four repetitions: Functionally Fair One to two repetitions: Functionally Poor Zero repetitions: Nonfunctional
Sitting	Scapular depression	Five repetitions: Functional Three to four repetitions: Functionally Fair One to two Repetitions: Functionally Poor Zero repetitions: Nonfunctional

Source: Palmer ML, Epler M: Clinical Assessment Procedures in Physical Therapy. Philadelphia, PA, JB Lippincott, 1990.

TABLE 7-22 The Simple Shoulder Test

1. Is your shoulder comfortable with your arm at rest by your side?
2. Does your shoulder allow you to sleep comfortably?
3. Can you reach the small of your back to tuck in your shirt with your hand?
4. Can you place your hand behind your head with the elbow straight out to the side?
5. Can you place a coin on a shelf at the level of your shoulder without bending your elbow?
6. Can you lift 1 pound (a full pint container) to the level of your shoulder without bending your elbow?
7. Can you lift 8 pounds (a full gallon container) to the level of the top of your head without bending your elbow?
8. Can you carry 20 pounds at your side with the affected extremity?
9. Do you think you can toss a softball underhand 10 yards with the affected extremity?
10. Do you think you can throw a softball overhand 20 yards with the affected extremity?
11. Can you wash the back of your opposite shoulder with the affected extremity?
12. Would your shoulder allow you to work full time at your usual job?

Source: Matsen FH III, Lippitt SB, Sidles JA, et al.: Evaluating the shoulder. In Matsen FH III, Lippitt SB, Sidles JA (eds): Practical Evaluation of Management of the Shoulder, pp 1–17. Philadelphia, PA, WB Saunders, 1994.

- *Posterior glide of the G-H joint.* The clinician palpates and stabilizes the coracoid process and the lateral one-third of the clavicle. With the hypothenar eminence of the same hand, the clinician palpates the anterior aspect of the humeral head (Figure 7-11). With the other hand, the clinician gently grasps the distal end of the humerus (Figure 7-11). From this position, the clinician glides the humerus posteriorly at the G-H joint, parallel to the anterior-posterior plane of the glenoid fossa. The quantity of motion is noted and compared with the other side.
- Passive accessory motion testing of the acromioclavicular joint
  - Anterior and posterior rotation of the clavicle (Figure 7-12) and anterior and posterior glide of the A-C joint (Figure 7-13)
- Passive accessory motion testing of the sternoclavicular joint
  - Anterior and inferior glide
  - Superior glide (Figure 7-14)

TABLE 7-23 Glenohumeral Joint Motions and Their Appropriate Axis and Accessory Motions

Plane/axis of motion	Physiologic motion	Accessory motion
Sagittal/medial-lateral	Flexion/extension	Spin
Coronal/anterior-posterior	Abduction	Inferior glide
	Adduction	Superior glide
Transverse/longitudinal	Internal rotation	Posterior glide
	External rotation	Anterior glide

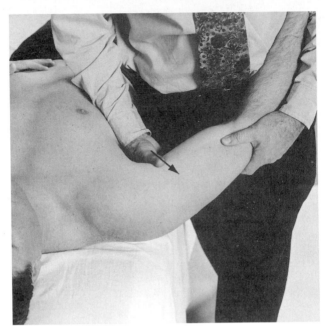

FIG. 7-9 Distraction of the G-H joint.

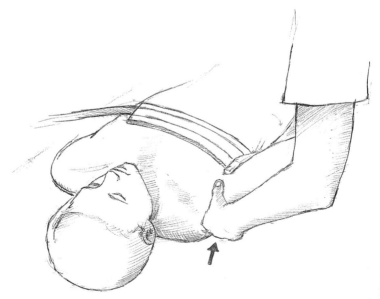

FIG. 7-10 Inferior glide of the G-H joint.

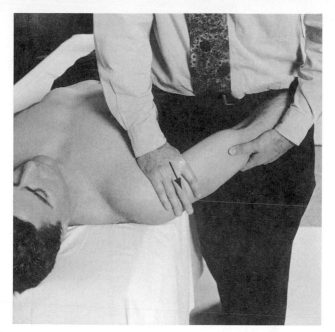

FIG. 7-11 Posterior glide of the G-H joint.

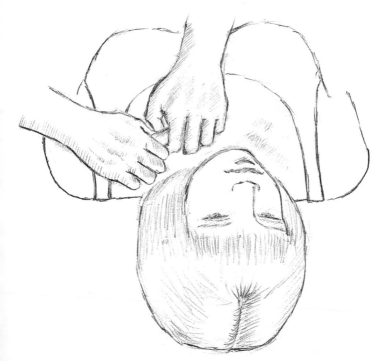

FIG. 7-12 Anterior and posterior rotation of the clavicle.

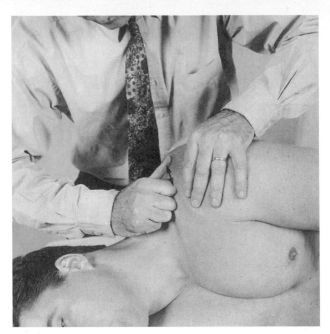

FIG. 7-13   Anterior and posterior glide of the A-C joint.

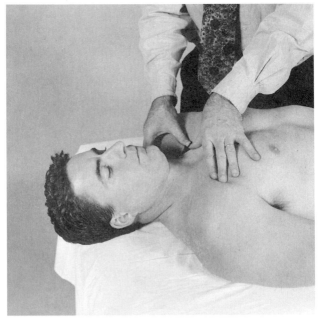

FIG. 7-14   Superior glide of the S-C joint.

Passive Accessory Motion Testing of the Scapulothoracic Joint   The patient is positioned in side lying. His or her head is sufficiently supported to maintain the cervical spine in neutral. The clinician stands in front of the patient. Using one hand the clinician grasps the inferior and medial border of the uppermost scapula. The other hand grasps the anterior aspect of the shoulder. The clinician gently brings both hands together, lifting the scapula (Figure 7-15). This position is held until the muscles are felt to relax. Once the muscle relaxation has occurred, the clinician moves the scapula diagonally into the proprioceptive neuromuscular facilitation (PNF) patterns for the scapula.

Special Tests of the Shoulder Complex

The special tests for the shoulder are provocative maneuvers designed to assess various structures or confirm a diagnosis (Table 7-24). Selection for their use is at the discretion of the clinician and is based on a complete patient history.

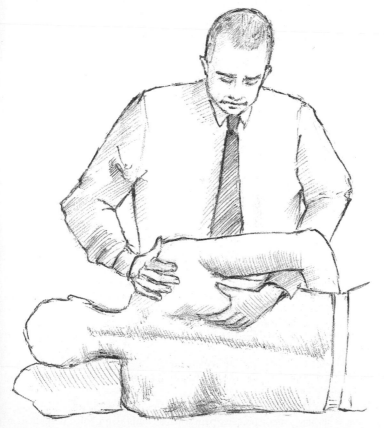

FIG. 7-15   Passive accessory motion testing of the scapulothoracic joint.

TABLE 7-24 Special Tests Used and the Significance of Their Positive Findings

Test	Maneuver	Diagnosis suggested by positive result
Apley scratch	Patient touches superior and inferior aspects of opposite scapula	Loss of range of motion: rotator cuff problem
Neer's sign	Arm in full flexion	Subacromial impingement
Hawkins-Kennedy	Forward flexion of the shoulder to 90° and internal rotation	Supraspinatus tendon impingement
Drop-arm	Arm lowered slowly to waist	Rotator cuff tear
Cross-arm	Forward elevation to 90° and active adduction	Acromioclavicular joint arthritis
Spurling's	Spine extended with head rotated to affected shoulder while axially loaded	Cervical nerve root disorder
Apprehension	Anterior pressure on the humerus with external rotation	Anterior glenohumeral instability
Relocation	Posterior force on humerus while externally rotating the arm	Anterior glenohumeral instability
Sulcus sign	Pulling downward on elbow or wrist	Inferior glenohumeral instability
Yergason	Elbow flexed to 90° with forearm pronated	Biceps tendon instability or tendinitis
Speed's maneuver	Elbow flexed 20°–30° and forearm supinated	Biceps tendon instability or tendinitis
"Clunk" sign	Rotation of loaded shoulder from extension to forward flexion	Labral disorder

Source: Woodward TW, Best TM: The painful shoulder: Part I. Clinical evaluation. Am Fam Phys 2000;61:3079–3088.

Rotator Cuff Integrity and Subacromial Impingement Tests

Impingement sign, commonly referred to as impingement syndrome, is a mechanical impingement of the rotator cuff between the coracoacromial arch and the humeral head (see *Orthopaedic Examination, Evaluation, and Intervention*, pp 427–430). Anything that decreases the volume of this space such as calcifications in the acromioclavicular ligament and anterior acromial spur formation can cause impingement. Hypertrophy of the acromioclavicular joint secondary to arthritis has also been implicated in the cause of impingement.

Arm positions that cause the humeral greater tuberosity to impinge against the inferior aspect of the acromion will reproduce pain in patients with impingement syndrome.

Subacromial Impingement Tests Patients with subacromial impingement syndrome usually perceive pain when a compressing force is applied on the greater tuberosity and rotator cuff region.[33] Pain may also be elicited with shoulder abduction in internal or external rotation.[33] These maneuvers constitute the basis of the Hawkins-Kennedy test and the Neer test.[34]

Neer Impingement Sign Test   While scapular rotation is prevented with one hand of the clinician, the arm of the patient is passively forced into elevation at an angle between flexion and abduction, by the clinician's other hand. Overpressure (in neutral, internal rotation, external rotation) is applied (Figure 7-16).

Hawkins-Kennedy Impingement Test[35]   The arm of the patient is passively flexed up to 90° in the plane of the scapula. The elbow is stabilized and the arm is forced into internal rotation (Figure 7-17).

Yocum Test   The patient lifts the elbow to shoulder height when resting the hand on the opposite shoulder (Figure 7-18).

Crossover Impingement/Horizontal Adduction Test   The patient's arm is positioned in 90° of glenohumeral flexion. The clinician passively moves the patient's arm into horizontal adduction, and applies over pressure (Figure 7-19). Although the crossover impingement/horizontal adduction test provokes compressing forces on rotator cuff tendons that are localized under the acromioclavicular joint (A-C joint), it is a test more likely to be used to investigate A-C joint dysfunction.[36–39]

Lock Test[40,41]   The Lock test is used to help differentiate the cause of symptoms when the patient complains of localized catching shoulder pain and pain or restricted movement when attempting to abduct the arm. Since

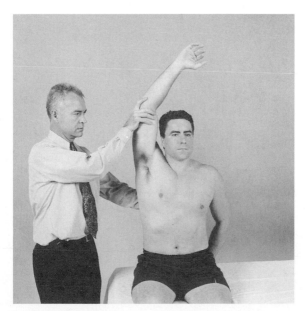

FIG. 7-16   Neer impingement test.

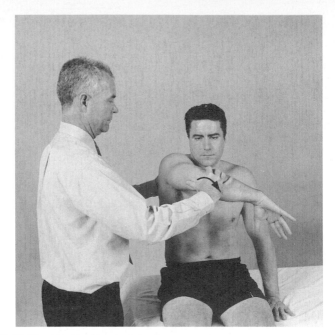

FIG. 7-17   Hawkins-Kennedy impingement test.

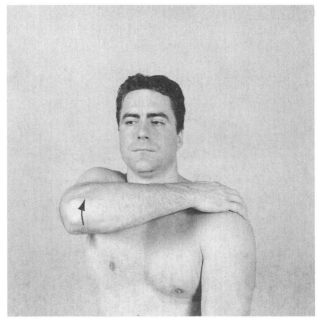

FIG. 7-18   Yocum test.

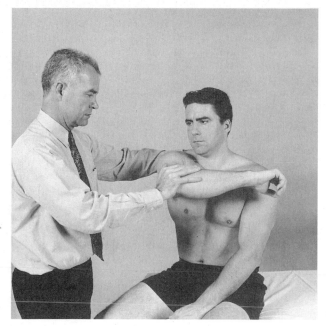

FIG. 7-19   Crossover impingement test.

the clinician controls the motion, this test can be a very sensitive test to help confirm the presence of an impingement of the supraspinatus tendon (Figure 7-20).

Positive findings for this test include reproduction of the patient's symptoms and a decrease in range of motion compared to uninvolved shoulder.

Dropping Sign*[42]   The "dropping sign" is performed with the patient in sitting or standing. The clinician places the patient's elbow in 90° of flexion with the arm by the side. The shoulder is externally rotated to 45° and the patient is then asked to externally rotate the shoulder against resistance. If the patient is unable to maintain the externally rotated position, the arm drops back to the neutral position of shoulder rotation. This is called the "dropping sign."

Rotator Cuff Rupture Tests

Drop Arm Test   The clinician passively raises the patient's arm to an overhead position. The patient is asked to lower his or her arm with the palm down. If at any point in the descent, the patient's arm drops, this is indicative of a full thickness tear.

Biceps and Superior Labral Tears   The long head of biceps tendon runs up the bicipital groove under the transverse ligament, through the shoulder joint, and attaches to the superior glenoid via the superior labrum. The biceps tendon and superior labrum can be involved in various pathologic processes including bicipital tendinitis, biceps rupture, biceps tendon subluxation or dislocation, and tears of the superior labrum.[43]

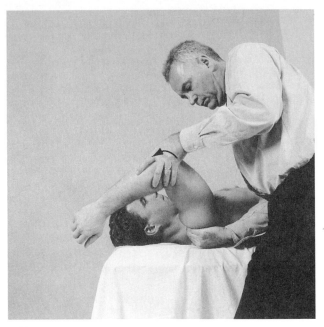

FIG. 7-20   Lock test.

Clunk Test   The Clunk test is the traditional test for diagnosing labral tears. The patient is positioned in supine. One hand of the clinician is placed on the posterior aspect of the shoulder over the humeral head, while the other hand grasps the humerus above the elbow. The clinician fully abducts the arm over the patient's head. Using the hand placed posterior to the humeral head, the clinician pushes anteriorly, while the other hand externally rotates the humerus. A clunk-like sensation may be felt if a free labral fragment is caught in the joint.[43]

Crank Test   The "crank test"[44] is performed with the patient positioned in supine. The patient's arm is elevated to 160° in the scapular plane of the body and is in maximal internal or external rotation. The clinician then applies an axial load along the humerus. A positive test is indicated by the reproduction of a painful click in the shoulder during the maneuver.

Speed's Test   The patient's arm is positioned in shoulder flexion, full external rotation, full elbow extension, and full forearm supination. The clinician applies manual resistance in a downward direction. The test is positive if localized pain at the bicipital groove is reproduced.

The Speed's test suggests a superior labral tear when resisted forward flexion of the shoulder causes bicipital groove pain.[4,45] The Speed's test is also used to detect bicipital tendinitis (see Yergason's test).[36,46]

Yergason's Test[47]   The patient's arm is positioned in 90° of elbow flexion. The patient is asked to supinate his or her forearm, and externally rotate the arm against the manual resistance of the clinician (Figure 7-21).

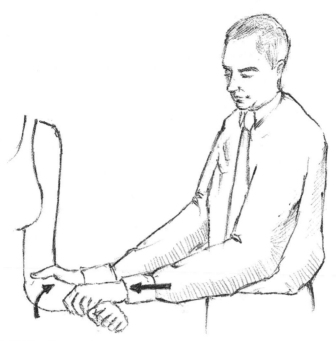

FIG. 7-21   Yergason's test.

O'Brien Test   The O'Brien test is a two-part active compression test. The test is performed with the patient's arm adducted 10° in the front of the chest with the shoulder flexed to 90° and fully internally rotated. In this position, the arm is flexed upward against the clinician's downward-directed force. The test is then repeated in the same manner except that the arm is positioned in maximum external rotation. Pain with this maneuver is typical in patients with superior labral tears.[4]

Biceps Load Test   The biceps load test was designed and has been tested on patients with recurrent anterior dislocations.[48] The test was performed on 75 patients (64 men, 11 women) with an age range of 16 to 41 years; the average age was about 25 years. The biceps load test demonstrated a sensitivity of 90.9%; a specificity of 96.9%; a positive predictive value of 83%; and a negative predictive value of 98%, with a kappa coefficient of 0.85.[48] It is important to remember that this subpopulation may respond differently than patients without a history of dislocation; therefore, extrapolation beyond this population is probably not recommended. The test is performed with the patient supine. The clinician sits on same side and abducts the shoulder to 90° while maintaining the forearm in a supinated position. The patient is allowed to relax, and an apprehension test is performed. When the patient becomes apprehensive with external rotation, the clinician stops externally rotating, and the patient is then asked to flex the elbow against the resistance of the clinician. The patient is asked if he or she feels any difference with the contraction. If the patient feels less apprehensive or more comfortable, the test is negative for a superior labrum tear. If the patient feels no change or the shoulder becomes more painful, the test is positive for a superior labrum tear. The authors recommend repeating the test if positive.[48]

The remaining tests are reserved for when the clinician needs to differentiate the structure causing the symptoms, when the provocation of symptoms during the examination has been minimal, or to rule out the possibility of instability.

Stability Testing

Instability patterns of the shoulder include anterior, posterior, inferior, and a combination of all three referred to as multidirectional instability. The most common direction of instability is anterior. The examination is used to assess possible directions of instability and to correlate these with apprehension and symptom reproduction. The clinician notes the amount of passive translation between the humeral head and the glenoid fossa and any reproduction of symptoms and apprehension when stressing the shoulder.[5] It is important to remember that there is no correlation between the amount of joint laxity/mobility and joint instability at the shoulder.[49] Joint stability is more likely a function of connective tissue support and an intact neuromuscular system.[50] A clicking or grinding detected with translation is a nonspecific sign that may suggest labral pathology, such as a Bankart or a superior labrum anterior to posterior (SLAP) lesion.[5] The stability tests can be performed with the patient seated or supine.

Glenohumeral—Load and Shift Test   The clinician's index finger is placed across the anterior G-H joint line and humeral head, and the long finger over the coracoid process. The clinician then applies a "load and shift" of the humeral head across the stabilized scapula in an anterior-medial direction to assess anterior stability and in a posterior-lateral direction to assess posterior instability. The normal motion anteriorly is half of the distance of the humeral head. Although attempts have been made to grade or quantify the degree of instability more specifically, the literature supports no consistency in the grading to date.[51–55]

Apprehension Test   The patient is positioned in supine with arm in 90° of abduction and full external rotation. The clinician holds the patient's wrist with one hand, while the other hand stabilizes the patient's elbow (Figure 7-22). The clinician applies over pressure into external rotation. Patient apprehension from this maneuver, rather than pain, is considered a positive test for anterior instability. Pain with this maneuver, but without apprehension, may indicate pathology other than instability, such as posterior impingement of the rotator cuff.

Sulcus Sign for Inferior Instability   The patient's arm is positioned in 20°–50° of abduction and neutral rotation.[56,57] An inferior traction force is applied to the shoulder. Excessive inferior translation of the humeral head with this maneuver is manifested by a dimpling of the overlying skin (sulcus sign), which is the result of a widening of the space between the acromion and humeral head. The sulcus sign can be observed as a depression greater than a finger width between the lateral acromion and the head of the humerus (Figure 7-23) when longitudinal traction is applied to the dependent arm in more than one position.[58]

The sulcus sign can be graded by measuring the distance from the inferior margin of the acromion to the humeral head. A distance of less than 1 cm is graded as 1+ sulcus, 1–2 cm as a 2+ sulcus, and greater than 2 cm as a grade 3+ sulcus.[59]

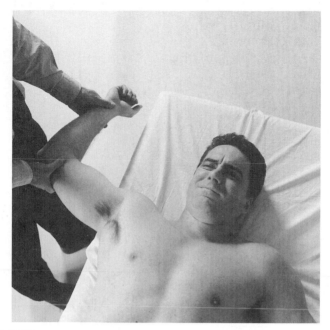

FIG. 7-22   Apprehension test.

Jobe Subluxation/Relocation Test   The clinician grasps the patient's forearm with one hand to maintain the testing position and grasps the humeral head with the other hand. The clinician gently applies an anterior push to the posterior aspect of the subluxed humeral head. Pain and apprehension from the patient indicate a positive test for a superior labral tear.[4] After pushing the humeral head anteriorly and demonstrating pain and apprehension, the clinician should then push the humeral head posteriorly while maintaining the shoulder in the same position (relocation part of the test). Reduction of pain and apprehension further substantiates the clinical finding of anterior instability and may indicate a positive test.

***Rockwood Test for Anterior Instability*[60]**   The patient is seated with the clinician standing behind. With the arm by the patient's side, the clinician passively externally rotates the shoulder. The patient then abducts the arm to approximately 45° and the test is repeated. The same maneuver is again repeated with the arm abducted to 90° and then 120°, in order to assess the different stabilizing structures. A positive test is indicated when apprehension is noted in the latter three positions (45°, 90°, and 120°).

***Anterior Release Test*[61]**   The anterior release test is performed with the patient in supine and his or her shoulder positioned in 90° of abduction and maximally externally rotated while a posteriorly directed force is applied to the proximal humerus. A positive test produces an increase or reproduction in the patient's symptoms on release of the posteriorly directed force on the humerus.

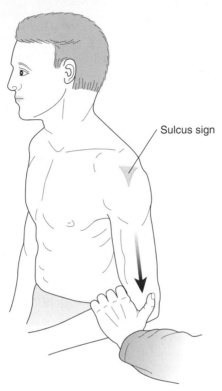

Sulcus sign

FIG. 7-23 Sulcus sign.

Spurling's Test In a patient with neck pain or pain that radiates below the elbow, a useful maneuver to further evaluate the cervical spine is Spurling's test. The patient's cervical spine is placed in extension and the head rotated toward the affected shoulder. An axial load is then placed on the spine (Figure 7-24). Reproduction of radicular type pain to the ipsilateral side is a positive test. This position closes down the neural foramina, and can compress the cervical nerve roots as they exit the foramen. With a herniated nucleus pulposus or foraminal stenosis, any decrease in foraminal space is likely to reproduce radicular type pain.

Reproduction of the patient's shoulder or arm pain with this maneuver warrants further evaluation of the bony and soft tissue structures of the cervical spine.

Neurologic Examination

If a scanning examination is not performed, a thorough sensory examination of all upper extremity dermatomes and the deep tendon reflexes of all extremities should be assessed in those situations where the patient is complaining of neck or arm pain or both, and also when the clinician has been unable to reproduce the symptoms with the shoulder examination.[7] A small number of patients, particularly athletes, have an entirely normal physical examination, but continue to complain of pain. In such cases the clinician should look for training errors in

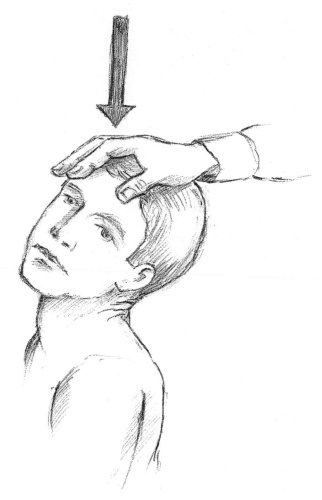

FIG. 7-24   Spurling's test.

the athlete's program or chronic overuse injury. Alternatively, pain may be a normal adaptation to increasing loads placed on the shoulder as it accommodates new demands. It should be stressed that repeated physical examinations over time, particularly with highly competitive athletes, are needed to evaluate changing pain patterns, which may highlight the real diagnostic culprit.

Vascular Examination

A thorough vascular examination is critical in trauma cases and is important in patients complaining of vague aching, heaviness, or fatigue radiating down the arm.[5] The vascular status of the upper extremity can be assessed by palpation of the distal arteries with the arm in various positions.[7] These tests can include those for thoracic outlet syndrome (see *Orthopaedic Examination, Evaluation, and Intervention*, pp 1066–1068). In addition, an inspection of the skin color, temperature, hair growth, and alteration in sensation should routinely be assessed.[5]

Diagnostic Studies

An A-P view (anterior-posterior view with the humerus in internal rotation and a second anterior-posterior view with the humerus in external rotation) of the G-H joint may show calcific tendinitis of the cuff and superior migration of the humeral head, which should prompt further imaging studies if the clinician suspects a rotator cuff tear. However, the conclusions on the radiology reports concerning single plane views should be treated with caution as they have been well documented to result in misdiagnosis.[62]

The "scapular-Y" view, obtained by tilting the x-ray beam approximately 60° relative to the A-P view, provides good visualization of the glenohumeral alignment.[63]

Arthrography aids in the diagnosis of full thickness rotator cuff tears (Table 7-25).[64] Bone scans are rarely used in the diagnosis of shoulder pain, but a computed tomographic (CT) scan report can be useful in confirming the clinical findings in some cases (Table 7-25).[4] The MRI is very reliable in

Table 7-25 Imaging Studies of the Shoulder

Imaging modality	Advantages	Disadvantages
MRI	Ninety-five percent sensitivity and specificity in detecting complete rotator cuff tears, cuff degeneration, chronic tendinitis, and partial cuff tears No ionizing radiation	Often identifies an apparent "abnormality" in an asymptomatic patient
Arthrography	Good at identifying complete rotator cuff tear or adhesive capsulitis (frozen shoulder)	Invasive Relatively poor at diagnosing a partial rotator cuff tear
Ultrasonography	Accurately diagnoses complete rotator cuff tears	Less useful in identifying partial cuff tears Operator-dependent interpretation
MRI arthrography	Reliably identifies full-thickness rotator cuff tears and labral tears	Invasive
CT scanning	May be useful in diagnosis of subtle dislocation	Ionizing radiation

MRI = magnetic resonance imaging; CT = computed tomographic.
Source: Woodward TW, Best TM: The painful shoulder: Part II. Acute and chronic disorders. Am Fam Phys 2000;61:3291–3300.

TABLE 7-26 Differential Diagnosis for Common Causes of Shoulder Pain

Condition	Approximate patient age	Mechanism of injury	Area of symptoms	Symptoms aggravated by	Observation	AROM	PROM	End-feel	Pain with resisted	Tenderness with palpation
Rotator cuff tendinitis										
Acute	20–40	Microtrauma/macrotrauma	Anterior and lateral shoulder	Overhead motions	Swelling—anterior shoulder	Limited abduction	Limited abduction	—	Abduction ER	Pain below anterior acromial rim
Chronic	30–70	Microtrauma/macrotrauma	Anterior and lateral shoulder	Overhead motions	Atrophy of scapular area Atrophy of shoulder area	Limited abduction and flexion	Pain on IR and ER at 90° abduction	—	Abduction ER IR	Anterior shoulder Pain below anterior acromial rim
Bicipital tendinitis	20–45	Microtrauma	Anterior shoulder	Overhead motions	Swelling—anterior shoulder	Limited ER when arm in 90° abduction Pain on full flexion from full extension	Pain on combined extension of shoulder and elbow	—	Elbow flexion	Over bicipital groove
Rotator cuff rupture	40+	Macrotrauma	Posterior/superior shoulder	Arm elevation	Atrophy of scapular area	Limited abduction	Full and pain free	—	Abduction ER	Pain below anterolateral acromial rim
Adhesive capsulitis	35–70	Microtrauma/macrotrauma	Shoulder and upper arm—poorly localized	All motions	Atrophy of shoulder area	Pain with or without restriction All motions limited especially ER and abduction	All motions limited especially ER and abd	Capsular	Most/all	Varies

(Continued)

195

TABLE 7-26 Differential Diagnosis for Common Causes of Shoulder Pain (Continued)

Condition	Approximate patient age	Mechanism of injury	Area of symptoms	Symptoms aggravated by	Observation	AROM	PROM	End-feel	Pain with Resisted	Tenderness with Palpation
A-C joint sprain	Varies	Macrotrauma	Point of shoulder	Horizontal adduction	Step/bump at point of shoulder	Limited abduction Limited horizontal adduction	Limited abduction Pain with horizontal adduction Pain on IR at 90° abduction	—	ER Flexion	Point of shoulder Soft tissue thickening at point of shoulder
Subacromial bursitis	Varies	Microtrauma	Anterior and lateral shoulder	Overhead motions	Often unremarkable	Limited abduction and IR May have full range but pain in mid-range of flexion/abd	Pain only in mid-range abduction and flexion	—	Most/all	Pain below anterolateral acromial rim
Chronic Instability	20–40	Microtrauma	Anterior and lateral shoulder, and upper arm	Extremes of motion	Often unremarkable	Full and pain free	Full and pain free	Excessive joint play	Weakness rather than pain	Poorly localized
Glenohumeral arthritis	50+	Gradual onset, but can be traumatic	Poorly localized	Arm activity	Possible posterior positioning of humeral head	Capsular pattern (ER > abduction > IR)	Pain	Capsular	Weakness of rotator cuff, rather than pain	Poorly localized

Condition	Age	Onset	Pain location	Aggravating	Inspection/Position	ROM		Strength/Neuro	Palpation
"SICK" (scapula, medial border prominence and scapular dyskinesis) scapula	20–40	Microtrauma	Anterior/superior shoulder Posterosuperior scapular Arm, forearm, hand	Overhead activities	Scapular malposition Inferior medial border prominence Dyskinesia of scapular movement	Decreased forward flexion, which diminishes when clinician manually repositions the scapula into retraction and posterior tilt	Normal	—	Weakness rather than pain
Cervical radiculopathy	Varies	Typically none but can be traumatic	Upper back, below shoulder	Cervical extension, cervical side bending and rotation to ipsilateral side, full arm elevation	May have lateral deviation of head away from painful side	Decreased cervical flexion, cervical side bending and rotation to ipsilateral side. Decreased arm elevation on involved side	Painful into restricted active range of motions Positive Spurling's test	Empty	Weakness rather than pain Other neurologic changes

Medial coracoid Superomedial angle of scapula

Varies. May have numbness over dermatomal area

detecting lesions of the capsule, and labrum, as well as associated rotator cuff tears (Table 7-25). It can generally indicate the approximate size of a rotator cuff tear and may also indicate whether the critically important subscapularis tendon is torn.[4,65,66]

EXAMINATION CONCLUSIONS—THE EVALUATION

Following the examination, and once the clinical findings have been recorded, the clinician must determine a specific diagnosis or a working hypothesis, based on a summary of all the findings. This diagnosis can be structure related (medical diagnosis) (Table 7-26), or a diagnosis based on the preferred practice patterns as described in the *Guide to Physical Therapist Practice* (see *Orthopaedic Examination, Evaluation, and Intervention*, pp 196–205).[67]

REFERENCES

1. Aufranc OE, Barr JS, Rowe CR: The upper extremity. In AAOC Instructional Course Lectures, 1957. St Louis, MO, Mosby, p. 72–79.
2. Jobe FW, Pink M: Classification and treatment of shoulder dysfunction in the overhead athlete. J Orthop Sports Phys Ther 1993;18:427–431.
3. Woodward TW, Best TM: The painful shoulder: Part I. Clinical evaluation. Am Fam Phys 2000;61:3079–3088.
4. Burkhart SS: A 26-year-old woman with shoulder pain. JAMA 2000;284 (12):1559–1567.
5. Boublik M, Hawkins RJ: Clinical examination of the shoulder complex. J Orthop Sports Phys Ther 1993;18:379–385.
6. Hawkins RJ, Bokor DJ: Clinical evaluation of shoulder problems. In Rockwood CA, Matsen FA (eds): The Shoulder. Philadelphia, PA, WB Saunders, 1990.
7. Yocum LA: Assessing the shoulder. History, physical examination, differential diagnosis, and special tests used. Clin Sports Med 1983;2:281–289.
8. Spindler K, Dovan T, McCarty E: Clinical cornerstone. Excerpta Med 2001;3:26–37.
9. Cappel K, et al.: Clinical examination of the shoulder. In Tovin BJ, Greenfield B (eds): Evaluation and Treatment of the Shoulder—an Integration of the Guide to Physical Therapist Practice, pp 75–131. Philadelphia, PA, FA Davis, 2001.
10. Davies GJ, DeCarlo MS: Examination of the shoulder complex. In Bandy WD (ed): Current Concepts in the Rehabilitation of the Shoulder. Sports Physical Therapy Section—Home Study Course. LaCrosse, WI, Sports Physical Therapy Section, APTA, 1995.
11. Minter WW: A shoulder hand syndrome in coronary disease. J Med Assoc GA 1967;56:45–49.
12. Silliman FJ, Hawkins RJ: Clinical examination of the shoulder complex. In Andrews JR, Wilk KE, (eds): The Athlete's Shoulder. New York, Churchill Livingstone, 1994.
13. Sahrmann SA: Movement impairment syndromes of the shoulder girdle. In Sahrmann SA (ed): Movement Impairment Syndromes, pp 193–261. St Louis, MO, Mosby, 2001.
14. Mattingly GE, Mackarey PJ: Optimal methods for shoulder tendon palpation: a cadaver study. Phys Ther 1996;76:166–174.
15. Cyriax J: Textbook of Orthopaedic Medicine, Diagnosis of Soft Tissue Lesions, 8th ed. London, Bailliere Tindall, 1982.
16. Davies GJ, Dickhoff-Hoffman S: Neuromuscular testing and rehabilitation of the shoulder complex. J Orthop Sports Phys Ther 1993;18:449–458.
17. Kessel L, Watson M: The painful arc syndrome: Clinical classification as a guide to management. J Bone Joint Surg Br 1977;59:166–172.
18. Warner JJ, Navarro RA: Serratus anterior dysfunction. Recognition and treatment. Clin Orthop 1998;349:139–148.

19. Daigneault J, Cooney LM Jr: Shoulder pain in older people. J Am Geriatr Soc 1998;46(9):1144–1151.
20. Codman EA: The Shoulder, Rupture of the Supraspinatus Tendon and Other Lesions in or About the Subacromial Bursa. Boston, MA, Thomas Todd, 1934.
21. Post M, Mayer J: Suprascapular nerve entrapment: Diagnosis and treatment. Clin Orthop 1987;223:126–130.
22. Cohen RB, Williams GR Jr: Impingement syndrome and rotator cuff disease as repetitive motion disorders. Clin Ortho Related Res 1998;351:95–101.
23. Cuomo F: Diagnosis, classification, and management of the stiff shoulder. In Iannotti JP, Williams GR (eds): Disorders of the Shoulder: Diagnosis and Management, pp 397–417. Philadelphia, PA, Williams & Wilkins, 1999.
24. Kamkar A, Irrgang JJ, Whitney S: Non-operative management of secondary shoulder impingement syndrome. J Orthop Sports Phys Ther 1993;17(5):212–224.
25. Kuhn JE, Plancher KD, Hawkins RJ: Scapular winging. J Am Acad Orthop Surg 1995;3:319–325.
26. Paine RM, Voight M: The role of the scapula. J Orthop Sports Phys Ther 1993;18:386–391.
27. Dunleavy K: Relationship between the shoulder and the cervicothoracic spine. Independent Home Study Course: Solutions to shoulder disorders, pp 1–25. La Crosse, WI, Orthopedic Section, APTA, 2001.
28. Gerber C, Krushell RJ: Isolated rupture of the tendon of the subscapularis muscle: Clinical features in 16 cases. J Bone Joint Surg 1991;73B:389–394.
29. Babyar SR: Excessive scapular motion in individuals recovering from painful and stiff shoulders: causes and treatment strategies. Phys Ther 1996;76:226–247.
30. Miniaci A, Salonen D: Rotator cuff evaluation: imaging and diagnosis. Orthop Clin North America 1997;28:43–58.
31. Safee-Rad R, et al.: Normal functional range of motion of upper limb joints during performance of three feeding activities. Arch Phys Med Rehab 1990;71:505–509.
32. Pearl ML, et al.: A system for describing positions of the humerus relative to the thorax and its use in the presentation of several functionally important arm positions. J Shoulder Elbow Surg 1992;1:113–118.
33. Calis M, et al.: Diagnostic values of clinical diagnostic tests in subacromial impingement syndrome. Ann Rheum Dis 2000;59(1):44–47.
34. Frieman BG, Albert TJ, Fenlin JM: Rotator cuff disease: a review of diagnosis, pathophysiology and current trends in treatment. Arch Phys Med Rehabil 1994;75:604–609.
35. Hawkins RJ, Kennedy JC: Impingement syndrome in athletics. Am J Sports Med 1980;8:151–163.
36. Hermann B, Rose DW: Stellenwert von Anamnese und klinischer Untersuchung beim degenerativen Impingement Syndrom im Vergleich zu operativen Befunden-eine prospektive Studie. Z Orthop Ihre Grenzgeb 1996;134:166–170.
37. Warren RF: Shoulder pain. In Paget S, Pellicci P, Beary JF (eds): Manual of Rheumatology and Outpatient Orthopaedic Disorders, pp 99–109. Boston, MA, Little, Brown, 1993.
38. Akgün K: Kronik subakromiyal sikisma sendromunun konservatif tedavisinde ultrasonun etkinligi. Istanbul, University of Istanbul, 1993. Proficiency Thesis.
39. Akgün K et al.: Subakromiyal sikisma sendromu klinik tanisinda sikisma (Neer) testinin înemi. Fizik Tedavi ve Rehabilitasyon Dergisi 1997;22:5–7.
40. Maitland G: Peripheral Manipulation, 3rd ed. London, Butterworth, 1991.
41. Mullen F: Locking and quadrant of the shoulder: Relationships of the humerus and scapula during locking and quadrant. In Proceedings of the Sixth Biennial Conference, Manipulative Therapist Association of Australia. Adelaide, Australia, 1989.
42. Neer CS: Anatomy of shoulder reconstruction. In Neer CS (ed): Shoulder Reconstruction, pp 1–39. Philadelphia, PA, WB Saunders, 1990.
43. Clarnette RG, Miniaci A: Clinical exam of the shoulder. Med Sci Sports Exerc 1998;30(4 Suppl):1–6.
44. Liu SH, Henry MH, Nuccion SL: A prospective evaluation of a new physical examination in predicting glenoid labral tears. Am J Sports Med 1996;24:721–725.

45. Field LD, Savoie FH: Arthroscopic suture repair of superior labral detachment lesions of the shoulder. Am J Sports Med 1993;21:783–791.
46. Magee DJ: Shoulder. In Orthopedic Physical Assessment, pp 90–142. Philadelphia, PA, WB Saunders, 1992.
47. Yergason RM: Rupture of biceps. J Bone Joint Surg 1931;13:160.
48. Kim SH, Ha KI, Han KY: Biceps load test: a clinical test for superior labrum anterior and posterior lesions (SLAP) in shoulders with recurrent anterior dislocations. Am J Sports Med 1999;27:300–303.
49. Engebretsen L, Craig EV: Radiographic features of shoulder instability. Clin Orthop 1993;291:29–44.
50. Jenkins WL: Relationship of overuse impingement with subtle hypomobility or hypermobility. Home Study Course—Solutions to Shoulder Disorders. La Crosse, WI, Orthopaedic Section, APTA, 2001.
51. Bigliani LU: The Unstable Shoulder. Rosemont, IL, AAOS, 1995.
52. Gerber C, Ganz R: Clinical assessment of instability of the shoulder. J Bone Joint Surg 1984;66B:551.
53. Glousman R, Jobe FW, Tibone JE: Dynamic EMG analysis of the throwing shoulder with glenohumeral instability. J Bone Joint Surg 1988;70:220–226.
54. Hawkins RJ, et al.: Translation of the glenohumeral joint with the patient under anesthesia. J Shoulder Elbow Surg 1996;5:286–292.
55. Hanyman DT, et al.: Translation of the humeral head on the glenoid with passive glenohumeral motion. J Bone Joint Surg 1990;72A:1334.
56. Pagnani MJ, Galinat BJ, Warren RF: Glenohumeral instability. In DeLee JC, Drez D (eds): Orthopaedic Sports Medicine: Principles and Practice. Philadelphia, PA, WB Saunders, 1993.
57. Callanan M, et al.: Shoulder instability. Diagnosis and management. Aust Fam Physician 2001;30:655–661.
58. Jobe FW, Bradley JP: The diagnosis and nonoperative treatment of shoulder injuries in athletes. Clin Sports Med 1989;8:419–439.
59. Neer CSI, Foster CR: Inferior capsular shift for involuntary inferior and multidirectional instability of the shoulder. J Bone Joint Surg 1980;62A:897–908.
60. Rockwood CA: Subluxations and dislocations about the shoulder. In Rockwood CA, Green DP (ed): Fractures in Adults—I. Philadelphia, PA, JB Lippincott, 1984.
61. Gross ML, Distefano MC: Anterior release test: a new test for occult shoulder instability. Clin Orth Rel Res 1997;339:105–108.
62. Rockwood CA Jr, et al.: X-ray evaluation of shoulder problems. In Rockwood CA Jr, Matsen FA III, (eds): The Shoulder, pp 178–207. Philadelphia, PA, WB Saunders, 1990.
63. Rubin SA, Gray RL, Green WR: The scapular "Y" view: a diagnostic aid in shoulder trauma. A technical note. Radiology 1974;110:725–726.
64. Swen WA, et al.: Is sonography performed by the rheumatologist as useful as arthrography executed by the radiologist for the assessment of full thickness rotator cuff tears? J Rheum 1998;25:1800–1806.
65. Kneeland JB: Magnetic resonance imaging: General principles and techniques. In Iannotti JP, Williams GR (eds): Disorders of the Shoulder: Diagnosis and Management, pp 911–925. Philadelphia, PA, Williams & Wilkins, 1999.
66. Tirman PF, et al.: Association of glenoid labral cysts with labral tears and glenohumeral instability: radiologic findings and clinical significance. Radiology 1994;190:653–658.
67. Guide to physical therapist practice. Phys Ther 2001;81:S13–S95.

8 | The Elbow and Forearm

OVERVIEW

The elbow serves as the central link in the kinetic chain of the upper extremity. The examination of elbow pain can be challenging because of the complexity of the joint and its location. This location provides a myriad of potential causes for elbow symptoms and requires a thorough appreciation of the anatomy and biomechanics of the elbow to diagnose the cause of these symptoms correctly (see *Orthopaedic Examination, Evaluation, and Intervention*, pp 520–532).

The movements of the elbow complex, produced by muscle action (Table 8-1), include flexion and extension of the elbow, and pronation and supination of the forearm. Stability of the elbow complex during these movements is provided by the osseous relationships, the joint capsule, and by medial and lateral ligament complexes (Table 8-2).

The elbow has complex innervation (Tables 8-1, 8-3). All of the major peripheral nerves that cross the elbow are subject to entrapment (see *Orthopaedic Examination, Evaluation, and Intervention*, pp 557–562). The median nerve crosses the elbow medially and passes through the two heads of the pronator teres, which is a potential site of entrapment. The ulnar nerve passes along the medial arm and posterior to the medial epicondyle through the cubital tunnel, a likely site of compression. The radial nerve descends the arm laterally. It divides into the superficial (sensory) branch and the deep (motor or posterior interosseous) branch. The deep branch must then pass through the arcade of Fröhse, a fibrous arch formed by the proximal margin of the superficial head of the supinator muscle, where it is most susceptible to injury.

EXAMINATION

With a sound knowledge of elbow and forearm anatomy and differential diagnosis, coupled with good history taking, most elbow conditions can be identified (see *Orthopaedic Examination, Evaluation, and Intervention*, pp 532–544).

History

The initial aspect of the examination is the history. The nature of the complaint together with its chronicity is essential in forming a working hypothesis and guiding the physical examination.[1] Hand dominance and alleviating or aggravating factors are also important to establish.

During the history, the clinician must determine the chief complaint and whether there is a specific mechanism of injury. If the injury is traumatic in origin, a mechanism should be determined. One of the most common traumatic injuries to the elbow is the FOOSH (Fall On the Out Stretched Hand) (Table 8-4). In addition to information regarding a specific mechanism, the clinician should seek information about recreational and occupational activities involving a repetitive load that could initiate a cycle of microtrauma, chronic inflammation, tissue degeneration, necrosis, and ultimately tendon rupture (Table 8-5).[2]

TABLE 8-1 Muscles of the Elbow and Forearm: Their Actions, Nerve Supply, and Nerve Root Derivation

Action	Muscles acting	Nerve supply	Nerve root deviation
Elbow flexion	1. Brachialis	Musculocutaneous	C5-6, (C7)
	2. Biceps brachii	Musculocutaneous	C5-6
	3. Brachioradialis	Radial	C5-6, (C7)
	4. Pronator teres	Median	C6-7
	5. Flexor carpi ulnaris	Ulnar	C7-8
Elbow extension	1. Triceps	Radial	C7–8
	2. Anconeus	Radial	C7-8, (T1)
Forearm supination	1. Supinator	Posterior inter-osseous (radial)	C5-6
	2. Biceps brachii	Musculocutaneous	C5-6
Forearm pronation	1. Pronator quadratus	Anterior inter-osseous (median)	C8, T1
	2. Pronator teres	Median	C6-7
	3. Flexor carpi radialis	Median	C6-7
Wrist extension	1. Extensor carpi radialis longus	Radial	C6-7
	2. Extensor carpi radialis brevis	Posterior inter-osseous (radial)	C7-8
	3. Extensor carpi ulnaris	Posterior inter-osseous (radial)	C7-8
Wrist flexion	1. Flexor carpi radialis	Median	C6-7
	2. Flexor carpi ulnaris	Ulnar	C7-8

Source: Magee DJ (ed): Orthopedic physical assessment. Philadelphia, PA, WB Saunders, 2002.

Pain is the most common presenting symptom, but may not be the only one. It is important to determine the type and location of all the symptoms (Table 8-6, Figure 8-1) as this may assist in the diagnosis:[2]

- *Anterior elbow pain.* Anterior elbow pain with a history of repetitive elbow flexion and forearm supination may indicate the presence of biceps tendinosis. Further confirmation may be provided if resisted elbow flexion and forearm supination increases the symptoms. If the anterior elbow pain is associated with distal paresthesias, pronator syndrome (anterior interosseous branch of the median) should be suspected, especially if resisted forearm pronation increases the symptoms. Further confirmation may be provided if there is weakness of the index and middle flexor digitorum profundus (FDP), the flexor pollicis longus (FPL), and the pronator quadratus. Reports of repetitive hyperextension should lead the clinician to suspect an anterior capsular strain, torn brachialis with associated myositis.
- *Posterior elbow pain.* Posterior elbow pain with a history of repetitive elbow extension may indicate triceps tendinosis. Further confirmation may be provided if there is tenderness of the triceps tendon just superior to its attachment on the olecranon. Posterior elbow pain associated with clicking or locking of the elbow with terminal extension is suggestive of olecranon

TABLE 8-2 Articular and Ligamentous Contributions to Elbow Stability

Stabilization	Elbow extended	Elbow flexed 90°
Valgus stability	Anterior capsule UCL and bony articular (proximal half of sigmoid notch) *equally divided*	UCL (ulnar [medial] collateral ligament) proves 55% 0% anterior capsule and bony articulation (proximal half of sigmoid notch)
Varus stability	Anterior capsule (32%) Joint articulation (55%) RCL (radial [lateral] collateral ligament) (14%)	Joint articulation (75%) Anterior capsule (13%) RCL (9%)
Anterior displacement	Anterior oblique ligament Anterior joint capsule Trochlea-olecranon articulation (minimal)	
Posterior displacement	Anterior capsule Radial head against the capitellum Coracoid against the trochlea	
Distraction	Anterior capsule (85%) RCL (5%) UCL (5%) Triceps, biceps, brachialis, brachioradialis, and forearm muscles	RCL (10%) UCL (78%) Capsule (8%)

Source: Sobel J, Nirschl RP: Elbow injuries. In Zachazewski JE, Magee DJ, Quillen WS (eds): Athletic Injuries and Rehabilitation, pp 543–583. Philadelphia, PA, WB Saunders, 1996.

impingement or an olecranon stress fracture. This latter condition is often associated with increased pain on resisted elbow extension. Olecranon bursitis is another cause of posterior elbow pain. This condition is often associated with a localized swelling and tenderness over the posterior aspect of the elbow.

- *Lateral elbow and forearm pain.* The most common cause of lateral elbow pain is lateral epicondylitis (tennis elbow), a degenerative tendinosis of the extensor carpi radialis brevis muscle. Typically, this condition worsens with grasping activities and resisted wrist extension. Compression of the deep branch of the radial nerve as it passes through the radial tunnel is a less common cause of lateral elbow and forearm pain. This condition tends to worsen with activities involving repetitive pronation and supination. Lateral elbow pain associated with a history of a repetitive valgus loading and compression of the elbow may indicate radiocapitellar chondromalacia. The typical presenting symptoms are catching, locking, and lateral elbow pain with active use of the elbow. Swelling and localized tenderness are noted at the affected site. An axial load applied with passive supination and pronation often provokes pain and can be helpful in differentiating radiocapitellar chondromalacia from lateral tennis elbow.

TABLE 8-3 Nerve Innervation of the Elbow Complex and Injury Consequences

Nerve	Motor loss	Sensory loss	Functional loss
Median nerve (C6-8, T1)	Pronator teres Flexor carpi radialis Palmaris longus Flexor digitorum superficialis Flexor pollicis longus Lateral half of flexor digitorum profundus Pronator quadratus Thenar eminence Lateral two lumbricals	Palmar aspect of hand with thumb, index, middle, and lateral half of ring finger Dorsal aspect of distal third of index, middle, and lateral half of ring finger	Pronation weakness Wrist flexion and abduction weakness Loss of radial deviation at wrist Inability to oppose or flex thumb Thumb abduction weakness Weak grip Weak or no pinch (ape hand deformity)
Anterior interosseous nerve (branch of median nerve)	Flexor pollicis longus Lateral half of flexor digitorum profundus Pronator quadratus Thenar eminence muscles Lateral two lumbricals	None	Pronation weakness especially at 90° elbow flexion Weakness of opposition and thumb flexion Weak finger flexion Weak pinch (no tip-to-tip) Weak wrist flexion
Ulnar nerve (C7-8, T1)	Flexor carpi ulnaris Medial half of flexor digitorum profundus Palmaris brevis Hypothenar eminence Adductor pollicis Medial two lumbricals All interossei	Dorsal and palmar aspect of little and medial half of ring finger	Loss of ulnar deviation at wrist Loss of distal flexion of little finger Loss of abduction and adduction of fingers Inability to extend second and third phalanges of little and ring fingers (benediction hand deformity) Loss of thumb adduction

Redial nerve (C5-8, T1)	Anconeus Brachioradialis Extensor carpi radialis longus and brevis Extensor digitorum Extensor pollicis longus and brevis Abductor pollicis longus Extensor carpi ulnaris Extensor indices Extensor digiti minimi	Dorsum of hand (lateral two-thirds) Dorsum and lateral aspect of thumb Proximal two-thirds of dorsum of index, middle, and half of ring finger	Loss of supination Loss of wrist extension (wrist drop) Inability to grasp Inability to stabilize wrist Loss of finger extension Inability to abduct thumb
Posterior interosseous nerve (branch of ulnar nerve)	Extensor carpi radialis brevis Extensor digitorum Extensor pollicis longus and brevis Abductor pollicis longus Extensor carpi ulnaris Extensor indices Extensor digiti minimi	None	Weak wrist extension Weak finger extension Difficulty stabilizing wrist Difficulty with grasp Inability to abduct thumb

Source: Magee DJ (ed): Orthopedic physical assessment. Philadelphia, PA, WB Saunders, 2002.

TABLE 8-4 FOOSH Injury History

Description	Possible injury
Fell forward and landed on outstretched hand	Distal radial fracture
Fell forward on hand, and sprained wrist	Scaphoid fracture
Landed on hand with arm outstretched behind	Distal humerus fracture
Landed on outstretched hand with elbow locked	Supracondylar fracture

Source: Dent S: Befuddled by a FOOSH? FR Report 2000;6:9.

TABLE 8-5 Activities Commonly Associated with Overuse Elbow Injuries

Activity	Injuries
Bowling	Biceps tendinosis, radial tunnel syndrome
Boxing	Triceps tendinosis
Friction in football, wrestling, or basketball	Olecranon bursitis
Golf	Golfer's elbow (trailing arm), radial tunnel syndrome
Gymnastics	Biceps tendinosis, triceps tendinosis
Posterior dislocation	Posterolateral rotatory instability
Racquet sports	Pronator syndrome, triceps tendinosis, olecranon stress fracture, lateral tennis elbow, radial tunnel syndrome, golfer's elbow, ulnar nerve entrapment
Rowing	Radial tunnel syndrome
Skiing	Ulnar nerve entrapment
Swimming	Radial tunnel syndrome
Throwing	Pronator syndrome, triceps tendinosis, olecranon impingement, olecranon stress fracture, radio-capitellar chondromalacia, ulnar collateral ligament sprain, golfer's elbow, ulnar nerve entrapment
Weight lifting	Biceps tendinosis, triceps tendinosis, anterior capsule strain, radial tunnel syndrome, ulnar nerve entrapment

Source: Chumbley EM, O'Connor FG, Nirschl RP: Evaluation of overuse elbow injuries. Am Fam Phys 2000;61:691–700.

TABLE 8-6 The Location of Elbow Pain and Possible Causes

Anterior elbow	Posterior elbow	Lateral elbow	Medial elbow
Biceps tendinosis	Triceps tendinosis	Lateral epicondylitis (tennis elbow)	Medial epicondylitis (golfer's elbow)
Pronator syndrome	Olecranon impingement	Radial tunnel syndrome	Ulnar collateral ligament sprain
Anterior capsule strain	Olecranon stress fracture	Radiocapitellar chondromalacia	Ulnar nerve entrapment
	Olecranon bursitis	Posterolateral rotatory instability	

Source: Chumbley EM, O'Connor FG, Nirschl RP: Evaluation of overuse elbow injuries. Am Fam Phys 2000;61:691–700.

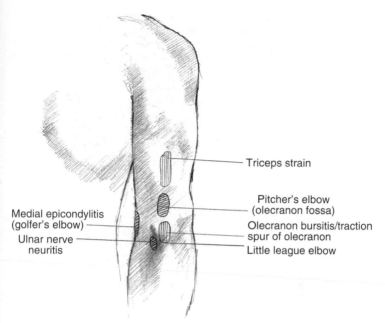

FIG. 8-1 Pain locations on the posterior elbow and their possible causes.

- *Medial elbow pain.* The most common causes of medial elbow pain include medial epicondylitis (golfer's elbow), a tendinosis of the elbow flexor/forearm pronator group, ulnar collateral ligament sprain, and ulnar nerve entrapment. Medial epicondylitis is associated with complaints with activities that require rapid wrist flexion and forearm pronation. An ulnar collateral ligament sprain is characterized by an insidious onset of medial elbow pain that becomes worse with activity. The presenting symptom of ulnar nerve entrapment is medial elbow pain accompanied with distal paresthesias along the ulnar aspect of the forearm and hand and weakness of the grip.

  The severity, duration, timing, and nature of the pain (intermittent or constant) should be ascertained:

- *Severity.* The severity of symptoms can be judged by whether they occur only after activity (chronic), with activity (subacute), or at rest (acute).
- *Duration.* Symptoms that have been present for weeks or months point to overuse, once the more insidious reasons for prolonged pain are ruled out. Information about the patient's occupational and recreational activities can help differentiate (see Table 8-5). It is important to identify the specific musculotendinous structures that are at risk for overuse or have been injured through overuse.
- *Timing.* The timing of the onset of symptoms can often be helpful in identifying the offending activity and thus the tissues at risk for overuse.

- *Nature.* Mechanical symptoms, such as clicking with motion, locking in extension and, catching are indicative of intra-articular pathology. Sharply localized pain is often a result of extra-articular pathology, such as tennis elbow.[3] Pain arising from the elbow itself is frequently of a "deep" nature and can extend into the extensor compartment.[3] Referred pain is more often diffuse.

In addition to pain, reported decreases in function can be caused by weakness or stiffness. It is particularly important to identify symptoms that are the result of neurologic compromise. This can be determined using questions about neck pain and previous neck injury, and questions that attempt to establish a relationship between head and neck movements and symptom reproduction. Symptoms that originate from the neck and radiate below the elbow are suggestive of a cervical spine disorder.[4] Weakness or paresthesias can also be clues to peripheral nerve entrapment syndromes (see Table 8-3). It is worth remembering that the reported loss of function may only occur with vigorous activity, either at work or during sports and may therefore be difficult to reproduce.[1]

Finally, adaptations to dysfunction should be noted because disability can be compensated for by enlisting the other extremity or by increasing motion at adjacent joints.[1]

Systems Review

The clinician should be able to determine the suitability of the patient for physical therapy. Co-existing medical problems, medications, and prior medical and surgical histories should be noted. If the clinician is concerned with any signs or symptoms of a visceral, vascular, psychogenic, spondylogenic, or systemic disorder that is out of the scope of physical therapy, the patient should be referred to an appropriate health care provider (see *Orthopaedic Examination, Evaluation, and Intervention*, p 534). Given its location, a thorough investigation of elbow pain requires ruling out referred symptoms from the neck, shoulder, wrist, and hand. Neurogenic pain usually responds well to physical therapy.

Tests and Measures

A systematic examination of the elbow includes observation, palpation, range of motion testing, neurologic assessment, the use of pertinent special tests, and the assessment of related areas[2] (see *Orthopaedic Examination, Evaluation, and Intervention*, pp 532–544). These related areas include, but are not limited to, the neck, the shoulder and the wrist.

Observation

At the elbow joint complex, observation and inspection are extremely important, as much of the structures are subcutaneous. For an accurate and thorough examination of the elbow, the clinician must be able to visualize both arms. The involved elbow should be inspected for scars, redness, nodules, atrophy, deformities, and swelling. The earliest sign of elbow effusion is a loss of the elbow dimples. Sudden swelling of the elbow in the absence of trauma suggests infection, inflammation, or gout.

Observation of the elbow should be from all views. To ensure this, the observation should be systematically divided into anterior, lateral, posterior, and medial aspects.[1,3]

Anterior Aspect

Anterior joint effusion is an evidence of significant swelling. The axial alignment of the elbow should be assessed. With the elbow extended and the forearm positioned in supination, the humerus and forearm should normally be in valgus.[1] This angle is referred to as the *carrying angle* and varies from 13° to 16° for females, and from 11° to 14° for males.[5,6,7] Any difference in the carrying angle of the elbow is more obvious when the elbow is in extension. The carrying angle of the involved elbow should be compared to the other side before any conclusions are drawn. It is important to note that an accurate assessment of the carrying angle is difficult if a significant fixed flexion deformity of the elbow joint is present. The most common cause of an altered carrying angle is past trauma or epiphyseal growth disturbances. A valgus deformity is typically caused by nonunion of a fractured lateral condyle and may be associated with tardy ulnar nerve palsy.[3] A varus deformity (Gunstock) can follow malunion of a supracondylar fracture.[3]

Posterior Aspect

The olecranon tip is normally visible subcutaneously. Gradual swelling over the posterior tip of the elbow, which can sometimes be golf ball-sized but may not be tender to palpation, could be caused by an inflammation or infection of the olecranon bursa or by a traction spur of the olecranon (see Figure 8-1).[1] Sudden swelling over this area accompanied with a history of trauma is more likely the result of a posterior ulnar subluxation or a rupture of the triceps tendon.[1] A diminished tip of the olecranon could result from a prior partial olecranon excision or an anterior elbow subluxation or dislocation.[1] The triangular relationship of the epicondyles and the olecranon at 90° of elbow flexion and full extension is often disrupted in the presence of a fracture, dislocation, or degeneration. At 90° of flexion the three bony landmarks form an isosceles triangle, and when the arm is extended, they form a straight line.[8,9]

Nodules on the extensor surface of the elbow may indicate the presence of a rheumatoid disease, gout, or other systemic processes.[1]

Medial Aspect

The medial epicondyle is usually visible on the medial aspect of the elbow. Behind this is the ulnar nerve, which is palpable (Figure 8-2). In certain cases of ulnar neuritis the ulnar nerve may appear enlarged.[3] Ulnar nerve involvement can be determined using the Tinel's test (see Special tests) or motion and joint play tests. A combination of sustained flexion and a restriction in joint-play decreases the overall volume within the cubital tunnel, which can increase the symptoms of ulnar nerve compression.[10,11]

Lateral Aspect

Most swelling appears beneath the lateral epicondyle. Fullness in the region of the lateral infracondylar process indicates synovial proliferation if on palpation the swelling has a boggy consistency.[3] If the swelling can be completely obliterated with pressure, and particularly if cross-fluctuation is present, an increase in synovial fluid is present.[3] Bony hard swelling in this region is often associated with radial heal pathology, such as a previous fracture or posterior subluxation.[3]

Palpation

Because they are superficial, most of the elbow structures are easily palpable, making it easier for the clinician to pinpoint the specific area of pain. However, in cases wherein the pain is more diffuse, the diagnosis becomes somewhat more difficult. A logical sequence based on surface anatomy is outlined below.

Bony and Ligamentous Structures

Bony structures feel hard, whereas ligamentous structures feel firm.

Medial and Lateral Epicondyle   The lateral and medial epicondyles should be palpated for tenderness or effusion. The medial epicondyle (see Figure 8-2) can be palpated on the medial aspect of the distal humerus, while

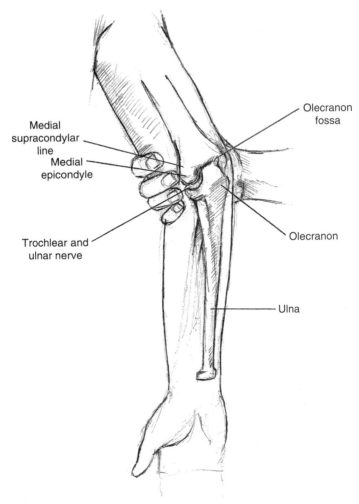

FIG. 8-2   Palpation points on the medial aspect of the elbow.

the lateral epicondyle (Figure 8-3) is more difficult to palpate. Tenderness of the medial epicondyle is a common finding with medial epicondylitis (Golfer's elbow) (see Figure 8-1). Tenderness of the lateral epicondyle is commonly found with lateral epicondylitis (Tennis elbow) (Figure 8-4), especially over the origin of the extensor carpi radialis brevis.

The Humeroulnar Joint Line   The joint line is located at a point approximately 2 cm distal to an imaginary line joining the two epicondyles (see Figure 8-2), which passes medially and inferiorly. The joint lines are firm on palpation, and lie between two structures that are harder.[9]

Supracondylar Ridges   (see Figures 8-2, 8-3) By asking the patient to make a fist with the wrist in slight extension, the extensor carpi radialis longus (ECRL) can be felt on the lateral supracondylar ridge, which is just superior to the lateral epicondyle.[9]

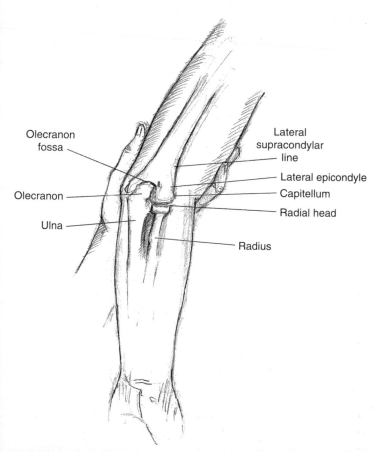

FIG. 8-3 Palpation points on the lateral aspect of the elbow.

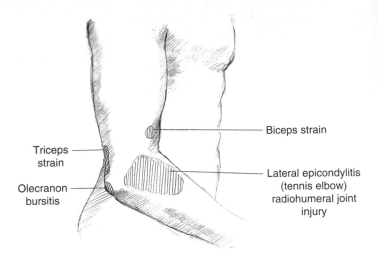

FIG. 8-4 Pain locations on the lateral elbow and their possible causes.

Olecranon The olecranon (see Figure 8-3) should be easy to locate. The olecranon ends distally in a point. Just distal to this point, the posterior border of the ulna can be palpated along its entire length (see Figure 8-2).

Head of the Radius To palpate the radial head (see Figure 8-3) at the humeroradial joint, the clinician places the index finger on the lateral humeral epicondyle. From here, the index finger slides posteriorly and distally between the humerus and the radial head.[9]

Radial Tuberosity The radial tuberosity can be difficult to palpate. It serves as the attachment for the biceps brachii tendon.

Annular Ligament This ligament is located distal to the lateral epicondyle, and applying passive supination and pronation of the forearm, can facilitate its palpation.

Lateral (Radial) Collateral Ligament This ligament can be palpated as a cordlike structure that passes from the lateral epicondyle of the humerus to the annular ligament and lateral surface of the ulna.

The ulnar nerve also should be palpated in the ulnar groove (see Figure 8-2) to elicit paresthesias that would suggest nerve entrapment.

Muscles

The muscles of the forearm can be divided into compartments according to location (Table 8-7).

Biceps The short head of the biceps is located at the coracoid process (together with the coracobrachialis muscle).[9] The long head of the biceps cannot be palpated at its origin, but it is palpable in the intertubercular groove. The muscle belly of the biceps is easily identifiable, especially with resisted elbow flexion and forearm supination.

Brachialis The origin of the brachialis can be palpated posterior to the deltoid tuberosity. Its insertion can be palpated at a point medial to the

TABLE 8-7 Muscle Compartments of the Forearm

Compartment	Principal muscles
Anterior	Pronator teres
	Flexor carpi radialis
	Palmaris longus
	Flexor digitorum superficialis
	Flexor digitorum profundus
	Flexor pollicis longus
	Flexor carpi ulnaris
	Pronator quadratus
Posterior	Abductor pollicis longus
	Extensor pollicis brevis
	Extensor pollicis longus
	Extensor digitorum communis
	Extensor digitorum proprius
	Extensor digiti quinti
	Extensor carpi ulnaris
Mobile wad	Brachioradialis
	Extensor carpi radialis longus
	Extensor carpi radialis brevis

musculotendinous junction of the biceps, at the proximal border of the bicipital aponeurosis.[9]

Brachioradialis   The brachioradialis can be palpated from the radial border of the cubital fossa distally to the radial styloid process.

Common Flexor Origin   This is located at the medial epicondyle, and the flexor-pronator mass is located at the medial aspect of the elbow.

Common Extensor Origin   This is located at the lateral epicondyle.

Supinator   The borders of the supinator within the cubital fossa are formed by the brachioradialis (radially), pronator teres (ulnarly), and tendon of the biceps (proximally).[9]

Triceps   Palpation of the triceps can be simplified by having the patient abduct the arm to 90°. The lateral head of the triceps borders directly on the brachial muscle, whereas the medial head runs underneath both the long and lateral heads of the triceps. These two heads of the triceps can be palpated until their common insertion at the olecranon.[9]

Anconeus   This small muscular triangle can be palpated between the olecranon, the posterior border of the ulna, and the lateral epicondyle.

Neurovascular Structures

If the radial tuberosity is palpable, the posterior interosseous nerve is usually located no closer than 2 centimeters from the tuberosity in a dorsal direction with the forearm pronated. The brachial artery can be palpated anteriorly to the elbow and the pulse palpated and compared bilaterally.

Active Range of Motion with Passive Overpressure

The patient with elbow pain should have a detailed assessment of his or her motion (Figures 8-5, 8-6). It is important to determine how much range of motion is necessary for the patient to perform his or her job and recreational activities. Most activities of daily living may be accomplished with

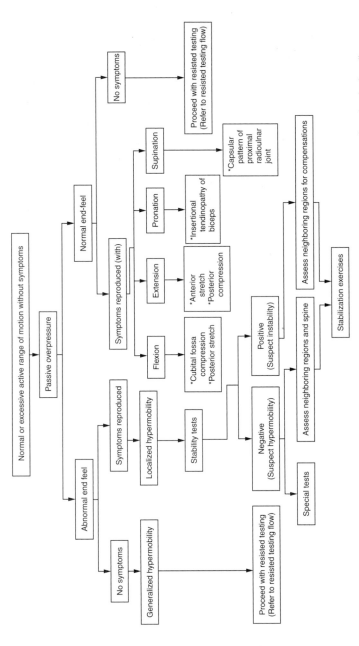

FIG. 8-5 Examination sequence in the presence of symptoms with normal or excessive active range of motion in the elbow.

214

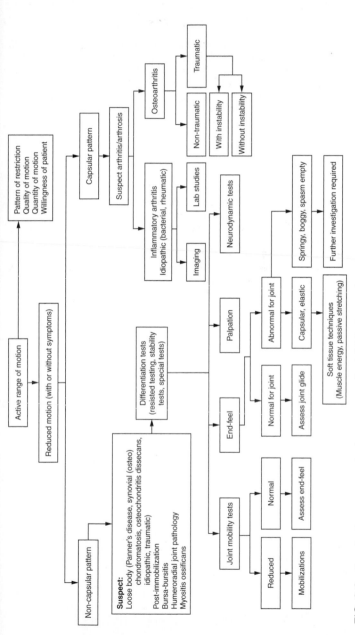

FIG. 8-6 Examination sequence in the presence of painful flexion and/or extension at the elbow.

a functional arc of 100° from 30° to 130°.[12] In addition to assessing the following elbow and forearm motions, the various motions that occur at the wrist (flexion, extension, radial deviation, and ulnar deviation must also be assessed, refer to Chapter 9).

Range of motion of the elbow and forearm can be assessed with the patient seated, although elbow extension is better evaluated with the patient standing. The patient is asked to perform active flexion, extension (Figure 8-7), pronation, and supination (Figure 8-8) of the elbow, and the ranges are recorded. Normal ranges of motion at the elbow complex are 140° to 150° of flexion, 0° to 10° of extension/hyperextension, 90° of supination, and 80° to 90° of pronation. Supination and pronation should be tested with the elbow flexed to 90° (see Figure 8-8). If symptoms are not reproduced with the single plane motions, combined motions of the elbow are tested (see next section). Capsular or noncapsular patterns should be determined. The capsular patterns at the elbow are depicted in Table 8-8. Active movement often accentuates any crepitus during motion, which can be caused by articular surface damage, a loose body, or an osteophyte.[3] Nerve injury typically decreases active but not passive motion.[1]

The end-feels of elbow motion should be classified as either compliant, suggesting soft tissue restriction, or rigid, suggesting a mechanical bony limit. Passive elbow flexion (Figure 8-9) should have an end-feel of soft tissue approximation. Passive flexion may aggravate an ulnar nerve neuropathy.[13] Passive elbow extension (Figure 8-10) should have a bony end-feel. A springy end-feel with passive elbow flexion may indicate a loose body. Elbow extension is usually the first motion to be limited, and the last to be restored with

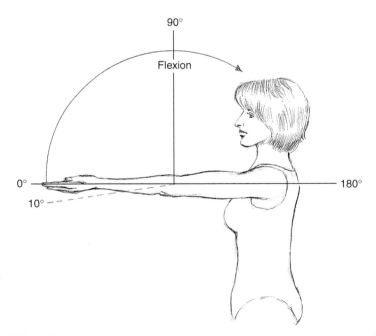

FIG. 8-7   Elbow flexion, extension.

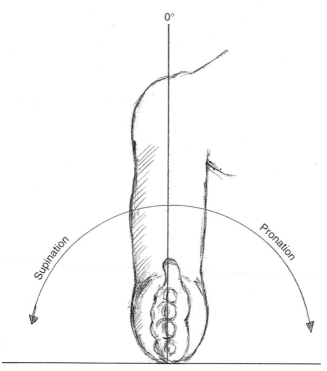

FIG. 8-8   Forearm pronation and supination.

intrinsic joint problems.[13,14] Thus it serves as the most sensitive barometer of injury and of recovery of the elbow.[1] Even minor swelling or effusion prevents full extension of the elbow. The clinician should be particularly careful of the elbow that has lost a gross amount of extension post trauma, especially if accompanied by a painful weakness of elbow extension, as this may indicate an olecranon fracture. A significant loss of motion, with no accompanying weakness, could indicate myositis ossificans. Pain that occurs at the limit(s) of motion suggests bony impingement. The clinician should also note the degree of ulnar adduction or abduction that occurs with the elbow motions.

TABLE 8-8 Capsular Patterns of Restriction at the Elbow

Joint	Limitation of motion (passive angular motion)
Humeroulnar	Flexion > Extension (±4:1)
Humeroradial	No true capsular pattern; possible equal limitation of pronation and supination
Superior radioulnar	No true capsular pattern; possible equal limitation of pronation and supination with pain at end ranges
Inferior radioulnar	No true capsular pattern; possible equal limitation of pronation and supination with pain at end ranges

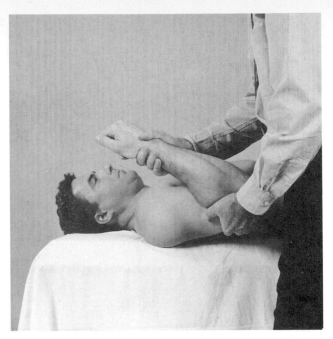

FIG. 8-9   Passive elbow flexion (*Reproduced with permission from Dutton M: Orthopaedic Examination, Evaluation, and Intervention, p 537 (Fig. 15–16). New York, McGraw-Hill, 2004.*)

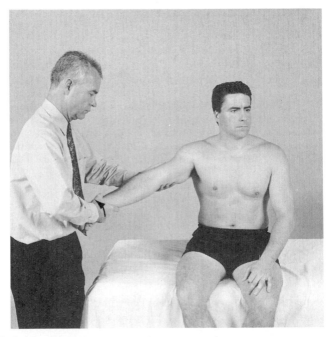

FIG. 8-10   Passive elbow extension.

Pain throughout the central arc of flexion and extension, or pronation and supination, implies degeneration of the humeroulnar or proximal radioulnar joints, respectively. The predominant cause of fixed flexion contractures can be determined by applying passive overpressure into extension and noting the site of pain. Posterior pain indicates that posterior impingement is the likely culprit, whereas anterior pain indicates that anterior capsule adaptive shortening is the principal cause.[3]

Passive pronation and supination are applied by grasping the proximal aspect of the forearm. Passive overpressure is superimposed at the end of the available ranges, using the appropriate conjunct rotations. A decrease in pronation or supination can represent pathology at either the proximal or distal radioulnar joint, bony deformity of the radius or ulna, or contractures of the interosseous membrane.[1] For example, decreased supination and pronation are frequent sequelae of a Colles' fracture, advanced degenerative changes, dislocations, and fractures of the forearm and elbow. Of particular interest is the acute limitation of supination and extension in children, which likely results from a "pulled elbow."

Combined Motions

Combined movement testing is used to assess the patient who has full range of motion, yet has complaints of pain. The following combinations are assessed:

- Elbow flexion, adduction, and forearm pronation
- Elbow flexion, abduction, and forearm supination
- Elbow extension, abduction, and forearm pronation
- Elbow extension, adduction, and forearm supination
- Elbow flexion combined with supination should have a capsular end-feel, whereas elbow flexion combined with pronation should have a bony end-feel.

Resistive Testing

In addition to all the shoulder muscles that insert at or near the elbow (biceps, brachialis, triceps), the clinician must also test the other muscles responsible for elbow flexion and extension, in addition to the muscles involved with forearm supination, pronation, and wrist flexion and extension (see Table 8-1). Elbow flexion strength is normally 70% greater than extension strength.[3] Supination strength is normally 15% greater than pronation strength.[3]

Elbow Flexion

Resisted elbow flexion is tested with the forearm in pronation, then supination, and then neutral rotation (Figure 8-11). Pain with resisted elbow flexion most frequently implicates the biceps, especially if resisted supination is also painful. The brachialis is implicated if resisted elbow flexion with the forearm in full pronation is painful. The brachioradialis is rarely involved. Weakness of elbow flexion could suggest median nerve or C5-8 nerve root compromise. Both sides are tested for comparison.

Elbow Extension

Resisted elbow extension is tested (Figure 8-12). Both sides are tested for comparison. Pain with resisted elbow extension implicates the triceps muscle, although the anconeus muscle could also be involved. Weakness of elbow extension could suggest radial nerve or C7-8 nerve root compromise.

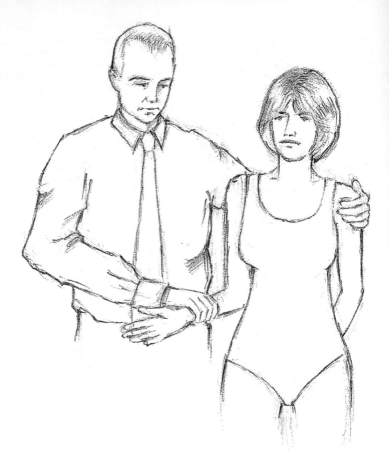

FIG. 8-11 Resisted elbow flexion.

Forearm Pronation/Supination

The clinician should test the strength of the forearm muscles by grasping the patient's hand in a handshake. The patient should be asked to exert maximum pressure to turn the palm first up (using supinators) then down (using pronators). Weakness in the supinators may indicate tendinitis, a rupture, or a subluxation of the biceps tendon at the shoulder. It may also indicate a C5-6 nerve root lesion, radial nerve lesion (supinator), or musculocutaneous nerve (C5-6) lesion (biceps). The supinator muscle is rarely injured.

Pronator weakness is associated with rupture of the pronator teres from the medial epicondyle, fracture of the medial elbow, and lesions of the C6-7 or median nerve roots. Pronator quadratus weakness, which is tested with the elbow held in a flexed position to neutralize the humeral head of the pronator teres muscle, could indicate a lesion of the anterior interosseous nerve. The pronator teres or quadratus are rarely injured. Individuals with medial or

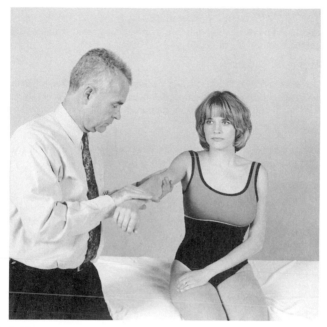

FIG. 8-12   Resisted elbow extension.

lateral epicondylitis will also find the aforementioned maneuvers painful, and resisted wrist flexion and extension can be used to help differentiate the former and latter respectively.

Wrist Flexion

The flexor carpi ulnaris is the strongest wrist flexor. To test the flexors, the clinician stabilizes the patient's mid-forearm with one hand while placing the fingers of the other hand in the patient's palm, with the palm facing the patient. The patient's attempt to flex the wrist with the elbow flexed must be resisted. Weakness is evident in rupture of the muscle origin, lesions involving the ulnar (C8, T1) or median nerve (C6, 7), or tendinitis at the medial elbow.

Wrist Extension

The most powerful wrist extensor is the extensor carpi ulnaris. To test the extensors, the clinician's hands are placed in the same position as in the preceding test, with the patient's palm facing the clinician. The patient is asked to extend the wrist with the elbow flexed. Rupture of the extensor origin, lesions of the C6-8 nerve root, or lateral tennis elbow can cause weakness.

Radial Deviation

Resisted radial deviation is tested with the elbow at 90° of elbow flexion, and at full elbow extension. Pain with resisted radial deviation is usually the result of a tennis elbow.

Ulnar Deviation

Resisted ulnar deviation, although rarely affected, is tested with the fingers in full flexion, and then in full extension.

Extension of Fingers 2–5

For resisted extension of the fingers 2–5, the elbow is positioned in full extension, the wrist in neutral, and the metacarpophalangeal (MCP) joints at 90° of flexion. Pain here usually the result of extensor digitorum tendinitis, or tennis elbow.

Extension of Fingers 2–3

For resisted extension of the fingers 2–3, the patient is positioned as above. Pain with resistance implicates tennis elbow.

Functional Assessment

The elbow, like the shoulder serves to position the hand for functional activities. A number of tests have been designed to assess elbow function (see *Orthopaedic Examination, Evaluation, and Intervention*, p 540). Table 8-9 outlines one such test. The essential arc of motion required for daily activities is 30°–130°.[3]

TABLE 8-9 Functional Testing of the Elbow

Starting position	Action	Functional test
Sitting, cuff weight attached to wrist	Elbow flexion	5-pound weight: Functional 3- to 4-pound weight: Functionally fair Active flexion (0 pound): Functionally poor Cannot flex elbow: Nonfunctional
Standing	Elbow extension with wall push-up	Five repetitions: Functional Three to four repetitions: Functionally fair One to two repetitions: Functionally poor Zero repetition: Nonfunctional
Standing facing door	Turning door knob into supination	Five repetitions: Functional Three to four repetitions: Functionally fair One to two repetitions: Functionally poor Zero repetition: Nonfunctional
Standing facing door	Turning door knob into pronation	Five repetitions: Functional Three to four repetitions: Functionally fair One to two repetitions: Functionally poor Zero repetition: Nonfunctional

Sources: Magee DJ (ed): Orthopedic physical assessment. Philadelphia, PA, WB Saunders, 2002.
Palmer ML, Epler M: Clinical assessment procedures in physical therapy. Philadelphia, PA, JB Lippincott, 1990.

Passive Physiologic Articular Motion Testing

The accessory motions can be used for examination and intervention purposes, with the latter incorporating graded glides.

Ulnohumeral Joint

The patient is positioned in supine with his or her head supported on a pillow. The clinician sits or stands facing the patient.

Distraction/Compression   The clinician stabilizes the humerus with one hand and wraps the fingers of the other hand around the proximal one-third of the forearm (Figure 8-13). The clinician applies a longitudinal force through the proximal forearm and along the line of the humerus to distract the ulnohumeral joint. The quality and quantity of motion is noted. The test is repeated on the opposite extremity and the findings compared.

Medial Glide   The clinician, using the medial aspect of the MCP joint of the index finger of the medial hand, palpates and stabilizes the medial aspect of the distal humerus (Figure 8-14). Using the other hand, the clinician palpates the lateral aspect of the olecranon with the MCP joint of the index finger (see Figure 8-14). The elbow is extended to the limit of physiologic range of motion. From this position, the clinician glides the ulna medially on the fixed humerus along the medial-lateral plane of the joint line. The quality and quantity of motion is noted. The test is repeated on the opposite extremity and the findings compared.

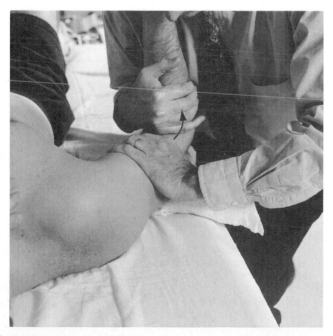

FIG. 8-13   Ulnohumeral distraction.

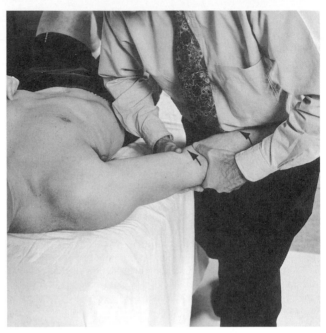

FIG. 8-14   Medial glide of ulnohumeral joint.

Lateral Glide   The clinician, using the MCP joint of the index finger of the medial hand, palpates and stabilizes the lateral aspect of the distal humerus. Using the other hand, the clinician palpates the medial aspect of the olecranon with the MCP joint of the index finger. The elbow is flexed to the limit of physiologic range of motion. From this position, the clinician glides the ulna laterally on the fixed humerus along the medial-lateral plane of the joint line. The quality and quantity of motion is noted. The test is repeated on the opposite extremity and the findings compared.

Radiohumeral Joint

The joint glides for the radiohumeral joint are performed with elbow positioned in 70° flexion and 35° of supination. The patient is in supine position with his or her hand cradled by the clinician. The following tests are performed:[15,16]

- *Distraction.* The clinician places a thumb of the stabilizing hand between the radial head and the lateral epicondyle. With the other hand, the clinician grasps the radius and applies a longitudinal distraction force along the length of the radius (Figure 8-15). A longitudinal compression force can be applied using the same patient–clinician position.
- *Motion testing of the radial head.* Once located, the clinician grasps the radial head between the thumb and index finger (Figure 8-16). The radial head is moved in an anterior and posterior direction, and any restriction of motion is noted. The posterior glide of the radius is coupled with pronation/extension, and anterior glide is coupled with supination/flexion. The most common dysfunction of the radial head is a posterior radial head, which is accompanied with a loss of the anterior glide.

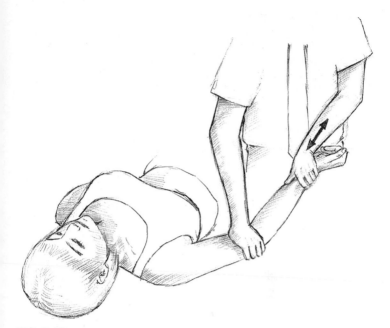

FIG. 8-15 Distraction of radius.

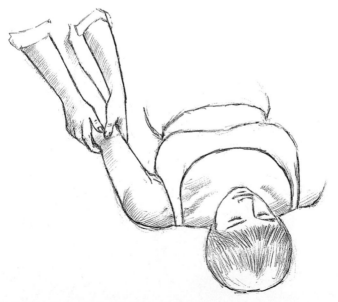

FIG. 8-16 Anterior-posterior glide of radial head.

Proximal Radioulnar Joint

Anterior-Posterior Glide   The clinician palpates and stabilizes the proximal one-third of the ulna with one hand. With a pinch grip of the index finger and thumb, the clinician palpates the head of the radius with the other hand (Figure 8-17). From this position, the clinician glides the head of the radius anteriorly-posteriorly at the proximal radioulnar joint, in an obliquely anterior-medial/posterior-lateral direction. The quality and quantity of motion is noted. The test is repeated on the opposite extremity and the findings compared.

Distal Radioulnar Joint

Anterior-Posterior Glide   The patient is positioned supine with his or her head resting on a pillow. The clinician palpates and stabilizes the distal one-third of the ulna with one hand. With a pinch grip of the fingers and thenar eminence of the other hand, the clinician palpates the distal one-third of the radius (Figure 8-18). From this position, the clinician glides the radius anteriorly/posteriorly at the distal radioulnar joint, in an obliquely anterior-medial/posterior-lateral direction. The quality and quantity of motion is noted. The test is repeated on the opposite extremity and the findings compared.

Stress Tests

Medial (Ulnar) Collateral Ligament (Valgus Test)

The clinician stabilizes the distal humerus with one hand and palpates the distal forearm with the other. The anterior band of the medial collateral ligament

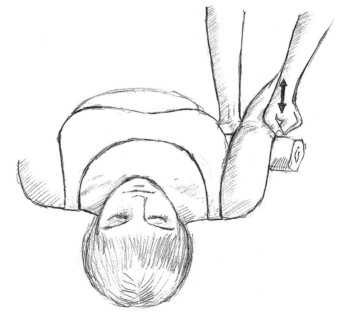

FIG. 8-17   Anterior-posterior glide of proximal radioulnar joint.

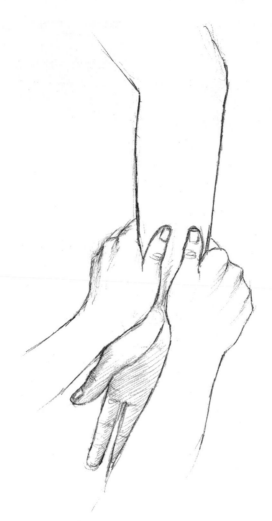

FIG. 8-18 Anterior-posterior glide of distal radioulnar joint.

(MCL) tightens in the ranges of 0°–90° of flexion, becoming lax in full extension, before tightening again in hyperextension to about 20°–30° of flexion. The posterior bundle is taut in flexion beyond 90°.[14,17–19]

The anterior band is tested with the sustained application of a valgus stress while flexing the elbow to between 15° and 30° (Figure 8-19).[20,21]

The posterior band is best tested using a "milking" maneuver. The patient is seated and his or her arm is positioned in shoulder flexion, elbow flexion beyond 90°, and forearm supination. The clinician pulls downward on the patient's thumb.[20] This maneuver generates a valgus stress on the flexed elbow. A positive sign is indicated by the reproduction of pain.

The tests are repeated on the opposite extremity and the findings compared.

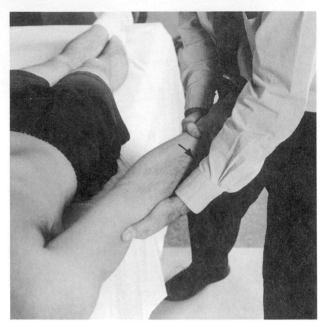

FIG. 8-19 Medial collateral ligament stress test.

Lateral Pivot Shift Apprehension Test The lateral pivot shift test is used in the diagnosis of posterolateral rotatory instability. The patient is positioned supine with the involved extremity overhead. The clinician grasps the patient's wrist and elbow. The elbow is supinated with a mild force at the wrist, and a valgus movement and compressive force is applied to the elbow during flexion.[22] This results in a typical apprehension response with reproduction of the patient's symptoms and a sense that the elbow is about to dislocate. Reproducing the actual subluxation, and the clunk that occurs with reduction, usually can only be accomplished with the patient under general anesthesia or occasionally after injecting local anesthetic into the elbow.

Lateral (Radial) Collateral Ligament (Varus Test)

The lateral collateral ligament (LCL) is tested with the elbow positioned in 15° to 30° short of full extension. The clinician stabilizes the humerus and adducts the ulnar, producing a varus force at the elbow (Figure 8-20). The end-feel is noted and compared with the results from the same test at the other elbow.

Special Tests

Tennis Elbow

A number of tests exist for tennis elbow (lateral epicondylitis). Two are described here:

- *Cozen's test.* The clinician stabilizes the patient's elbow with one hand and the patient is asked to pronate the forearm, extend and radially deviate the

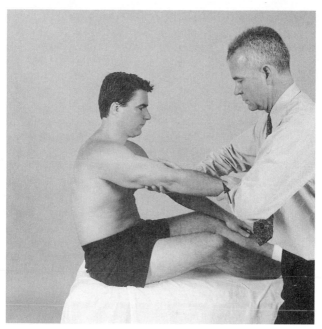

FIG. 8-20   Lateral collateral ligament stress test.

wrist against the manual resistance of the clinician (Figure 8-21). A reproduction of pain in the area of the lateral epicondyle indicates a positive test.
- *Mill's test.* The clinician palpates the patient's lateral epicondyle with one hand, while pronating the patient's forearm, fully flexing the wrist, and extending the elbow. A reproduction of pain in the area of the lateral epicondyle indicates a positive test.

Golfer's Elbow (Medial Epicondylitis)

The clinician palpates the medial epicondyle with one hand, while supinating the forearm, and extending the wrist and elbow with the other hand. A reproduction of pain in the area of the medial epicondyle indicates a positive test.

Elbow Flexion Test for Cubital Tunnel Syndrome

The patient is positioned sitting. The patient is asked to depress both shoulders, flex both elbows maximally, supinate the forearms, and extend the wrists.[23] This position is maintained for 3–5 minutes. Tingling or paresthesia in the ulnar distribution of the forearm and hand indicates a positive test.

Pressure Provocative Test for Cubital Tunnel Syndrome

With the elbow held in 20° of flexion and the forearm in supination, the clinician applies pressure proximal to the cubital tunnel.[24]

Tinel's Sign (at the Elbow)

The clinician locates the groove between the olecranon process and the medial epicondyle through which the ulnar nerve passes. This groove is

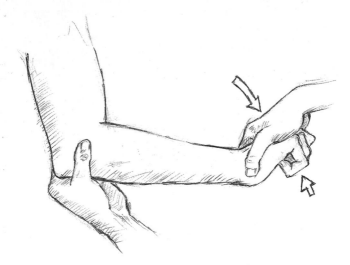

FIG. 8-21 Cozen's test.

tapped by the index finger of the clinician. A positive sign is indicated by a tingling sensation in the ulnar distribution of the forearm and hand distal to the tapping point.

Imaging Studies*[2]   Standard radiographs of the elbow include the straight anteroposterior view and the true lateral view. The radial head normally articulates with the capitellum, and a line bisecting the proximal radial shaft should always pass through the capitellum on any radiographic view. Special views include axial projections to evaluate the olecranon fossa, oblique views to assess the radial head, and stress views to evaluate joint stability.[25]

Bone scanning is sensitive but not specific for detecting stress fractures, healing fractures, infections, and tumors. Computed tomographic (CT) scanning is useful for delineating complex osseous anatomy. For example, these tests are useful in demonstrating if impingement from the olecranon or coranoid process is present, and are also useful in determining the presence of loose bodies.[3] Magnetic resonance imaging (MRI) can be helpful in identifying soft tissue masses, articular cartilage anatomy, ligament ruptures, and chondral defects. Arthrography may be useful for defining articular surfaces and identifying loose bodies or capsular defects.[26]

Electromyography and nerve conduction studies are used to evaluate suspected nerve compression syndromes.

EXAMINATION CONCLUSIONS—THE EVALUATION

Following the examination, and once the clinical findings have been recorded, the clinician must determine a specific diagnosis or a working hypothesis, based on a summary of all the findings. This diagnosis can be structure related (medical diagnosis) (Table 8-10), or a diagnosis based on the preferred practice patterns as described in the *Guide to Physical Therapist Practice*.[27]

TABLE 8-10 Differential Diagnosis for Common Causes of Elbow Pain

Condition	Patient age	Mechanism of injury	Area of symptoms	Symptoms aggravated by	Observation	AROM	PROM	End-feel	Resisted	Special tests	Tenderness with palpation
Bicipital tendinitis	20–50	Repetitive hyperextension of the elbow with pronation, or repetitive stressful pronation/supination	Anterior aspect of the distal part of the arm	Elbow extension and shoulder extension	Unremarkable	Possible pain with elbow flexion	Pain with passive shoulder and elbow extension		Pain on elbow flexion and supination		Distal biceps belly. The musculotendinous portion of the biceps Bicipital insertion of the radial tuberosity
Triceps tendinitis	20–50	Overuse of the upper arm and elbow, especially in activities like throwing and hammering	Posterior aspect of elbow	Activities involving elbow extension or full elbow flexion	Possible swelling near the point of the elbow	Elbow extension Possible pain with extreme elbow flexion	Pain with passive shoulder and elbow flexion		Pain on elbow extension		Posterior aspect of elbow

(Continued)

231

TABLE 8-10 Differential Diagnosis for Common Causes of Elbow Pain (*Continued*)

Condition	Patient age	Mechanism of injury	Area of symptoms	Symptoms aggravated by	Observation	AROM	PROM	End-feel	Resisted	Special tests	Tenderness with palpation
Lateral epicondylitis	35–55	Gradual overuse	Lateral aspect of elbow	Activities involving wrist extension/grasping	Possible swelling (over lateral elbow)	Possible pain on wrist flexion with elbow extension	Pain on wrist flexion with the forearm pronated and the elbow extended		Pain on resisted wrist extension and radial deviation, with the elbow extended	Cozen's	Lateral elbow (over the extensor carpi radialis brevis [ECRB] and ECRL)
Medial epicondylitis	35–55	Gradual overuse	Anteromedial aspect of elbow	Activities involving wrist flexion	Possible swelling (over medial elbow)	Pain on wrist extension	Pain on combined wrist extension and forearm supination		Pain on finger extension. Pain on pronation with wrist flexion	Mill's. Passive supination of the forearm, and extension of the wrist and elbow	Anteromedial elbow
Olecranon bursitis	20–50	Trauma	Posterior aspect of elbow	Contact with posterior elbow	Swelling over posterior elbow	Possible pain with extreme elbow flexion	Pain on full elbow flexion		Strong and pain free		Posterior elbow

232

Ulnar collateral ligament Injury	20–45	Excessive valgus force to medial compartment of the elbow	Ulnar aspect of the elbow	Valgus stress of the elbow, throwing, pitching	May have ecchymosis over ulnar aspect	Pain with full extension possible	Passive extension of the elbow, valgus stress	Depends on severity	Usually unremarkable	Valgus stress with elbow flexed at approx 25° and humerus in external rotation	Ulnar aspect of elbow
Ulnar nerve entrapment	20–40	Gradual overuse / Trauma	Medial elbow, forearm, and hand / Medial 1 1/2 fingers	Activities involving elbow and wrist extension	Atrophy of hand muscles if chronic	Inability to fully close hand	Full and pain free		Weakness of grip	Elbow flexion and pressure provocative test Tinel's at elbow Wartenberg's sign Froment's sign	Anteromedial elbow
Radial nerve entrapment	Varies	Can be overuse, direct trauma	Lateral elbow	Varies	Usually unremarkable	Usually unremarkable	Usually unremarkable		Pain with resisted forearm supination, resisted extension of middle finger		Maximal tenderness is usually elicited over the radial tunnel if radial tunnel syndrome

(Continued)

233

TABLE 8-10 Differential Diagnosis for Common Causes of Elbow Pain (Continued)

Condition	Patient age	Mechanism of injury	Area of symptoms	Symptoms aggravated by	Observation	AROM	PROM	End-feel	Resisted	Special tests	Tenderness with palpation
Median nerve entrapment	20–40	Gradual overuse	Anterior forearm	Activities involving full elbow extension or pronation of the forearm	Atrophy of anterior forearm and hand muscles if chronic	Pain on forearm pronation	Full and pain free		Weakness on pronation, wrist flexion, and thumb opposition	Benediction sign	Over the pronator teres 4 centimeter distal to the cubital crease with concurrent resistance against pronation, elbow flexion, and wrist flexion—Pronator syndrome
			Lateral 3½ fingers							Inability to perform "OK" sign (anterior interosseous syndrome) Resisted supination (compression of the lacertus fibrosis)	

REFERENCES

1. Colman WW, Strauch RJ: Physical examination of the elbow. Ortho Clin N Am 1999;30:15–20.
2. Chumbley EM, O'Connor FG, Nirschl RP: Evaluation of overuse elbow injuries. Am Fam Phys 2000;61:691–700.
3. Bell S: Examination of the elbow. Aust Fam Physician 1988;17:391–392.
4. Woodward TW, Best TM: The painful shoulder: Part I. Clinical evaluation. Am Fam Phys 2000;61:3079–3088.
5. An KN, Morrey BF: Biomechanics of the elbow. In Morrey BF (ed): The Elbow and Its Disorders, pp 53–73. Philadelphia, PA, WB Saunders, 1993.
6. An K-N, Morrey BF, Chao EY: The carrying angle of the human elbow joint. J Orthop Res 1984;1:369–378.
7. Beals RK: The normal carrying angle of the elbow. Clin Orthop 1976;119:194.
8. AAOS: Orthopedic knowledge update 4: home study syllabus. Rosemont, IL, American Academy of Orthopedic Surgeons, 1992.
9. Winkel D, Matthijs O, Phelps V: Examination of the elbow. In Diagnosis and Treatment of the Upper Extremities, pp 207–233. Gaithersburg, MD, Aspen, 1997.
10. Pecina M, Krmpotic-NemanicJ, Markiewitz A: Tunnel Syndromes. Boca Raton, FL, CRC, 1991.
11. Vennix MJ, Werstsch JJ: Entrapment neuropathies about the elbow. J Back Musculoskel Rehabil 1994;4:31–43.
12. Morrey BF, Askew LJ, Chao EYS: A biomechanical study of normal functional elbow motion. J Bone Joint Surg 1981;63A:872–877.
13. Hammer WI: Functional Soft Tissue Examination and Treatment by Manual Methods. Gaithersburg, MD, Aspen, 1991.
14. Morrey BF, An KN, Chao EYS: Functional evaluation of the elbow. In Morrey BF (ed): The Elbow and Its Disorders, pp 86–97. Philadelphia, PA, WB Saunders, 1993.
15. Kaltenborn FM: Manual Mobilization of the Extremity Joints: Basic Examination and Treatment Techniques, 4th ed. Oslo, Norway, Olaf Norlis Bokhandel, Universitetsgaten, 1989.
16. Maitland G: Peripheral Manipulation, 3rd ed. London, Butterworth, 1991.
17. Morrey BF: Applied anatomy and biomechanics of the elbow joint. Inst Course Lect 1986;35:59–68.
18. Morrey BF, An KN: Articular and ligamentous contributions to the stability of the elbow joint. Am J Sports Med 1983;11:315–319.
19. Morrey BF, An KN: Functional anatomy of the ligaments of the elbow. Clin Orthop 1985;201:84–90.
20. Jobe FW, Kvitne RS: Elbow instability in the athlete. Inst Course Lect 1991. 40:17–23.
21. Conway JE, et al.: Medial instability of the elbow in throwing athletes: treatment by repair or reconstruction of the ulnar collateral ligament. J Bone Joint Surg 1992;74A:67–83.
22. O'Driscoll SW, Bell DF, Morrey BF, Posterolateral rotatory instability of the elbow. J Bone Joint Surg 1991;73A:440–446.
23. Buehler MJ, Thayer DT: The elbow flexion test: a clinical test for cubital tunnel syndrome. Clin Orthop 1988;233:213–216.
24. Novak CB, et al.: Provocative testing for cubital tunnel syndrome. J Hand Surg – [Am] 1994;19:817–820.
25. Tamisiea DF: Radiologic aspects of orthopedic diseases. In Mercer LR (ed): Practical Orthopedics, pp 327–418. St Louis, MO, Mosby, 1995.
26. Tung GA, Brody JM: Contemporary imaging of athletic injuries. Clin Sports Med 1995;16:393–417.
27. Guide to physical therapist practice. Phys Ther 2001;81:S13–S95.

9 | The Wrist and Hand

OVERVIEW

The importance of normal hand function cannot be underestimated—the hand accounts for about 90% of upper limb function.[1] While the shoulder, elbow, and wrist serve to position the hand, it is only the hand that is capable of producing a remarkable level of dexterity and precision. This dexterity and precision depends on a number of factors including patient motivation and the exact synchronization of the joints and muscles that comprise the hand.

The thumb, which is involved in 40–50% of hand function, is the more functionally important of the digits.[1] The index finger, involved in about 20% of hand function, is the second most important, and the ring finger the least important. The middle finger, which accounts for about 20% of all hand function, is the strongest finger, and is important for both precision and power functions. Proper diagnosis and management of wrist and hand injuries are vital to maintaining proper function of the hand and preventing permanent disability.

Chapter 16 of the *Orthopaedic Examination, Evaluation, and Intervention* describes the respective bones, joints, soft tissues, and nerves, of the hand and wrist detailing both their individual and collective functions.

EXAMINATION

The examination of the wrist and hand requires a sound knowledge of surface anatomy and differential diagnosis, and must include an examination of the entire upper kinetic chain, and the cervical and thoracic spine. Most hand and wrist problems can be diagnosed by carefully considering three factors: anatomy, mechanism of injury, and epidemiology.

History

The examination of the wrist and hand begins by recording a detailed history, which helps focus the examination. All relevant information must be gathered about the site, nature, behavior, and onset of the current symptoms. This should include information about the patient's age, hand dominance, avocational activities, and occupation. Activities or occupations that involve sustained nonneutral positions of the hand and wrist subject nerves to prolonged stretch and periods of high pressure.[2] In addition, these positions place muscles at inefficient length-tension relationships,[3] resulting in decreased transmission of contractile forces to the fingers.[3,4]

The history should include questions about the following:

- How did the injury occur? If the problem is trauma related, the clinician should ascertain:
  - The forces applied. If the patient describes the mechanism of injury as a FOOSH (fall on the out stretched hand) injury, the history can provide some important clues (see Table 8-4).[5]
  - Where and when did the injury occur?
  - The position of the wrist and hand at the time of the trauma.

- Whether the environmental conditions at the time of injury were clean or dirty. The environment in which the injury took place as well as the inflicting instrument help determine the level of contamination and therefore the risk of infection.[6] In cases of potential contamination, it is well worth checking the patient's tetanus status.
- Whether there was an accompanying "pop" or "click." The presence of pops and clicks at the time of injury could indicate a fracture or ligamentous tear.
- Whether swelling occurred and if so, how and where. Refer to *Observation* section.
- Are there any local areas of tenderness? Determining the location of the pain can provide some clues as to the cause (Figure 9-1).
- When did the injury occur?
- Are they any associated medical factors? Factors such as medications, malnutrition, diabetes, and immunosuppression may inhibit the healing process.[6]
- Whether radiologic films were taken.
- The sequence of symptoms, the level of functional impairment, the progression of symptoms, the time of day the symptoms are worse, and whether the symptoms appear to be posture, or work-related.

If the problem is non-trauma related, the onset of pain or sensory change, swelling, or contracture should be ascertained. Knowledge of the past behavior of previous wrist, hand and finger disorders, and their interventions can help in assessing the nature of the patient's current problem.

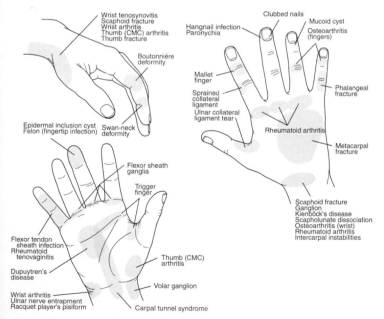

FIG. 9-1 Pain locations of the wrist and hand, and possible causes. (*Reproduced with permission from Dutton M: Orthopaedic Examination, Evaluation, and Intervention, p 255 (Fig. 9-4). New York, McGraw-Hill, 2004.*)

The patient's goals should be ascertained. Dysfunction of the hand can be very disabling, so inquiries concerning the functional demands of the patient must be made, and the intervention tailored accordingly.

Systems Review

A complete review of the medical history and general health of the patient should be included along with a review of systems, and the presence of other orthopedic, neurological or cardiopulmonary conditions. An upper quarter scanning examination is performed to provide an overview of the upper extremity, the direction for a more detailed examination, and to rule out referral from the cervical, thoracic, shoulder girdle, and elbow joints.

The clinician must be able to determine the suitability of the patient for physical therapy. All inflammatory conditions, whether infectious or not, are accompanied by diffuse pain or tenderness with movement. Rheumatoid arthritis (RA) often affects this region with more severity and frequency than elsewhere. Therefore, questions concerning other joint involvement and general debility must be asked. The presence of carpal tunnel syndrome, which is usually felt at night, may also indicate RA.

If the clinician is concerned with any signs or symptoms of a visceral, vascular, neurogenic, psychogenic, spondylogenic or systemic disorder that is out of the scope of physical therapy (see *Orthopaedic Examination, Evaluation, and Intervention*, pp 608–610), the patient should be referred back to their physician.

TESTS AND MEASURES

Observation

The physical examination of the wrist and hand should begin with a general observation of the patient's posture, especially the cervical and thoracic spine, and the position of hand in relation to the body. For example, the clinician should note whether the arm is held against the chest in a protective manner, or whether the arm swings normally during gait, or whether it just hangs loosely.

Rings and other jewelry should be removed if swelling has the potential to turn these objects into a tourniquet, even if the swelling appears to be remote.[6] The patient's hands can be highly informative (Table 9-1). The posture and alignment of the wrist and hand is examined:

- Wrist angulation into ulnar deviation increases shearing in the first dorsal compartment. This angulation can predispose the patient to De Quervain's syndrome.[7] A prominence of the distal ulna may indicate distal radioulnar joint instability.[8]
- The normal resting hand exhibits progressively increasing digital flexion as one progresses from the index to little fingers. An alteration in this normal cascade is often present in tendon injuries.[6] An indirect method of assessing the integrity of the flexor tendons is to apply digital pressure over the ulnar volar aspect of the forearm at the junction of the middle and distal thirds of the forearm. If the tendons are intact, the fingers will flex, especially the ulnar three.[6] Pressure over the radial aspect causes flexion of the thumb if the flexor pollicis longus tendon is intact.[6]
- The contour of the palmar surface, including the arches, should be examined. If a finger is involved, its attitude should be observed. Digital deformities are the hallmark of rheumatoid arthritis.[9]

TABLE 9-1 Outline of Physical Findings of the Hand

I. Variations in size and shape of hand

  A. Large, blunt fingers (spade hand)
    1. Acromegaly
    2. Hurler's disease (gargoylism)

  B. Gross irregularity of shape and size
    1. Paget's disease of bone
    2. Maffucci's syndrome
    3. Neurofibromatosis

  C. Spider fingers, slender palm (arachnodactyly)
    1. Hypopituitarism
    2. Eunuchism
    3. Ehlers-Danlos syndrome, pseudoxanthoma elasticum
    4. Tuberculosis
    5. Asthenic habitus
    6. Osteogenesis imperfecta

  D. Sausage-shaped phalanges
    1. Rickets (beading of joints)
    2. Granulomatous dactylitis (tuberculosis, syphilis)

  E. Spindliform joints (fingers)
    1. Early rheumatoid arthritis
    2. Systemic lupus erythematosus
    3. Psoriasis
    4. Rubella
    5. Boeck's sarcoidosis
    6. Osteoarthritis

  F. Cone-shaped fingers
    1. Pituitary obesity
    2. Frohlich's dystrophy

  G. Unilateral enlargement of hand
    1. Arteriovenous aneurysm
    2. Maffucci's syndrome

  H. Square, dry hands
    1. Cretinism
    2. Myxedema

  I. Single, widened, flattened distal phalanx
    1. Sarcoidosis

  J. Shortened fourth and fifth metacarpals (bradymetacarpalism)

  K. Shortened, incurved fifth finger (symptom of DuBois)
    1. Mongolism
    2. Gargoylism (broad, short, thick-skinned hand)

  L. Malposition and abduction, fifth finger
    1. Turner's syndrome (gonadal dysgenesis, webbed neck, etc.)

  M. Syndactylism
    1. Congenital malformations of the heart, great vessels
    2. Multiple congenital deformities
    3. Laurence-Moon-Biedl syndrome
    4. In normal individuals as an inherited trait

  N. Clubbed fingers
    1. Subacute bacterial endocarditis
    2. Pulmonary causes
      a. Tuberculosis
      b. Pulmonary arteriovenous fistula
      c. Pulmonic abscess
      d. Pulmonic cysts
      e. Bullous emphysema
      f. Pulmonary hypertrophic osteoarthropathy
      g. Bronchogenic carcinoma

(Continued)

TABLE 9-1 Outline of Physical Findings of the Hand (*Continued*)

    3. Alveolocapillary block
       a. Interstitial pulmonary fibrosis
       b. Sarcoidosis
       c. Beryllium poisoning
       d. Sclerodermatous lung
       e. Asbestosis
       f. Miliary tuberculosis
       g. Alveolar cell carcinoma
    4. Cardiovascular causes
       a. Patent ductus arteriosus
       b. Tetralogy of Fallot
       c. Taussig-Bing complex
       d. Pulmonic stenosis
       e. Ventricular septal defect
    5. Diarrheal states
       a. Ulcerative colitis
       b. Tuberculous enteritis
       c. Sprue
       d. Amebic dysentery
       e. Bacillary dysentery
       f. Parasitic infestation (gastrointestinal tract)
    6. Hepatic cirrhosis
    7. Myxedema
    8. Polycythemia
    9. Chronic urinary tract infections (upper and lower)
       a. Chronic nephritis
   10. Hyperparathyroidism (telescopy of distal phalanx)
   11. Pachydermoperiostosis (syndrome of Touraine, Solente, and Gole)
  O. Joint disturbances
    1. Arthritides
       a. Osteoarthritis
       b. Rheumatoid arthritis
       c. Systemic lupus erythematosus
       d. Gout
       e. Psoriasis
       f. Sarcoidosis
       g. Endocrinopathy (acromegaly)
       h. Rheumatic fever
       i. Reiter's syndrome
       j. Dermatomyositis
    2. Anaphylactic reaction-serum sickness
    3. Scleroderma
II. Edema of the hand
  A. Cardiac disease (congestive heart failure)
  B. Hepatic disease
  C. Renal disease
    1. Nephritis
    2. Nephrosis
  D. Hemiplegic hand
  E. Syringomyelia
  F. Superior vena caval syndrome
    1. Superior thoracic outlet tumor
    2. Mediastinal tumor or inflammation
    3. Pulmonary apex tumor
    4. Aneurysm

(*Continued*)

TABLE 9-1 Outline of Physical Findings of the Hand (*Continued*)

    G. Generalized anasarca, hypoproteinemia
    H. Postoperative lymphedema (radical breast amputation)
     I. Ischemic paralysis (cold, blue, swollen, numb)
    J. Lymphatic obstruction
       1. Lymphomatous masses in axilla
    K. Axillary mass
       1. Metastatic tumor, abscess, leukemia, Hodgkin's disease
    L. Aneurysm of ascending or transverse aorta, or of axillary artery.
    M. Pressure on innominate or subclavian vessels.
    N. Raynaud's disease
    O. Myositis
    P. Cervical rib
    Q. Trichiniasis
    R. Scalenus anticus syndrome

III. Neuromuscular effects
    A. Atrophy
       1. Painless
          a. Amyotrophic lateral sclerosis
          b. Charcot-Marie-Tooth peroneal atrophy
          c. Syringomyelia (loss of heat, cold, and pain sensation)
          d. Neural leprosy
       2. Painful
          a. Peripheral nerve disease
             (1) Radial nerve (wrist drop)
          b. Lead poisoning, alcoholism, polyneuritis, trauma
          c. Diphtheria, polyarteritis, neurosyphilis, anterior poliomyelitis
             (1) Ulnar nerve (benediction palsy)
          d. Polyneuritis, trauma
             (1) Median nerve (claw hand)
          e. Carpal tunnel syndrome
             (1) Rheumatoid arthritis
             (2) Tenosynovitis at wrist
             (3) Amyloidosis
             (4) Gout
             (5) Plasmacytoma
             (6) Anaphylactic reaction
             (7) Menopause syndrome
             (8) Myxedema
    B. Extrinsic pressure on the nerve (cervical, axillary, supraclavicular, or brachial)
       1. Pancoast tumor (pulmonary apex)
       2. Aneurysms of subclavian arteries, axillary vessels, or thoracic aorta
       3. Costoclavicular syndrome
       4. Superior thoracic outlet syndrome
       5. Cervical rib
       6. Degenerative arthritis of cervical spine
       7. Herniation of cervical intervertebral disk
    C. Shoulder-hand syndrome (complex regional pain syndrome)
       1. Myocardial infarction
       2. Pancoast tumor
       3. Brain tumor
       4. Intrathoracic neoplasms
       5. Discogenetic disease
       6. Cervical spondylosis
       7. Febrile panniculitis
       8. Senility

(*Continued*)

TABLE 9-1 Outline of Physical Findings of the Hand (*Continued*)

      9. Vascular occlusion
     10. Hemiplegia
     11. Osteoarthritis
     12. Herpes zoster
  D. Ischemic contractures (sensory loss in fingers)
      1. Tight plaster cast applications
  E. Polyarteritis nodosa
  F. Polyneuritis
      1. Carcinoma of lung
      2. Hodgkin's disease
      3. Pregnancy
      4. Gastric carcinoma
      5. Reticuloses
      6. Diabetes mellitus
      7. Chemical neuritis
        a. Antimony, benzene, bismuth, carbon tetrachloride, heavy metals, alcohol, arsenic lead, gold, emetine
      8. Ischemic neuropathy
      9. Vitamin B deficiency
     10. Atheromata
     11. Arteriosclerosis
     12. Embolic
  G. Carpodigital (carpopedal spasm) tetany
      1. Hypoparathyroidism
      2. Hyperventilation
      3. Uremia
      4. Nephritis
      5. Nephrosis
      6. Rickets
      7. Sprue
      8. Malabsorption syndrome
      9. Pregnancy
     10. Lactation
     11. Osteomalacia
     12. Protracted vomiting
     13. Pyloric obstruction
     14. Alkali poisoning
     15. Chemical toxicity
        a. Morphine, lead, alcohol
  H. Tremor
      1. Parkinsonism
      2. Familial disorder
      3. Hypoglycemia
      4. Hyperthyroidism
      5. Wilson's disease (hepatolenticular degeneration)
      6. Anxiety
      7. Ataxia
      8. Athetosis
      9. Alcoholism, narcotic addiction
     10. Multiple sclerosis
     11. Chorea (Sydenham's chorea, Huntington's disease)

Sources: Berry TJ: The Hand as a Mirror of Systemic Disease, 193–204. Philadelphia, PA, FA Davis, 1963.
Judge RD, Zuidema GD, Fitzgerald FT: General appearance. In Judge RD, Zuidema GD, Fitzgerald FT (eds): Clinical Diagnosis, pp 29–47. Boston, MA, Little, Brown and Company, 1982.

- Any wrist and finger deformities should be noted. For example, a wrist deformity of radial deviation with a prominent ulna could suggest a Colles fracture. Finger deformities include mallet finger, swan-neck deformity, and boutonniere deformity, in addition to those caused by fractures and dislocations (Table 9-2).

The clinician should observe how the patient appears to relate to the involved hand, and how the patient attempts to use the hand.[10] The clinician inspects the wrist and hands for evidence of lacerations, surgical scars, masses, localized swelling, or erythema. Scars should be examined for their degree of adherence, degree of maturation, hypertrophy (excess collagen within boundary of wound), and keloid (excess collagen that no longer conforms to wound boundaries). The location and type of edema should be noted. A determination is made as to whether the swelling is generalized or localized, hard or soft. Swellings on the dorsal aspect can be highlighted by passively flexing the wrist. Localized swellings can suggest the presence of a ganglion. Anterior effusion over the flexor tendons at the wrist may indicate rheumatoid tenovaginitis. Swelling following trauma for more than a few days probably suggests a carpal fracture. Localized swelling, accompanied with redness and tenderness may indicate an infection.

The nails should be inspected to see if they are healthy and pink (Table 9-3). Local trauma to the nails seldom involves more than one or two digits. The nails should be checked for hangnail infection, or whether they appear ridged, which could indicate an RA dysfunction. Clubbed nails are an indication of hypertrophy of underlying structures. The presence of a paronychia or a pale paronychia should prompt the clinician to probe the axilla and neck lymph nodes for tenderness and swelling. Beau's lines are transverse furrows that begin at the lunula and progress distally as the nail grows. They result from a temporary arrest of growth of the nail matrix occasioned by trauma or systemic stress.[11] Spoon nails (koilonychias) may occur in a form of iron deficiency anemia, coronary disease, and with the use of strong detergents.[11] Clubbing of the nails, characterized by a bulbous enlargement of the distal portion of the digits, may occur in association with cardiovascular disease, subacute endocarditis, advanced cor pulmonale, and pulmonary disease.[11]

Finger color should be observed. Fingers that are white in appearance might indicate Raynaud's disease. Blotchy or red fingers might indicate liver disease. Blue fingers may indicate a circulatory problem.

Muscle atrophy in the hand likely indicates a nerve compression syndrome. Atrophy of the thenar eminence suggests median nerve involvement, while atrophy of the hypothenar eminence suggests ulnar nerve involvement.

Active Range of Motion, Then Passive Range of Motion with Overpressure

The uninvolved wrist and hand should always be examined first. This allows for a determination of the normal function, allays the patient's anxiety, and allows for a true comparison of function.[12] The gross motions of wrist, hand, finger, and thumb flexion, extension, and radial and ulnar deviation are tested, first actively and then passively (Table 9-4). Any loss of motion compared with the contralateral, nonsymptomatic wrist and hand should be noted. Palpation may be performed with the range of motion tests or separately (refer to Palpation section).

During flexion of the fingers, the overall area of the fingers should converge to a point on the wrist corresponding to the radial pulse. This can only

TABLE 9-2 Hand and Finger Deformities and Their Possible Causes

Deformity	Possible cause
MCP joint flexion	Rupture of the extensor tendon just proximal to the MCP joint
Hyperextension of the MCP joint	Paralysis of the interossei
Deepening of the palmar gutter, and an inability to fully stretch out the palm	Tightness of the palmar aponeurosis
Wasting of the hypothenar eminence and a clawed hand with flexion of the fourth and fifth digits (Hand of benediction)	Ulnar nerve palsy
Wrist drop with increased flexion of the wrist, flexion of the MCP joint and extension of the DIP joints	Radial nerve lesion
Isolated thenar atrophy	Arthritis of the carpometacarpal joint
	Median nerve lesion
	C8, or the T1 nerve root lesion
Ape-hand deformity with a wasting of the thenar eminence, and an inability to oppose or flex the thumb or abduct it in its own plane[a]	Median nerve palsy
Z-deformity of the wrist	Pattern of deformity in the rheumatoid hand[b]
Atrophy of the hand intrinsics	Pancoast tumor
Claw hand deformity	Loss of the ulnar nerve motor innervation to the hand, with resultant paralysis of the interosseous muscles, and muscle atrophy of the hypothenar eminence. This deformity is more severe in lesions distal to innervation of the FDP muscle, as this muscle adds to the flexion force on the IP joints.[c]
PIP hyperextension and slight flexion of the DIP	Rupture or paralysis of the flexor digitorum superficialis (FDS)
A fixed flexion deformity of the MCP and proximal interphalangeal joints, especially in the ring or little finger	Dupuytren's contracture
A hook-like contracture of the flexor muscles, which is worse with wrist extension as compared to flexion	Volkmann's ischemic contracture

[a]Onieal M-E: The hand: Examination and diagnosis. In American Society for Surgery of the Hand. New York, Churchill Livingstone, 1990.
[b]Feldon P, Millender LH, Nalebuff EA: Rheumatoid arthritis in the hand and wrist. In Green DP (ed): Operative Hand Surgery, 3rd ed., pp 1587–1690. New York, Churchill Livingstone, 1993.
[c]Wadsworth CT: Anatomy of the hand and wrist. In Manual Examination and Treatment of the Spine and Extremities, pp 128–138. Baltimore, MD, Williams & Wilkins, 1988.

TABLE 9-3 Glossary of Nail Pathology

Condition	Description	Occurrence
Beau's lines	Transverse lines or ridges marking repeated disturbances of nail growth	Systemic diseases, toxic or nutritional deficiency states of many types, trauma (from manicuring)
Defluvium unguium (onychomadesis)	Complete loss of nails	Certain systemic diseases such as scarlet fever, syphilis, leprosy, alopecia areata, and exfoliative dermatitis
Diffusion of lunula unguis	"Spreading" of lunula	Dystrophies of the extremities
Eggshell nails	Nail plate thin, semitransparent bluish-white, with a tendency to curve upward at the distal edge	Syphilis
Fragilitas unguium	Friable or brittle nails	Dietary deficiency, local trauma
Hapalonychia	Nails very soft, split easily	Following contact with strong alkalis; endocrine disturbances, malnutrition, syphilis, chronic arthritis
Hippocratic nails	"Watch-glass nails associated with drumstick fingers"	Chronic respiratory and circulatory diseases, especially pulmonary tuberculosis; hepatic cirrhosis
Koilonychia	"Spoon nails"; nails are concave on the outer surface	Dysendocrinisms (acromegaly), trauma, dermatoses, syphilis, nutritional deficiencies, hypothyroidism
Leukonychia	White spots or striations or rarely the whole nail may turn white (congenital type)	Local trauma, hepatic cirrhosis, nutritional deficiencies, and many systemic diseases
Mees' lines	Transverse white bands	Hodgkin's granuloma, arsenic and thallium toxicity, high fevers, local nutritional derangement
Moniliasis of nails	Infections (usually paronychial) caused by yeast forms (Candida albicans)	Occupational (common in food-handlers, dentists, dishwashers, and gardeners)
Onychatrophia	Atrophy or failure of development of nails	Trauma, infection, dysendocrinism, gonadal aplasia, and many systemic disorders.

(*Continued*)

TABLE 9-3 Glossary of Nail Pathology (*Continued*)

Condition	Description	Occurrence
Onychauxis	Nail plate is greatly thickened	Mild persistent trauma, systemic diseases such as peripheral stasis, peripheral neuritis, syphilis, leprosy, hemiplegia, or at times may be congenital
Onychia	Inflammation of the nail matrix causing deformity of the nail plate	Trauma, infection, many systemic diseases
Onychodystrophy	Any deformity of the nail plate, nail bed, or nail matrix	Many diseases, trauma, or chemical agents (poisoning, allergy)
Onychogryposis	"Claw nails"—extreme degree of hypertrophy, sometimes with horny projections arising from the nail surface	May be congenital or related to many chronic systemic diseases (see onychauxis)
Onycholysis	Loosening of the nail plate beginning at the distal or free edge	Trauma, injury by chemical agents, many systemic diseases
Onychomadesis	Shedding of all the nails (defluvium unguium)	Dermatoses such as exfoliative dermatitis, alopecia areata, psoriasis, eczema, nail infection, severe systemic diseases, arsenic poisoning
Onychophagia	Nail biting	Neurosis
Onychorrhexis	Longitudinal ridging and splitting of the nails	Dermatoses, nail infections, many systemic diseases, senility, injury by chemical agents, hyperthyroidism
Onychoschizia	Lamination and scaling away of nails in thin layers	Dermatoses, syphilis, injury by chemical agents
Onychotillomania	Alteration of the nail structures caused by persistent neurotic picking of the nails	Neurosis
Pachyonychia	Extreme thickening of all the nails; the nails are more solid and more regular than in onychogryposis	Usually congenital and associated with hyperkeratosis of the palms and soles
Pterygium unguis	Thinning of the nail fold and spreading of the cuticle over the nail plate	Associated with vasospastic conditions such as Raynaud's phenomenon and occasionally with hypothyroidism

Sources: Berry TJ: The Hand as a Mirror of Systemic Disease, pp 179–191. Philadelphia, PA, FA Davis, 1963.
Judge RD, Zuidema GD, Fitzgerald FT: General appearance. In Judge RD, Zuidema GD, Fitzgerald FT (eds): Clinical Diagnosis, 4th ed., pp 29–47. Boston, MA, Little, Brown, 1982.

TABLE 9-4 Active Range of Motion Norms for the Forearm, Wrist, and Hand

Motion	Degrees
Forearm pronation	85–90
Forearm supination	85–90
Radial deviation	15–25
Ulnar deviation	30–45
Wrist flexion	80–90
Wrist extension	70–90
Finger flexion	MCP: 85–90; PIP: 100–115; DIP: 80–90
Finger extension	MCP: 30–45; PIP: 0; DIP: 20
Finger abduction	20–30
Finger adduction	0
Thumb flexion	CMC: 45–50; MCP: 50–55; IP: 85–90
Thumb extension	MCP: 0; IP: 0–5
Thumb adduction	30
Thumb abduction	60–70

occur if the index finger flexes in a sagittal plane and all the others in an increasing oblique plane. Malrotation is a rotary malalignment that can be seen in phalangeal or metacarpal fractures with this maneuver, as the involved finger will not converge with the others.[6] A skyline view of the knuckles is made. In full flexion, a dorsally subluxed capitate may be seen as a local swelling on the back and middle of the flexed wrist.

During measurement of motion, one must be aware that finger joint positions may affect wrist joint ranges (and vice versa) because of the constant length of the extrinsic tendons that cross multiple joints. For example, greater wrist flexion occurs with finger extension than with finger flexion because the extensor digitorum tendons are not stretched maximally. Thus, during the examination, the clinician should maintain all joints in a consistent position (usually neutral), except the one being measured. In addition, the clinician should identify wrist and finger joint position when measuring the strength of related muscles.

Fanning and folding of the hand is performed by palpating the palmar surface of the pisiform, scaphoid, hamate and trapezium with the index and middle fingers, and the dorsal surface of the capitate with the thumbs as the hand is alternately fanned and folded. During these motions, the clinician should note the quantity and quality of the conjunct rotations.

During active and passive testing, the presence of crepitus must be determined. The presence of crepitus with motion may indicate a tendon sheath synovitis or vaginitis.

Wrist

Pronation and supination of the wrist on the forearm will provisionally test the triangular fibrocartilage complex (TFCC), and the proximal and distal radioulnar joints. Full forced pronation–supination without evoking pain, essentially eliminates the distal radioulnar joint (DRUJ) and the TFCC as potential sources of the patient's complaints.[13]

Wrist flexion, extension, (Figure 9-2) ulnar deviation, and radial deviation (Figure 9-3) are assessed. Wrist extension can be tested bilaterally by asking the patient to place the palms together and then to lift up the elbows. Normal range for wrist extension is approximately 75°. Wrist flexion is

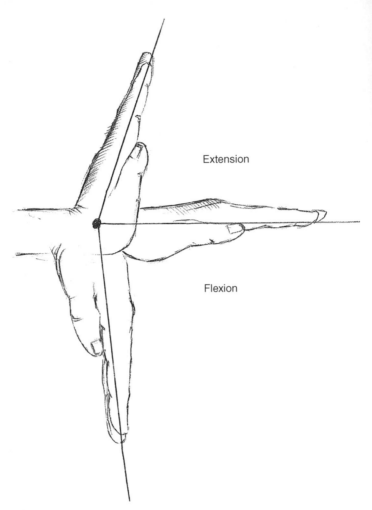

FIG. 9-2   Wrist flexion and extension.

tested bilaterally by asking the patient to place the dorsal aspect of the hand together and then dropping the elbows. Normal range for wrist flexion is approximately 85°. According to Watson,[13] any loss of passive wrist flexion is a sign of underlying organic carpal pathology. Radial and ulnar deviation are also assessed. Normal range for ulnar deviation is approximately 35°. Radial deviation should be tested in three positions: forearm pronation, forearm supination, and neutral. Normal range for radial deviation is approximately 20°.

If the single plane motions do not provoke symptoms, combined motions can be used. These include combining wrist extension with ulnar and then radial deviation, and combining wrist flexion with ulnar and radial deviation.

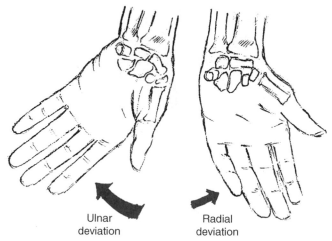

Ulnar
deviation

Radial
deviation

FIG. 9-3   Radial and ulnar deviation.

Thumb

The following motions are tested in varying degrees of wrist flexion and extension:

- First carpometacarpal (CMC) abduction, adduction, flexion, extension, opposition. During opposition (Figure 9-4), the clinician should observe for the conjunct rotation component of the motion.
- First metacarpophalangeal (MCP) (Figure 9-5), and interphalangeal (IP) flexion and extension (Figure 9-6).

Fingers

It should never be assumed that lack of full active flexion or extension of the proximal interphalangeal (PIP) is merely secondary to joint pain or fusion, because closed rupture of the middle slip of the extensor hood is easily missed until the appearance of a boutonniere deformity.[14] Total active motion of the fingers is the sum of all angles formed by the MCP, PIP, and distal interphalangeal (DIP) joints in simultaneous maximum active flexion, minus the total extension deficit at the MCP, PIP, and DIP joints (including hyperextension at the IP joints) in maximum active extension.

A normal value for total active range of motion in the absence of a normal contralateral digit for comparison is 260°, based on 85° of MCP flexion, 110° of PIP motion, and 65° of DIP motion.[15]

A comparison of active and passive motion indicates the efficiency of flexor and extensor excursion and/or degree of muscle strength within the available passive range of motion.[15] Instances of greater passive than active motion may indicate a limited tendon glide due to adherence of the tendon to surrounding structures, relative lengthening of the tendon caused by injury or surgery, weakness or pain.[15]

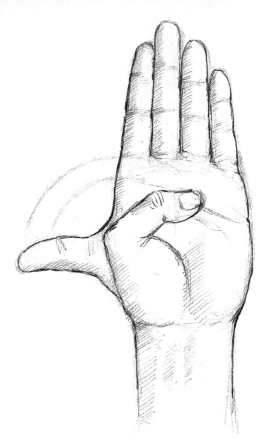

FIG. 9-4 Thumb opposition.

Due to the multitude of joints and multiarticular muscles found in the hand, the clinician may need to differentiate between various structures to determine the cause of a motion restriction. The soft tissue structures that may contribute to a motion restriction include:[15]

- *Hand intrinsics.* The Bunnell-Littler test is used to determine whether flexion restriction of the PIP is caused by tightness of the intrinsic muscles, or a restriction of the MCP joint capsule. The MCP joint is held by the clinician in a few degrees of extension with one hand, while the other hand attempts to flex the PIP joint. If the joint cannot flex, tightness of the intrinsics or a joint capsular contraction should be suspected.[16] From this position, the clinician now slightly flexes the MCP joint, thereby relaxing the intrinsics, and attempts to flex the PIP joint. If the joint can now flex, the intrinsics are tight. If the joint still cannot flex then restriction is probably caused by a capsular contraction of the joint. This test is also called the intrinsic-plus test.[17]
- *Oblique retinacular (Landsmeer's) ligament.* The Haines-Zancolli test is used to determine whether restricted flexion in the DIP joints is caused by

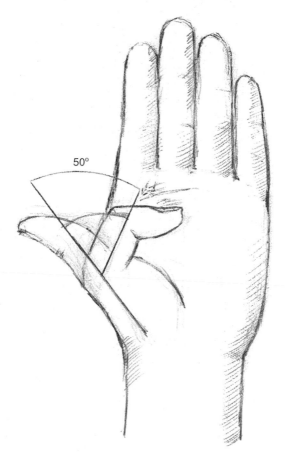

50°

FIG. 9-5   Flexion and extension of the first MCP joint.

a restriction of the PIP joint capsule, or tightness of the oblique retinacular ligament. The test for a contracture of this ligament is the same as the Bunnell-Littler test, only at the PIP and DIP joints. The clinician positions and holds the PIP joint in a neutral position with one hand, and attempts to flex the DIP joint with the other hand. If no flexion is possible, it can be a result of either a tight retinacular ligament or capsular contraction. The PIP joint is then slightly flexed to relax the retinacular ligament. If the DIP can now flex, the restriction is because of tightness in the retinacular ligament. If the DIP cannot flex then the restriction is because of a capsular contraction.

- *Extrinsic flexor and extensor tendons.* Adherence of the extrinsic flexors is tested by passively maintaining the fingers and thumb in full extension while passively extending the wrist. In the presence of flexor tightness, the increasing flexor tension that develops as the wrist is passively extended will pull the fingers into flexion. Adherence of the extensor tendons is simply a reverse process. The digits are passively maintained in full flexion,

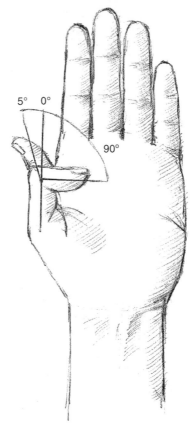

FIG. 9-6 Flexion and extension of the first IP joint.

while the wrist is passively flexed. If tension pulling the fingers into extension is detected by the clinician's hand as the wrist is brought into flexion, extrinsic extensor tightness exists.

Functional Screen

A number of motions can be used to quickly assess hand function, including:

- Opposition of the thumb and little finger
- Pad to pad mobility of thumb and other fingers. The majority of the functional activities of the hand require at least 5 centimeters of opening of the fingers and thumb.[18]
- The ability to make three different fists:
  - The hook fist (placing fingertips onto MCP joint)
  - Standard fist
  - Straight fist (placing fingertips on the thenar and hypothenar eminences). The ability to flex the fingers to within 1–2 centimeters of the distal palmar crease is an indication of functional range of motion for many hand activities.[18]

Palpation

Palpation of the following muscles, tendon, insertions, ligaments, capsules, and bones should occur *as indicated*, and be compared with the uninvolved side. Clinically important information about the course of the hand nerves can be provided using the cardinal line, which is an imaginary line drawn from the apex of the thumb-index web space across the palm parallel to the proximal palmar crease:[6,19]

- The radial borderline is drawn along the radial border of the long finger and intersects the cardinal line at the point where the motor branch of the median nerve enters the thenar musculature.
- The point where the thenar crease intersects the cardinal line is approximately over the point where the motor branch emerges from the median nerve.
- A line drawn between the two points of intersection described above approximates the course of the superficial nerve.
- A line drawn from the intersection of the cardinal line and the radial border of the index finger palmar digital crease approximates the course of the radial digital nerve to the index finger.
- The ulnar borderline is drawn along the ulnar border of the ring finger. It intersects the cardinal line over the hook of the hamate. A line drawn from this intersection to the ulnar border of the little finger palmar digital crease overlies the course of the ulnar digital nerve to the little finger

Radial Styloid Process

The radial styloid process (Figure 9-7) is larger and rounder than the ulnar styloid process. It is located at the most proximal point of the anatomic snuffbox (see below), during radial abduction of the thumb. With simultaneous radial deviation of the wrist, this prominence becomes visible. Tenderness over the styloid, especially with radial deviation, may indicate contusion, fracture, or radioscaphoid arthritis.[20]

Scaphoid

The scaphoid is palpated just distal to the radial styloid in the anatomic snuffbox (see Figure 9-7). The neck of the scaphoid is located on the floor of the anatomic snuffbox. Palpation can be made easier by positioning the wrist in ulnar deviation. The scaphoid may be grasped and moved passively, by firm pressure between an opposed index finger and thumb applied to the palmar surface and anatomic snuffbox simultaneously. In most individuals, the scaphoid is mildly tender to palpation, but those with scaphoid fracture, nonunion, or scaphoid instability have severe discomfort (see *Special Tests*).[13,21]

Trapezium

The trapezium is located immediately proximal to the base of the first metacarpal bone, just distal to the scaphoid (see Figure 9-7). The tubercle of the trapezium lies anteriorly at the base of the thenar eminence. It can be made more prominent by opposing the thumb to the little finger, and ulnarly deviating the wrist. Tenderness over this carpal may indicate scaphotrapezial arthritis secondary to scaphoid instability.[22]

Thumb CMC Joint

To examine the thumb CMC joint, the clinician palpates carefully along the shaft of the thumb metacarpal down to its proximal flair. Just proximal to this flair is a small depression where the CMC joint is located. By applying direct

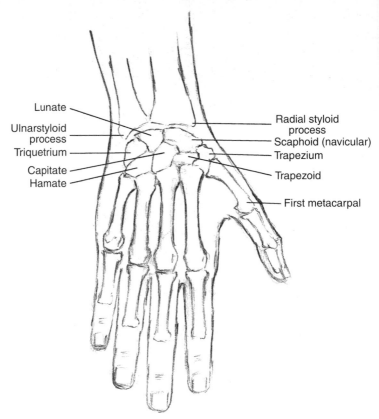

FIG. 9-7   Palpation points.

radial and ulnar stresses to the joint, the clinician can determine the overall stability of the joint, as compared to the other thumb. Tenderness here is usually indicative of degenerative arthritis.

EPB and APL Tendons

The extensor pollicis brevis (EPB) and abductor pollicis longus (APL) tendons make up the first extensor compartment on the dorsum of the wrist, and together form the radial border of the anatomic snuffbox. Extending and radially abducting the thumb can enhance prominence of these tendons. Tenderness over these tendons may indicate De Quervain's tenosynovitis.

Lister's Tubercle

This is a small bony prominence on the dorsal and distal end of radius. It is found by sliding a finger proximally from a point between the index and middle finger. Just distal to the Lister's tubercle is the joint line of the scaphoid and radius. The extensor carpi radialis longus (ECRL) and extensor carpi radialis brevis (ECRB) tendons travel radial to Lister's tubercle, and insert on the base of the second and third metacarpals. The extensor digitorum communis (EDC) tendon travels ulnar to Lister's tubercle.

Lunate

The lunate is located just distal and ulnar to Lister's tubercle with the wrist flexed, and is immediately proximal to, and in line with, the capitate (see Figure 9-7). The mobile lunate can be felt to glide dorsally with extension. It is the most commonly dislocated carpal and the scapholunate articulation is the most common area for carpal instability. Scapholunate synovitis (dorsal wrist syndrome) or a scapholunate ligament injury presents with tenderness or fullness in this region.[13] Tenderness specific to the lunate can indicate Kienböck's disease or avascular necrosis of the lunate.[23,24]

Capitate

The capitate (see Figure 9-7) is palpated proximally over the dorsal aspect of the third metacarpal until a small depression is felt. While palpating in this depression, as the wrist is flexed, the clinician should feel the capitate, the central bone of the carpus, move dorsally. Tenderness in this depression may indicate scapholunate or lunotriquetral instability, or capitolunate degenerative joint disease.

Second and Third Metacarpals

The base of the second and third metacarpals and the CMC joints are localized by palpating proximally along the dorsal surfaces of the index and long metacarpals to their respective bases.[8] A bony prominence found at the base of the second or third metacarpal may be a carpal boss, a variation found in some individuals as a result of hypertrophic changes of traumatic origin.[8]

Ulnar Head and Styloid Process

The ulnar head forms a rounded prominence on the ulnar side of the wrist, which is easily palpated with the forearm in pronation (see Figure 9-7).[8] The ulnar styloid process is ulnar, and distal, to the head of the ulna. It is best located with the forearm in supination.

Triangular Fibrocartilage Complex

The TFCC is located distal to the ulnar styloid, and proximal to the triquetrum. Tenderness over this structure indicates an injury to the TFCC.[12]

Hamate

The hook of the hamate is palpated just distal and radial (in the direction of the thumb web space) to the pisiform on the palmar aspect (see Figure 9-7). Locating the hamate can be made easier if the clinician places the middle of the distal phalanx of the thumb on the pisiform, with the thumb pointing between the web space between the index and long finger. Tenderness over this carpal is common, and so the clinician should compare findings with the other side. Severe tenderness could indicate a fracture of the hamate, especially if associated with a fall on the outstretched hand (FOOSH injury) or a missed hit swing of a racket or bat.[25]

Triquetrum

The triquetrum is located by radially deviating the wrist while palpating just distal to the ulnar styloid (see Figure 9-7). With ulnar deviation, the triquetrum articulates with the TFCC, which functions as a buffer between the styloid and the triquetrum. Tenderness and swelling in the triquetral hamate region are often present with midcarpal instability, which occurs when the palmar triquetral-hamate-capitate ligament is ruptured or sprained.[26]

Pisiform

The pisiform is located on the flexor aspect of the palm, on top of triquetrum, at the distal crease (Figure 9-8). Tenderness of this structure indicates pisotriquetral arthritis or inflammation of the flexor carpi ulnaris tendon.[12]

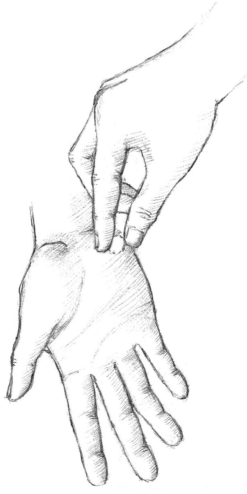

FIG. 9-8   Palpating the pisiform.

Tunnel of Guyon

The tunnel of Guyon is located in the space between the hamate and pisiform.[27] This tunnel serves as a passageway for the ulnar nerve and artery into the hand.

Carpal Tunnel

The distal wrist crease marks the proximal edge of the carpal tunnel. The boundaries of the carpal tunnel are:

- *Radial.* Palmar scaphoid tubercle and trapezium
- *Ulnar.* Pisiform and hamate
- *Dorsal.* The carpal bones
- *Palmar.* Transverse carpal ligament
- *Proximal.* Palmar antebrachial fascia
- *Distal.* Distal edge of retinaculum at CMC level, flexor carpi radialis (FCR), and scaphoid tubercle

Flexor Retinaculum

The flexor retinaculum transforms the carpal arch into the carpal tunnel. It is attached laterally to the tubercle of the scaphoid and tubercle of the trapezium, and attached medially to the pisiform and hook of the hamate. Its proximal edge is at the distal crease of the wrist.

Metacarpophalangeal Joint

The MCP joint lies distal to the palmar digital crease over the proximal phalanx in an imaginary line connecting the radial aspect of the proximal palmar crease to the ulnar aspect of the distal palmar crease.

Proximal Interphalangeal Joints

The PIP crease approximates the level of the PIP joint. Palpation of the PIP joint offers important information. Palpation of the joint over four planes (dorsal, palmar, medial, lateral) allows assessment of point tenderness over ligamentous origins and insertions that is highly suggestive of underlying soft-tissue disruption.[14] In cases in which the joint is grossly swollen and tender, this part of the examination may provide more accurate information several days after the injury.[14]

Distal Interphalangeal Joint

The DIP crease is just proximal to the level of the PIP joint.

Pain Provocation Tests

Radioulnar Ballottement Test

The radioulnar ballottement test is used to assess distal radioulnar joint instability. The patient's elbow is flexed and the clinician uses his or her thumb and index finger to stabilize the radius radially and the ulnar head ulnarly (Figure 9-9). Stress is applied in an anterior-posterior direction. Normally there is no movement in the anterior or posterior direction in maximum supination or pronation. Pain or mobility with this test is suggestive of radioulnar instability.

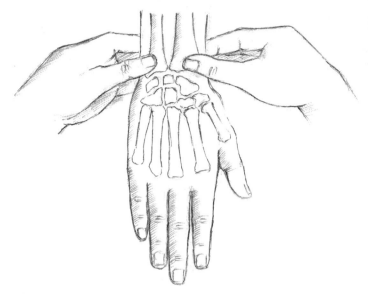

FIG. 9-9 Radioulnar ballottement test.

Pain with Wrist Flexion

To determine whether a painful wrist flexion is caused by a problem between scaphoid and radius, or scaphoid and the trapezium and trapezoid, the wrist is placed in full flexion, with the dorsal surface of the hand resting on the treatment table. The clinician pushes on the scaphoid and second metacarpal in a dorsal direction. An increase in pain with this maneuver may indicate a problem at the scaphoid-radius articulation.

If there is no increase in pain with this maneuver, the wrist is placed in a neutral position with regard to flexion and extension. The clinician stabilizes the trapezium and trapezoid, and pushes the scaphoid dorsally. An increase in pain with this maneuver may indicate a problem at the trapezium/trapezoid-scaphoid articulation.

To determine whether the painful wrist flexion is caused by a problem between the capitate and the lunate, or the lunate and the radius, the wrist is placed in full flexion. The clinician pushes the lunate in palmar direction. An increase in pain with this maneuver may indicate a problem at the capitate–lunate articulation. If the pain is not increased with this maneuver, the wrist is placed in full flexion and the clinician pushes the lunate in a dorsal direction. An increase in pain with this maneuver may indicate a problem at the lunate–radius articulation. A decrease in pain with this maneuver may indicate a problem at the capitate–lunate articulation.

Pain with Wrist Extension

To determine whether the pain with wrist extension is caused by a problem between the scaphoid and the radius, or the scaphoid and the trapezium/trapezoid, the wrist is positioned in full extension with the palm positioned on the table. The clinician pushes on the radius in a palmar direction thus increasing the amount of wrist extension. An increase in pain with this maneuver may indicate a problem at the scaphoid-radius articulation. If this maneuver does not increase pain, the wrist is positioned as before. The clinician now pushes on the radius in a dorsal direction. A decrease in pain with this maneuver may indicate a problem at the scaphoid-radius articulation. An increase in pain with this maneuver may indicate a problem at the scaphoid and trapezium/trapezoid articulation.

Placing the wrist as before in full extension and pushing on the scaphoid in a dorsal direction confirm this. A decrease in pain with this maneuver indicates a problem between the scaphoid and radius, whereas an increase in pain with this maneuver indicates the problem is between the scaphoid and the trapezium/trapezoid.

The clinician fixes the scaphoid and pushes the trapezium/trapezoid in a palmar direction. A decrease in pain with this maneuver may indicate a problem at the scaphoid–trapezium/trapezoid articulation. If the pain remains unchanged with this maneuver, the problem is likely to be at the scaphoid–radius articulation. To confirm this hypothesis, the scaphoid can be pushed in a palmar direction while the wrist is maintained in the position of full extension. This should increase the pain if the hypothesis is correct.

To determine whether pain is caused by a problem between capitate and lunate, or the lunate and radius, the wrist is positioned in full extension, with the palm of the hand on the table. The clinician pushes on the radius in a palmar direction. An increase in pain with this maneuver indicates a problem at the capitate–lunate articulation.

If pushing the lunate and capitate in a palmar direction increases the pain, this may indicate a problem at the lunate–radius articulation.

If fixing the lunate and pushing the capitate in a palmar direction (a relative motion of the lunate dorsally in relation to the capitate) increases the pain, the problem is likely at the capitate–lunate articulation.

Thumb CMC Grind Test

The grind test is used to assess the integrity of the thumb CMC joint by axially loading the thumb metacarpal into the trapezium.[28,29] The clinician grasps the thumb metacarpal using the thumb and index finger on one hand, and the proximal aspect of the thumb CMC joint with the other hand. An axial compressive force, combined with rotation, is applied to the thumb CMC joint. Reproduction of the patient's pain, and crepitus, is a positive test for arthrosis and synovitis.

Lichtman Test

The Lichtman test is a provocative test for midcarpal instability.[28] The patient's forearm is positioned in pronation and the hand is held relaxed and supported by the clinician. The clinician gently moves the patient's hand from radial to ulnar deviation while compressing the carpus into the radius. A positive test is when the midcarpal row appears to "jump" or "snap" from a palmarly subluxed position to the height of the proximal row.[28]

Linscheid Test

The Linscheid test is used to detect ligamentous injury and instability of the second and third CMC joints. The metacarpal shafts are supported and the metacarpal heads are then pressed distally in a palmar and dorsal direction.[8] A positive test produces pain localized to the CMC joints.[30]

Scapholunate Provocation Tests

Scapholunate Shear (Ballottement) Test   The patient is positioned in sitting with his or her forearm pronated. With one hand, the clinician places an index finger on the scaphoid tuberosity and the thumb on the dorsal aspect of the scaphoid (Figure 9-10). With the other hand, the clinician grasps the lunate between the thumb and index finger. The lunate and scaphoid are then sheared in a palmar and then dorsal direction.[13] Laxity and reproduction of the patient's pain are positive signs for this test.[28]

Watson's Test (Scaphoid Shift) for Carpal Instability   As the scaphoid plays a critical role in coordinating and stabilizing movements between the proximal and distal rows of the carpals, damage to the intrinsic and extrinsic ligaments that support the scaphoid can result in persistent pain and dysfunction with loading activities.[22,31,32]

The scaphoid shift maneuver examines the dynamic stability of the wrist, in particular the integrity of the scapholunate ligament.[22]

The patient is positioned with his or her elbow resting in the lap in approximately 90° of flexion. The forearm slightly pronated, and the wrist ulnarly deviated. The clinician stabilizes the scaphoid tubercle with the thumb (Figure 9-11). As the wrist is brought passively into radial deviation, the normal flexion of the proximal row forces the scaphoid tubercle into a palmar direction (into the clinician's thumb). The clinician attempts to prevent the palmar motion of the scaphoid. When the scaphoid is unstable, its proximal

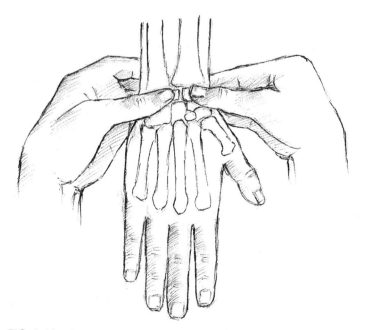

FIG. 9-10   Scapholunate shear (ballottement) test.

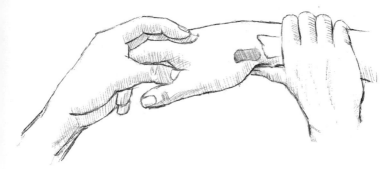

FIG. 9-11   Watson's test.

pole is forced to sublux dorsally (Figure 9-12).[28] Pain at the dorsal wrist or a clunk suggests instability.[33,34] The results are compared with the other hand.

The results from the scaphoid shift test should be used with caution as the test can be positive in up to one-third of uninjured individuals,[31] and has been found to have a sensitivity of 69%, and a specificity of 64–68%.[35,36]

Finger Extension Test   This test is used to demonstrate dorsal wrist syndrome, a localized scapholunate synovitis.[22] The clinician instructs the patient to fully flex the wrist, and then actively extend the digits at both the IP and MCP joints. The clinician then applies pressure on the fingers into flexion at the MCP joints while the patient continues to actively extend (Figure 9-13). A positive test occurs when there is production of central dorsal wrist pain and indicates the possibility of Kienböck's disease, carpal instability, joint degeneration or synovitis.[28]

Strength Testing

The muscles of the forearm, wrist, and hand are detailed in Table 9-5. Isometric tests are carried out in the extreme range, and if positive, in the neutral range. These isometric tests must include the interossei and lumbricales. The straight plane motions of wrist flexion, extension, ulnar, and radial deviation are tested initially. Pain with any of these tests requires a more thorough examination of the individual muscles.

Wrist

Flexor Carpi Radialis/Flexor Carpi Ulnaris   During the testing of these muscles, substitution by the finger flexors should be avoided by having patient not make a fist. The clinician applies the resistive force into extension and radial deviation for the flexor carpi ulnaris (FCU), and extension and ulnar deviation for the FCR.

Extensor Carpi Radialis Longus/Brevis   Any action of the EDC should be ruled out by having the patient make a fist while extending the wrist. The clinician applies the resistive force on the dorsum of the second and third metacarpals with the force directed into flexion and ulnar deviation.

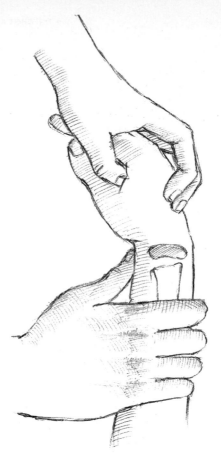

FIG. 9-12   Watson's test showing dorsally subluxed scaphoid.

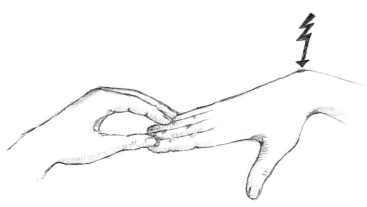

FIG. 9-13   Finger extension test.

TABLE 9-5 Muscles of the Forearm, Wrist, and Hand: Their Actions, Nerve Supply, and Nerve Root Derivation

Action	Muscles acting	Nerve supply
Forearm supination	Supinator	Posterior interosseous
	Biceps brachii	Musculocutaneous
Forearm pronation	Pronator quadratus	Anterior interosseous
	Pronator teres	Median
	Flexor carpi radialis	Median
Wrist extension	Extensor carpi radialis longus	Radial
	Extensor carpi radialis brevis	Posterior interosseous
	Extensor carpi ulnaris	Posterior interosseous
Wrist flexion	Flexor carpi radialis	Median
	Flexor carpi ulnaris	Ulnar
Ulnar deviation of wrist	Flexor carpi ulnaris	Ulnar
	Extensor carpi ulnaris	Posterior interosseous
Radial deviation of wrist	Flexor carpi radialis	Median
	Extensor carpi radialis longus	Radial
	Abductor pollicis longus	Posterior interosseous
	Extensor pollicis brevis	Posterior interosseous
Finger extension	Extensor digitorum communis	Posterior interosseous
	Extensor indices	Posterior interosseous
	Extensor digiti minimi	Posterior interosseous
Finger flexion	Flexor digitorum profundus	Anterior interosseous— lateral two digits Ulnar—medial two digits
	Flexor digitorum superficialis	Median
	Lumbricals	First and second: Median Third and fourth: Ulnar
	Interossei	Ulnar
	Flexor digiti minimi	Ulnar
Abduction of fingers	Dorsal interossei	Ulnar
	Abductor digiti minimi	Ulnar
Adduction of fingers	Palmar interossei	Ulnar
Thumb extension	Extensor pollicis longus	Posterior interosseous
	Extensor pollicis brevis	Posterior interosseous
	Abductor pollicis longus	Posterior interosseous
Thumb flexion	Flexor pollicis brevis	Superficial head: Median Deep head ulnar
Abduction of thumb	Flexor pollicis longus	Anterior interosseous
	Opponens pollicis	Median
	Abductor pollicis longus	Posterior interosseous
Adduction of thumb	Abductor pollicis brevis	Median
	Adductor pollicis	Ulnar
Opposition of thumb and little finger	Opponens pollicis	Median
	Flexor pollicis brevis	Superficial head: Median
	Abductor pollicis brevis	Median
	Opponens digiti minimi	Ulnar

Source: Magee DJ (ed): Orthopedic Physical Assessment. Philadelphia, PA, WB Saunders, 2002.

Extensor Carpi Ulnaris   Having patient make a fist in wrist extension, and the clinician applying the resistance on the ulnar dorsum of hand, with the force directed into flexion and radial deviation, tests the extensor carpi ulnaris (ECU).

Thumb

Abductor Pollicis Longus/Brevis   The forearm is positioned midway between pronation and supination, or in maximal supination. The MCP and IP joints are positioned in flexion. The muscles are tested with palmar abduction of the thumb in the frontal plane for the longus and in the sagittal plane for the brevis.

Opponens Pollicis   The forearm is positioned in supination and the dorsal aspect of the hand rests on the table. The patient is asked to tough the finger pads of the thumb and little finger together. Using one hand, the clinician stabilizes the first and fifth metacarpals and palm of the hand. With the other hand, the clinician applies a force in the opposite direction of opposition to the distal end of the first metacarpal.

Flexor Pollicis Longus/Brevis   The forearm is positioned in supination and supported by the table, and the hand is positioned so that the dorsal aspect rests on a table. The thumb is adducted. Applying resistance to the distal phalanx tests the longus, whereas resistance applied to the proximal phalanx tests both heads of the brevis.

Adductor Pollicis   This muscle is tested by having the patient hold a piece of paper between the thumb and radial aspect of the index finger's proximal phalanx while the clinician attempts to remove it. If weak or nonfunctioning, the IP joint of thumb flexes during this maneuver due to substitution by the flexor digitorum profundus (FDP) (Froment's sign).

Extensor Pollicis Longus/Brevis   Both of these muscles can be tested with the patient's hand flat on the table, palm down, and asking the patient to lift only the thumb off the table. To test each individually, resistance is applied to the dorsal aspect of the distal phalanx for the extensor pollicis longus (EPL), while stabilizing the proximal phalanx and metacarpal, and to the dorsal aspect of the proximal phalanx for the EPB while stabilizing the first metacarpal.

Intrinsics

Lumbricals   The four lumbricals are tested by applying resistance to the dorsal surface of the middle and distal phalanges, while stabilizing under the proximal phalanx of the finger being tested.

Palmar Interossei   The palmar and dorsal interossei act with the lumbricals to achieve MCP flexion coupled with PIP and DIP extension. The three palmar interossei also adduct the second, fourth, and fifth fingers to midline. Resistance is applied by the clinician to the radial aspect of the distal end of the proximal phalanx of the second, fourth, and fifth fingers, after first stabilizing the hand and fingers not being tested.

Dorsal Interossei/Abductor Digiti Minimi   The four dorsal interossei abduct the second, third, and fourth fingers from midline. The abductor digiti minimi abducts the fifth finger from midline.

The intrinsic muscles are tested in the frontal plane to avoid substitution by the extrinsic flexors and extensors. Resistance is applied by the clinician to the ulnar aspect of the distal end of the proximal phalanx of each of the four fingers, after first stabilizing the hand and fingers not being tested.

Fingers

Flexor Digitorum Profundus   This muscle is tested with DIP flexion of each digit, while the MCP and PIP are stabilized in extension and wrist neutral. Due to the variability of nerve innervation for this muscle group, each of the fingers can be tested to determine if a peripheral nerve lesion is present. The anterior interosseous nerve provides the nerve supply to the index finger, the main branch of the median nerve serves the middle finger, and the ulnar nerve serves the ring and little finger.

Flexor Digitorum Superficialis   There is normally one muscle tendon unit for each finger; however, an absent flexor digitorum superficialis (FDS) to the little finger is common. The clinician should only allow the finger to be tested to flex, by firmly blocking all joints of the nontested fingers, and wrist in neutral.

Extensor Digitorum/Extensor Indices Proprius/EDM   There is only one muscle belly for this four-tendon unit. These three muscles are the sole MCP joint extensors. With the wrist in neutral, the strength is tested with the metacarpals in extension and the PIP/DIP flexed. The extensor indices proprius (EIP) is isolated by positioning the index finger and hand, in the "number one" position—the index finger in extension with other fingers clenched in a fist. The extensor digiti minimi (EDM) is tested with resistance of little finger extension with the other fingers maintained in a fist.

To isolate intrinsic muscle function, the patient is asked to actively extend the MCP joint and then to attempt actively extend the PIP joint. Because the ED (extensor digitorum), EI, and EDM tendons are "anchored" at the MCP joint by active extension, only the intrinsic muscles can now extend the PIP joint. To test the terminal extensor tendon function, the clinician stabilizes the middle phalanx and asks the patient to extend the DIP joint.[10]

Flexor Digiti Minimi   The forearm is positioned in supination and the dorsal aspect of the hand rests on the table. The clinician stabilizes the fifth metacarpal and the palm with one hand, and then applies resistance to the palmar surface of the proximal phalanx of the fifth digit with the other hand.

Opponens Digit Minimi   The forearm is positioned in supination and the dorsal aspect of the hand rests on the table. The patient is asked to tough the finger pads of the thumb and little finger together. Using one hand, the clinician stabilizes the first and fifth metacarpals and palm of the hand. With the other hand, the clinician applies a force in the opposite direction of opposition to the distal end of the fifth metacarpal.

Grip Strength

A patient's grip strength is commonly used to assess hand function. A number of protocols using a sealed hydraulic dynamometer, such as the Jamar dynamometer (Asimow Engineering Co., Santa Monica, CA), have been shown to be accurate, reliable, and valid in measuring grip strength.[37]

It is probably wise to combine the results of different grip strength tests before making any decisions.[38]

The assessment of pinch strength is also used to assess function of the hand, using a pinch meter. Average values for the pulp-to-pulp pinch of each finger with the thumb are provided in Chapter 16 of *Orthopaedic Examination, Evaluation, and Intervention*.

Functional Assessment

The *functional position* of the wrist is the position in which optimal function is likely to occur.[39,40] This position involves wrist extension of between 20° and 35°, ulnar deviation of 10–15°, slight flexion of all the finger joints, midrange thumb opposition, and slight flexion of the thumb MCP and IP joints.[39] In this position, which minimizes the restraining action of the long extensor tendons, the pulps of the index finger and thumb are in contact.

The *functional range of motion* for the hand is the range in which the hand can perform most of its grip and other functional activities (Table 9-6).

The percentage losses of digital function are as follows: thumb, 40% to 50%; index finger, 20%; long finger, 20%; ring finger, 10%; little finger, 5%. Loss of the hand is 90% of the upper extremity and 54% of the whole person.[1]

Hand Disability Index[41]

The patient is asked to rate the following seven questions on a 0–3 scale, with 3 being the most difficult.

Unable to perform task = 0
Able to complete task partially = 1
Able to complete task but with difficulty = 2
Able to perform task normally = 3

TABLE 9-6 Functional Range of Motion of the Hand and Wrist[1–7]

Joint motion	Functional range of motion (degrees)
Wrist flexion	5–40
Wrist extension	30–40
Radial deviation	10–20
Ulnar deviation	15–20
MCP flexion	60
PIP flexion	60
DIP flexion	40
Thumb MCP flexion	20

Sources: Blair SJ, McCormick E, Bear-Lehman J, et al.: Evaluation of impairment of the upper extremity. Clin Orthop 1987;221:42–58.
Brumfield RH, Champoux JA: A biomechanical study of normal functional wrist motion. Clin Orth Rel Res 1984;187:23–25.
Palmer AK, Werner FW, Murphy D, et al.: Functional wrist motion: A biomechanical study. J Hand Surg 1985;10A:39–46.
Ryu J, Cooney WP, Askew LJ, et al.: Functional ranges of motion of the wrist joint. J Hand Surg 1991;16A:409–420.

Are you able to:

Dress yourself, including tying shoelaces and doing buttons?
Cut your meat?
Lift a full cup or glass to your mouth?
Prepare your own meal?
Open car doors?
Open jars that have previously been opened?
Turn taps on and off?

A variety of evaluation tools have been devised for the hand, which can be categorized into assessments of the neurovascular system, range of motion, sensibility, and function (see *Orthopaedic Examination, Evaluation, and Intervention*, pp 621–629).[18]

Grip and pinch measurements were outlined under *Grip Strength*. Dexterity tests include the following:

- *Minnesota rate of manipulation (MRMT)*. This test, which primarily measures gross coordination and dexterity, consists of five functions:

  1. Placing
  2. Turning
  3. Displacing
  4. One-hand turning and placing
  5. Two-hand turning and placing

  The activities are timed and compared with the time taken by the other hand, and then compared with normal values.[18,42]

- *Jebsen-Taylor hand-function test:*[43] This test, which requires the least amount of extremity coordination, measures prehension and manipulative skills, consists of seven subtests:

  a. Writing
  b. Card turning
  c. Picking up small objects
  d. Simulated feeding
  e. Stacking
  f. Picking up large, light objects
  g. Picking up large, heavy objects

  The subtests are timed and compared with the time taken by the other hand. The results are compared with normal values.[18,42]

- *Nine-hole peg test*. This assessed was designed to assess finger dexterity of each hand.[44] The patient is asked to use one hand to place nine 3.2-centimeter (1.3-inch) pegs in a 12.7 × 12.7 centimeter (5 × 5 inch) board, and is then asked to remove them. The task is timed and compared with the time taken by the other hand. The results are compared with normal values.[18,42]

- *Purdue pegboard test*.[45,46] This test evaluates finer coordination, requiring prehension of small objects, with measurement categories divided into:

  1. Right hand
  2. Left hand
  3. Both hands
  4. Right, left, and both hands
  5. Assembly

The subtests are timed and compared with normal values based on gender and occupation.[18,42]

- *Crawford small parts dexterity (CSPD) test.*[47] The CSPD test involves the use of tweezers and a screwdriver, and requires patients to control not only their hands, but also small tools. This test correlates positively with vocational activities that demand fine coordination skills.[18]

The problem with most of these tests and others is that the critical measure of function used is time, even though time is not an accurate measure of function.

Although not standardized, a few other simple tests can be used to assess hand dexterity. These include writing in a straight line, buttoning and unbuttoning different sized buttons, and zipping and unzipping using a variety of zipper sizes. The following scale can be used to grade these activities:

Unable to perform task = 0
Able to complete task partially = 1
Able to complete task but with difficulty = 2
Able to perform task normally = 3

Passive Physiologic Mobility Testing

In the following tests, the patient is positioned in sitting, and the clinician is standing/sitting, facing the patient. In each of the tests, the clinician notes the quantity of motion as well as the joint reaction. The tests are always repeated on, and compared to, the same joint in the opposite extremity. The closed and open packed positions of the wrist and hand are outlined in Table 9-7.

Wrist

Using one hand, the clinician palpates and stabilizes the distal aspect of the forearm, while using the other hand to grasp the patient's hand, distal to the wrist.

Flexion/Extension   The carpal bones are flexed and extended about the appropriate coronal axis through the midcarpal and radiocarpal joints.

Radial/Ulnar Deviation   The clinician radially and ulnarly deviates the carpal bones about the appropriate sagittal axis through the midcarpal and radiocarpal joints.

Fanning/Folding—Metacarpal   Using both hands, the clinician grasps the palmar and dorsal aspects of the thenar and hypothenar eminence, and then fans and folds the metacarpal bones about a longitudinal axis. This technique can also be used as a passive/active mobilization technique.

Phalanges

Using one hand, the clinician palpates and stabilizes the distal end of the metacarpal/phalanx close to the joint line, while using the other hand to palpate the proximal end of the adjacent phalanx.

Flexion/Extension   The clinician flexes and then extends the phalanx about the appropriate coronal axis through the MCP/IP joint.

Abduction/Adduction   The clinician abducts, and then adducts the phalanx about the appropriate sagittal axis through the MCP joint.

TABLE 9-7 The Open Pack and Close Pack Positions, and Capsular Patterns for the Articulations of the Wrist and Hand

Joint	Open pack	Close pack	Capsular pattern
Distal radioulnar	10° of supination	5° of supination	Minimal to no limitation with pain at the end ranges of pronation and supination
Radiocarpal (wrist)	Neutral with slight ulnar deviation	Extension	Equal limitation of flexion and extension
Intercarpal	Neutral or slight flexion	Extension	None
Midcarpal	Neutral or slight flexion with ulnar deviation	Extension with ulnar deviation	Equal limitation of flexion and extension
Carpometacarpal	*Thumb*—Midway between abduction and adduction and mid way between flexion and extension	*Thumb*—Full opposition	*Thumb*—Abduction then extension
	Fingers—Midway between flexion and extension	*Fingers*—Full flexion	*Fingers*—Equal limitation in all directions
Metacarpophalangeal	Slight flexion opposition *Fingers*—Full flexion	*Thumb*—Full extension	Flexion then extension
Interphalangeal	Slight flexion	Full extension	Flexion, extension

Passive Accessory Mobility Tests

In the following tests, the patient is positioned in sitting, and the clinician is standing or sitting, facing the patient. In each of the tests, the joint being tested is placed in its open packed position and the clinician notes the quantity of joint motion as well as the joint reaction to the test. The tests are always repeated on, and compared to, the same joint in the opposite extremity.

Radiocarpal Joint

- *Dorsal-palmar glide.* The patient's hand rests on the table with the wrist supported with a towel (Figure 9-14). Using one hand to stabilize the patient's distal forearm, the clinician grasps the patient's had with the other hand using the styloid processes and pisiform for landmarks. The proximal row of carpals is then moved dorsally and palmarly. The dorsal glide tests the joint's ability to extend, whereas the palmar glide assesses the ability of the joint to flex.
- *Ulnar and radial glide.* The patient's hand rests on the table with the wrist supported with a towel (Figure 9-15). Using one hand to stabilize the patient's distal forearm, the clinician grasps the patient's had with the other hand using the styloid processes and pisiform for landmarks. The proximal

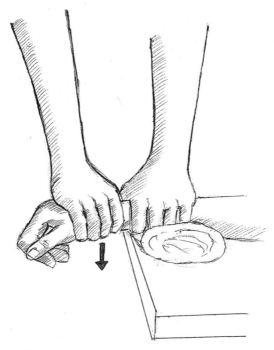

FIG. 9-14   Ventral glide of the radiocarpal (wrist) joint.

row of carpals is then moved dorsally and palmarly. The dorsal glide tests the joint's ability to extend, whereas the palmar glide assesses the ability of the joint to flex.

Intercarpal Joints

Example—Palmar glide of the scaphoid on the radius. The patient's hand rests on the table or is held forward by the clinician (Figure 9-16). The clinician grasps the patient's hand with both hands, with the index fingers placed on the proximal palmar surface of the radius, and the thumbs contacting the scaphoid dorsally (see Figure 9-16). The scaphoid is moved palmarly relative to the radius.

Carpal Motion Assessment

The Atkinson Method

Lateral Column   The clinician assesses the motion of the scaphoid in relation to the:

- Radius
- Capitate
- Lunate
- Trapezium
- Trapezoid

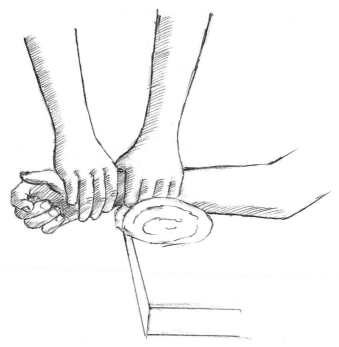

FIG. 9-15   Ulnar glide of the radiocarpal (wrist) joint.

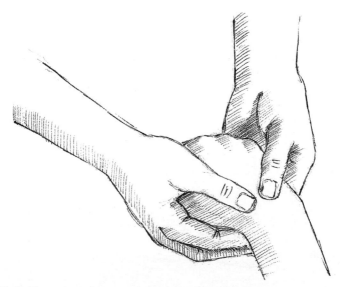

FIG. 9-16   Palmar glide of the scaphoid on the radius.

Central Column The clinician assesses the motion of the lunate in relation to the:

- Radius
- Capitate

Medial Column The clinician assesses the motion of the hamate in relation to the:

- Ulna
- Lunate
- Triquetrum

Carpometacarpal Joints

Using one hand, the clinician uses a pinch grip of the index finger and thumb to palpate and stabilize the carpal bone that articulates with the metacarpal bone being tested. With a pinch grip of the index finger and thumb of the other hand, the clinician palpates the metacarpal.

The first through fifth carpometacarpal joints are tested. The carpal bone is stabilized and the metacarpal is distracted (Figure 9-17) and glided posterior-anteriorly along the plane of the carpometacarpal joint. At the first carpometacarpal joint, radial and ulnar glides are also performed:

- *Ulnar glide.* The ulnar glide is used to assess the flexion glide of the joint. Using the thumb and index finger of one hand, the clinician stabilizes the trapezium and trapezoid as a unit (Figure 9-18). The thenar eminence of the other hand is placed on the first metacarpal of the patient's thumb, and the fingers wrap around the thumb to assist in maintaining the open packed position. The clinician applies a glide in an ulnar direction through the thenar eminence toward the radial aspect of the patient's metacarpal (see Figure 9-18).
- *Radial glide.* The radial glide is used to assess the extension glide of the joint. Using the thumb and index finger of one hand, the clinician stabilizes the trapezium and trapezoid as a unit. The thenar eminence of the other hand is placed on the first metacarpal of the patient's thumb, and the fingers wrap around the thumb to assist in maintaining the open packed position. The clinician applies a glide in a radial direction through the thenar eminence toward the ulnar aspect of the patient's metacarpal.

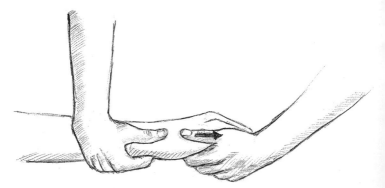

FIG. 9-17 Distraction of the carpometacarpal joint.

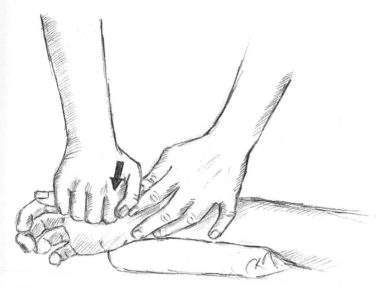

FIG. 9-18   Ulnar glide of the first carpometacarpal joint.

Intermetacarpal Joints

Although these joints between the metacarpal heads are not true synovial joints, motion does occur here during tasks involving grasping and releasing. The following example describes the technique to test the third and fourth intermetacarpal joint.

Using one hand, the clinician stabilizes the head and neck of the third metacarpal, while the other hand grasps the fourth metacarpal in a similar fashion (Figure 9-19). The head of the fourth metacarpal is then glided palmarly or dorsally with respect to the third metacarpal. The other metacarpals are tested similarly, with the third metacarpal always being the one stabilized as the third metacarpal serves as the center of movement during fanning and folding motions of the hand.

Metacarpophalangeal/Interphalangeal Joints

Using a pinch grip of the index finger and thumb of one hand, the clinician palpates and stabilizes the metacarpal/phalanx. With a pinch grip of the index finger and thumb of the other hand, the clinician palpates the adjacent phalanx.

Distraction   The clinician stabilizes the proximal bone, and then applies a long-axis distraction (Figure 9-20).

Posterior-Anterior Glide   The clinician stabilizes the proximal bone, and then glides the phalanx in a dorsal direction (Figure 9-21) and then ventral direction (Figure 9-22) along the plane of the joint.

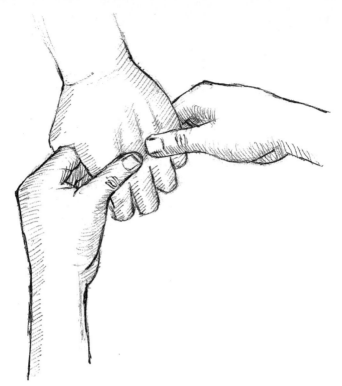

FIG. 9-19 Mobility testing of the third and fourth intermetacarpal joint.

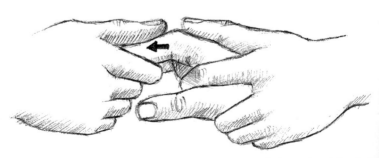

FIG. 9-20 Long axis distraction of the metacarpophalangeal or interphalangeal joints.

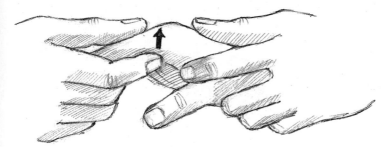

FIG. 9-21   Dorsal (posterior) glide of the metacarpophalangeal or interphalangeal joints.

Medial-Lateral (Radial-Ulnar Glide)   The clinician stabilizes the proximal bone, and then glides the phalanx medial-laterally along the plane of the joint (Figure 9-23).

Ligament Stability

The major ligaments of the wrist and hand are detailed in Table 9-8. A number of tests are available to evaluate the ligamentous stability of the forearm, wrist, hand, and finger joints. A nonspecific screening test for pseudoinstability involves holding the patient's hand with one hand and the patient's forearm in

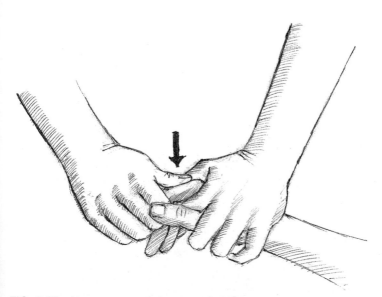

FIG. 9-22   Ventral (anterior) glide of the metacarpophalangeal or interphalangeal joints.

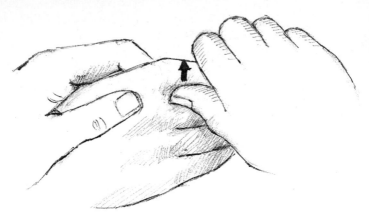

FIG. 9-23 Radial glide of the metacarpophalangeal or interphalangeal joints.

the other, while passively flexing and extending the patient's wrist. The presence of palpable clunks or shifts with this maneuver could suggest instability.

In the following specific tests, the patient is positioned in sitting, and the clinician is standing or sitting, facing the patient. The clinician must remember to perform these tests on the uninvolved sides to provide a basis for comparison.

Piano Key Test

The piano key test evaluates the stability of the distal radioulnar joint.[12] The clinician firmly stabilizes the distal radius with one hand and grasps the head of the ulna between the thumb and index fingers of the other hand. The ulnar head is depressed in an anterior direction (as in depressing a key on a piano).[28] The test is positive if there is excessive movement in a palmar direction, or if, on release of the ulna, the bone springs back into its high dorsal position. There may also be discomfort reported during the test.[8]

TABLE 9-8 Ligaments of the Wrist and Hand

Intrinsic		Extrinsic
Interosseous	Midcarpal	Radiocarpal/Ulnocarpal
Distal Row	*Dorsal*	*Dorsal*
Trapezium-trapezoid	Scaphotriquetral	Dorsal radiocarpal
Trapezoid-capitate	Dorsal intercarpal	
Capitohamate		
Proximal Row	*Palmar*	*Palmar*
Scapholunate	Scaphotrapeziotrapezoid	Radioscaphocapitate
Lunotriquetral	Scaphocapitate	Long radiolunate
Triquetrocapitate	Short radiolunate	
Triquetrohamate	Radioscapholunate	
	Ulnolunate	
	Ulnotriquetral	
	Ulnocapitate	
		Carpometacarpal

Lunotriquetral Shear (Reagan's) Test

The lunotriquetral shear maneuver, or Reagan's test,[48] assesses the stability of the lunotriquetral interosseous ligament.[12] The lunate is moved dorsally with the thumb of one hand, while the triquetrum is pushed palmarly by the index finger of the other hand. The wrist is placed in either radial or ulnar deviation. Stress is created between these two bones in the anterior-posterior plane (see Figure 9-24). Crepitation, clicks, or discomfort in this area suggests injury to the ligament.[28,49]

Pisotriquetral Shear Test

The pisotriquetral shear test assesses the integrity of the pisotriquetral articulation.[28] The clinician stabilizes the wrist with the fingers dorsal to the triquetrum, and the thumb over the pisiform. The pisiform is rocked back and forth in a medial and lateral direction (see Figure 9-25). A positive test is manifested with pain during this maneuver.

Pivot Shift Test of the Midcarpal Joint

The patient is positioned in sitting with the elbow flexed to 90°, resting on a firm surface, and the forearm supinated. The clinician uses one hand to stabilize the forearm, using the other hand to take the patient's hand into full radial deviation while maintaining the wrist in neutral with regard to flexion and extension. The patient's hand is then taken into full ulnar deviation. A positive test results if the capitate is felt to shift away from the lunate and indicates an injury to the anterior capsule and interosseous ligaments.[17]

Triangular Fibrocartilage Complex Load Test

This test can be used to detect an injury to the TFCC. It is performed by ulnarly deviating and axially loading the wrist and moving it dorsally and palmarly, or by rotating the forearm. A positive test elicits pain, clicking, or crepitus.[8]

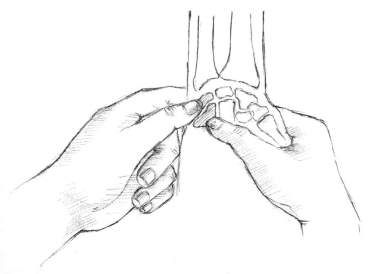

FIG. 9-24   The lunotriquetral shear maneuver, or Reagan's test.

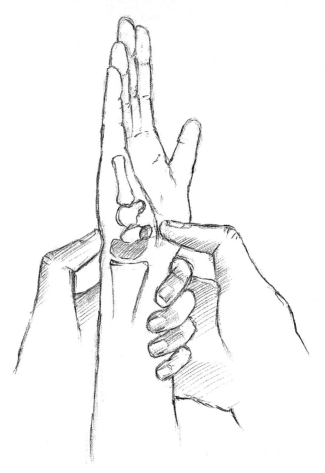

FIG. 9-25 The pisotriquetral shear test.

Neurovascular Status

A number of tests can be used to document the neurovascular status of the wrist and hand.

Allen Test

The Allen test is used to determine the patency of the vessels supplying the hand. The clinician compresses both the radial and ulnar arteries at the wrist, and then asks the patient to open and clench the respective fist, three to four times to drain the venous blood from the hand. The patient is then asked to hold the hand open while the clinician releases the pressure on the ulnar artery, and then the radial artery. The fingers and palm should be seen to regain their normal pink color. This procedure is repeated with the radial artery released and compression on the ulnar artery maintained. Normal filling time is usually less than 5 seconds. A distinct difference in the filling time suggests the dominance of one artery filling the hand.[49]

Tinel's Test for Carpal Tunnel Syndrome

The Tinel's test is used to assist in the diagnosis of carpal tunnel syndrome. The area over the median nerve is tapped gently at the palmar surface of the wrist. If this produces tingling in the median distribution, then the test is positive.[50] Tinel's sign has a sensitivity of 60% and a specificity of 67%.[51] The reliability and validity of the Tinel's test is moderately acceptable for use in clinical practice.[52–55]

Wartenberg's Sign

Wartenberg's sign is characterized by a position of abduction assumed by the little finger as a result of ulnar nerve paralysis.

Sensibility Testing

Sensation is the conscious perception of basic sensory input. Sensibility describes the neural events occurring at the periphery, nerve fibers, and nerve receptors. Sensation is what clinicians reeducate, whereas sensibility is what clinicians assess.[56]

The assessment of sensibility of the hand is an important component of every hand examination because sensation is essential for precision movements and object manipulation. Altered sensory perceptions can result from injuries to peripheral nerves or from spinal nerve root compression. The sensory system is described in Chapter 2. Two types of sensibility can be assessed:[57]

- *Protective.* This is evidenced by the ability to perceive pinprick, touch, and temperature.
- *Functional.* This is evidenced by a return of sensibility to a level that enables the hand to engage in full activities of daily living.

There exists a hierarchy of sensibility capacity:[57,58]

- *Detection.* This is the simplest level of function and requires that the patient be able to distinguish a single point stimulus from normally occurring atmospheric background stimulation.
- *Innervation density or discrimination.* This represents the ability to perceive that stimulus A differs from stimulus B.
- *Quantification.* This involves organizing tactile stimuli according to degree, texture, and so forth.
- *Recognition.* This is the most complicated level of function and involves the identification of objects with the vision occluded.

Stress Tests

Stress tests are those that combine the use of sensory tests with activities that provoke the symptoms of nerve compression. These tests are helpful in cases of patient reports of mild nerve compression when no abnormalities are detected by baseline sensory testing. Examples of stress tests include the Phalen's test, the Reverse Phalen's test, and the Hand Elevation test.

Phalen's Test for Carpal Tunnel Syndrome

For Phalen's[59,60] test, the patient sits comfortably with the wrists and elbows flexed. The test is positive if the patient experiences numbness or tingling within 45 seconds. For some patients, performance of this test recreates their wrist, thumb, or forearm ache.[61] Phalen's sign has a sensitivity of 75% and a specificity of 47%. The reliability and validity of Phalen's test is moderately acceptable for use in clinical practice.[53–55]

Reverse Phalen's Test for Carpal Tunnel Syndrome

For the Reverse Phalen's test, the patient sits comfortably with the wrists extended and elbows flexed.[62] Wrist extension has demonstrated a larger increase in intracarpal canal pressure when compared to wrist flexion.[50,63]

Hand Elevation Test for Carpal Tunnel Syndrome

The patient is seated or standing and is asked to elevate both arms above the head, and maintain them in this position for 2 minutes, or until the patient feels paresthesia or numbness in the hands.[64] In one study, this test was found to be more specific than Phalen's and Tinel's tests.[64]

Innervation Density Tests

These are a class of sensory tests that test the ability to discriminate between two identical stimuli placed close together on the skin. These tests are helpful in assessing sensibility after nerve repair and during nerve regeneration.[65]

Weber's (Moberg's) Two-Point Discrimination Test

Weber first introduced the two-point discrimination tests in 1953, using calipers, which were subsequently modified by Moberg for use with a paper clip in 1958.[65]

The clinician repeats the tests in an attempt to find the minimal distance at which the patient can distinguish between the two stimuli, decreasing or increasing the distance between the points depending on the response by the patient.[17] This distance is called the *threshold for discrimination*. Normal discrimination distance is less than 6 millimeters, although this can vary between individuals (see *Orthopaedic Examination, Evaluation, and Intervention*, p 628), and in the area of the hand, with normal fingertip scores occurring between 2 and 5 millimeters, and the finger surfaces scores between 3 and 7 millimeters.[66]

Special Tests

Carpal Shake Test

This test is used if intercarpal synovitis is suspected.[28] The clinician grasps the patient's distal forearm. The patient is asked to relax and the clinician shakes the wrist. Pain or resistance to this test indicates a positive test.

Sit to Stand Test

This test is used if synovitis of the wrist is suspected.[28] The patient is instructed to place both hands on the armrest of a chair and attempt to lift his or her body slightly off the chair. Pain or resistance to this test indicates a positive test.

Ulnar Impaction Test

This test is used to assess the articulation between the ulnar carpus and the triangular fibrocartilage.[28] The patient is positioned in sitting, with the elbow flexed to about 90° and the wrist positioned in ulnar deviation, and the fingers positioned in a slight fist. The clinician loads the wrist by applying a compressive force through the ring and small metacarpals. Pain with this test indicates a possible tear of the triangular fibrocartilage or ulnar impaction syndrome.

Finkelstein's Test[67]

This test is used to detect stenosing tenosynovitis of the APL and EPB. The clinician grasps the patient's thumb, stabilizes the forearm with one hand, and then deviates the wrist to the ulnar side with the other hand (Figure 9-26).

Flexor Digitorum Superficialis Test

This test is used to test the integrity of the FDS tendon. The clinician holds the patient's fingers in extension except for the finger being tested (this isolates the FDS tendon). The patient is instructed to flex the finger at the PIP joint. If this is possible, the FDS tendon is intact. Since this tendon can act independently because of the position of the finger, it is the only functioning tendon at the PIP joint. The DIP joint, motored by the FDP, has no power of flexion when the other fingers are held in extension.

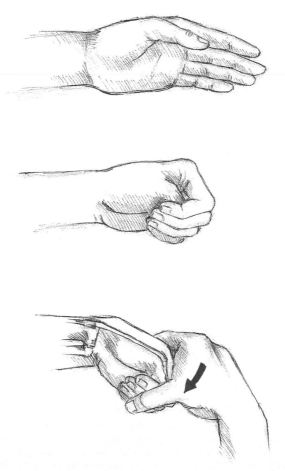

FIG. 9-26   Finkelstein's test.

Flexor Digitorum Profundus Test

These tendons work only in unison. To test the FDP, stabilize the PIP joint and the MCP joint in extension. Instruct patient to flex this finger at the DIP joint. If flexion occurs, the FDP is intact. If no flexion is possible the tendon is severed or the muscle denervated.

Extensor Hood Rupture

Elson[68] describes a test in which, from 90° of PIP flexion, the patient tries to extend the PIP joint against resistance. The absence of extension force at the PIP joint, and fixed extension at the distal joint, indicate complete rupture of the central slip.[14]

Froment's Sign

This is more of a sign than a test and may present as a complaint from the patient who reports an inability to pinch between the index finger and thumb without flexion at the DIP joint occurring.[69] A positive Froment's sign, which results from a weakness in the adductor pollicis and short head of the flexor pollicis brevis (FPB) muscles, indicates an ulnar nerve entrapment at the elbow or at the wrist.

Murphy's Sign

The patient is asked to make a fist. If the head of the third metacarpal is level with the second and fourth metacarpals, the sign is positive for the presence of a lunate dislocation.[70]

Wartenberg's Test

The Wartenberg test is used with patients who complain of pain over the distal radial forearm associated with paresthesias over the dorsal radial hand (Wartenberg syndrome). These patients frequently report symptom magnification with wrist movement or when tightly pinching the thumb and index digit together. The Wartenberg test involves tapping the index finger over the superficial radial nerve (similar to the Tinel test for carpal tunnel syndrome). A positive test is indicated by local tenderness and paresthesia with this maneuver. Hyperpronation of the forearm can also cause a positive Tinel sign.

Diagnostic Testing

Diagnostic testing of the forearm, wrist, and hand is limited to plain radiographs for most patients. Bony tenderness with a history of trauma or a suspicion of bone or joint disruption indicates a need for radiographs. Standard projections for the wrist are the posteroanterior, lateral, and oblique. For the patient with a suspicion of a scaphoid injury, a scaphoid view should be added.[12] Wrist conditions rarely require computed tomography (CT) scans and magnetic resonance imaging (MRI) scans.[49]

EXAMINATION CONCLUSIONS—THE EVALUATION

Following the examination, and once the clinical findings have been recorded, the clinician must determine a specific diagnosis or a working hypothesis, based on a summary of all the findings. This diagnosis can be structure related (medical diagnosis) (Table 9-9), or a diagnosis based on the preferred practice patterns as described in the *Guide to Physical Therapist Practice*.[71]

TABLE 9-9 Differential Diagnosis for Common Causes of Wrist and Hand Pain

Condition	Patient age	Mechanism of injury	Symptoms aggravated by	Observation	AROM	PROM	End-feel	Resisted	Special tests	Tenderness with palpation
Carpal tunnel syndrome	35–55	Gradual overuse Wide-variety of factors	Repetitive activities of wrist Sustained positioning of wrist in flexion	Thenar muscle atrophy (later stages)	Full and pain free			Weakness of grip on radial side (chronic) Strong and pain free (acute)	Tinel's Phalen's	Reproduction of symptoms with compression applied on anterior aspect of wrist
Wrist extensor tendinitis	20–50	Repetitive or prolonged activities, forceful exertion, awkward and static postures, vibration, and localized mechanical stress		Unremarkable		Wrist pain with finger flexion combined with radial or ulnar deviation		Pain with wrist extension		Anterior carpus
Wrist flexor tendinitis	20–50	Forceful gripping, rapid wrist movements, moving the wrist and fingers to the extremes of range	Activities involving wrist extension	Unremarkable	Wrist extension	Pain with combined wrist extension and elbow extension		Pain with wrist flexion		Pisiform In palm over base of second metacarpal

(Continued)

TABLE 9-9 Differential Diagnosis for Common Causes of Wrist and Hand Pain (Continued)

Condition	Patient age	Mechanism of injury	Symptoms aggravated by	Observation	AROM	PROM	End-feel	Resisted	Special tests	Tenderness with palpation
OA of first CMC joint	40–60	Repetitive trauma Degeneration	Repetitive use of thumb Strong gripping	Soft tissue thickening at base of thumb	Mid-limitation of all thumb movements	Pain with thumb rotation Pain on thumb extension and abduction		Weakness of grip on radial side (chronic)		Anatomic snuff box
Trigger finger	50+	Disproportion between the flexor tendon and its tendon sheath		Thickening/puckering of skin in palm	Decreased finger extension Clicking or jerking with movements	Full and pain free	Soft tissue resistance to finger extension	Strong and pain free		No pain, but snapping of flexor tendon felt with finger extension
De Quervains tenosynovitis	50+	Repetitive finger-thumb gripping combined with radial deviation	Overuse, repetitive tasks, which involve overexertion of the thumb	Swelling over lateral wrist/thumb	Decreased ulnar deviation Decreased thumb flexion	Pain on thumb flexion combined with ulnar deviation of wrist		Pain with abduction and extension of thumb	Finkelstein's	Lateral wrist and thumb

Dupuytren's contracture	40+	Multifactorial (alcohol, diabetes, epilepsy, smoking, trauma)		Thickening or puckering of skin in palm	Decreased finger extension	Soft tissue resistance to finger extension	Strong and pain free	Inability to place the palm of your hand completely flat on a hard surface	No tenderness, but thickening of soft tissues evident
Thumb ulnar collateral ligament injury	Varies	Forced hyperabduction and/or hyperextension stress of the thumb MCP joint	Extension of the thumb	Swelling at the ulnar side of the MCP joint	Usually unremarkable	Pain with passive hyperextension or hyperabduction	Usually unremarkable	Stress testing of the UCL	Ulnar side of the MCP joint of the thumb
Wrist sprain	20–40	Trauma (FOOSH injury)	Taking weight through the hand		Extremes of all ranges	Wrist pain with ulnar or radial deviation	Pain with strong resistance in any direction		Medial or lateral joint line

CMC = carpometacarpal; OA = osteoarthritis

REFERENCES

1. Hume MC, et al.: Functional range of motion of the joints of the hand. J Hand Surg 1990;15A:240–243.
2. Butler DS: Mobilization of the Nervous System. New York, Churchill Livingstone, 1992.
3. Kiser DM: Physiological and biomechanical factors for understanding repetitive motion injuries. Semin Occup Med 1987;2:11–17.
4. Keller K, Corbett J, Nichols D: Repetitive strain injury in computer keyboard users: pathomechanics and treatment principles in individual and group intervention. J Hand Ther 1998;11:9–26.
5. Dent S: Befuddled by a FOOSH? FR Report 2000;6:9.
6. Overton DT, Uehara DT: Evaluation of the injured hand. Emerg Med Clin North Am 1993;11:585–600.
7. Muckart RD: Stenosing tendovaginitis of abductor pollicis brevis at the radial styloid (de Quervain's disease). Clin Orthop 1964;33:201–208.
8. Skirven T: Clinical examination of the wrist. J Hand Ther 1996;9:96–107.
9. Nalebuff EA: The rheumatoid swan-neck deformity. Hand Clin 1989;5:215–214.
10. Wadsworth C: Wrist and hand. In Wadsworth C (ed): Current Concepts of Orthopedic Physical Therapy–Home Study Course, Orthopaedic Section. La Crosse, WI, APTA, 2001.
11. Judge RD, Zuidema GD, Fitzgerald FT: General appearance. In Judge RD, Zuidema GD, Fitzgerald FT (eds): Clinical Diagnosis, pp 29–47. Boston, MA, Little, Brown, 1982.
12. Onieal M-E: Common Wrist and Elbow Injuries in Primary Care. Lippincott's Primary Care Practice. Musculoskelet Cond 1999;3(4):441–450.
13. Watson HK, Weinzweig J: Physical examination of the wrist. Hand Clin 1997;13:17–34.
14. Freiberg A, et al.: Management of proximal interphalangeal joint injuries. J Trauma-Injury Infect Crit Care 1999;46(3):523–528.
15. Nicholson B: Clinical evaluation. In Stanley BG, Tribuzi SM (eds): Concepts in Hand Rehabilitation, pp 59–91. Philadelphia, PA, FA Davis, 1992.
16. Hoppenfeld S: Physical Examination of the Spine and Extremities. East Norwalk, CT, Appleton-Century-Crofts, 1976.
17. Tubiana R, Thomine J-M, Mackin E: Examination of the hand and wrist. London, Mosby, 1996.
18. Blair SJ, et al.: Evaluation of impairment of the upper extremity. Clin Orthop 1987;221:42–58.
19. Riordan DC, Kaplan EB: Kaplan's Functional and Surgical Anatomy of the Hand, 3rd ed. Philadelphia, PA, JB Lippincott, 1984.
20. Whipple TL: Preoperative evaluation and imaging. In Whipple TL (ed): Athroscopic Surgery: The Wrist, pp 11–36. Philadelphia, PA, JB Lippincott, 1992.
21. Osterman AL, Mikulics M: Scaphoid nonunion. Hand Clin 1988;14:437–455.
22. Watson HK, Ashmead D, Makhlouf MV: Examination of the scaphoid. J Hand Surg 1988;13A:657–660.
23. Alexander AH, Lichtman DM: Kienbock's disease. In Lichtman DM (ed): The Wrist and Its Disorders. Philadelphia, PA, WB Saunders, 1988.
24. Kienböck R: Concerning traumatic malacia of the lunate and its consequences: degeneration and compression fractures. Clin Orth Rel Res 1980;149:4–5.
25. Polivy KD, et al.: Fractures of the hook of the hamate—a failure of clinical diagnosis. J Hand Surg 1985;10A:101–104.
26. Rao SB, Culver JE: Triquetralhamate arthrodesis for midcarpal instability. J Hand Surg 1995;20A:583–589.
27. Wadsworth CT: Anatomy of the hand and wrist. In Manual Examination and Treatment of the Spine and Extremities, pp 128–138. Baltimore, MD, Williams & Wilkins, 1988.
28. Waggy C: Disorders of the wrist. In Wadsworth C (ed): Orthopaedic Physical Therapy Home Study Course—The Elbow, Forearm, and Wrist. Orthopaedic Section. La Crosse, WI, APTA, 1997.

29. Swanson A: Disabling arthritis at the base of the thumb: treatment by resection of the trapezium and flexible implant arthroplasty. J Bone and Joint Surg 1972;54A: 456.

30. Beckenbaugh RD: Accurate evaluation and management of the painful wrist following injury. Orthop Clin North Am 1984;15:289–306.

31. Wolfe SW, Gupta A, Crisco JJ, III: Kinematics of the scaphoid shift test. J Hand Surg 1997;22A:801–806.

32. Taleisnik J: Scapholunate dissociation. In Taleisnik J (ed): The Wrist, pp 239–278. New York, Churchill Livingstone, 1985.

33. Burton RI, Eaton RG: Common hand injuries in the athlete. Orthop Clin North [Am] 1973;4:809–838.

34. Taleisnik J: Classification of carpal instability. In Taleisnik J (ed): The Wrist, pp 229–238. New York, Churchill Livingstone, 1985.

35. LaStayo P, Howell J: Clinical provocative tests used in evaluating wrist pain: a descriptive study. J Hand Surg 1995;8:10–17.

36. Easterling KJ, Wolfe SW: Scaphoid shift in the uninjured wrist. J Hand Surg 1994;19A:604–606.

37. Mathiowetz V, et al.: Reliability and validity of grip and pinch strength evaluations. J Hand Surg 1984;9A:222–226.

38. Stokes HM, et al.: Identification of low effort patients through dynamometry. J Hand Surg 1995;20A:1047–1056.

39. Kapandji IA: The Physiology of the Joints, Upper Limb. New York, Churchill Livingstone, 1991.

40. Norkin C, Levangie P: Joint Structure and Function: A Comprehensive Analysis, pp 355–358. Philadelphia, PA, FA Davis, 1992.

41. Eberhardt K, Malcus Johnson P, Rydgren L: The occurrence and significance of hand deformities in early rheumatoid arthritis. Br J Rheum 1991;30:211–213.

42. Fess EE: The need for reliability and validity in hand assessment instruments. J Hand Surg 1986;11A:621–623 (editorial).

43. Jebsen RH, et al.: An objective and standardized test for hand function. Arch Phys Med Rehab 1969;50:311.

44. Beckenbaugh RD, et al.: Kienböck's disease: the natural history of Kienböck's disease and consideration of lunate fractures. Clin Orthop 1980;149:98–106.

45. Purdue Pegboard Test of Manipulative Dexterity. Chicago, IL, Service Research Assoc, 1968.

46. Tiffin J, Asker E: The Purdue pegboard: norms and studies of reliability and validity. J Appl Psychol 1948;32:324.

47. Crawford J: Crawford small parts dexterity test (CSPDT). In Psychological Corp (catalog): Tests, Products and Services for Business, Industry, and Government, p 32. Cleveland, OH, Harcourt Brace Jovanovich, 1985.

48. Reagan DS, Linscheid RL, Dobyns JH: Lunotriquetral sprains. J Hand Surg 1984;9A:502–514.

49. Onieal M-E: The hand: Examination and diagnosis. In American Society for Surgery of the Hand. New York, Churchill Livingstone, 1990.

50. Werner CO, Elmqvist D, Ohlin P: Pressure and nerve lesion in the carpal tunnel. Acta Orthop Scand 1983;54:312–316.

51. Stewart JD, Eisen A: Tinel's sign and the carpal tunnel syndrome. BMJ 1978;2:1125–1126.

52. Gellman H, et al.: Carpal tunnel syndrome: an evaluation of the provocative diagnostic tests. J Bone and Joint Surg 1986;68A:735–737.

53. Marx RG, et al.: The reliability of physical examination for carpal tunnel syndrome. J Hand Surg 1998;23B:499–502.

54. Golding DN, Rose DM, Selvarajah K: Clinical tests for carpal tunnel syndrome: an evaluation. Br J Rheum 1986;25:388–390.

55. Heller L, et al.: Evaluation of Tinel's and Phalen's signs in diagnosis of the carpal tunnel syndrome. Eur Neurol 1986;25:40–42.

56. Mackinnon SE, Dellon AL: Sensory rehabilitation after nerve injury. In Mackinnon SE, Dellon AL (eds): Surgery of the Peripheral Nerve, p 521. New York, Thieme Medical, 1988.

57. Anthony MS: Wounds. In Clark GL, et al. (eds): Hand Rehabilitation: A Practical Guide, pp 1–15. Philadelphia, PA, Churchill Livingstone, 1998.
58. Fess EE: Documentation: essential elements of an upper extremity assessment battery. In Hunter JM, Mackin EJ, Callahan AD (eds): Rehabilitation of the Hand: Surgery and Therapy, p 185. St Louis, MO, Mosby, 1995.
59. Phalen GS: The carpal tunnel syndrome: clinical evaluation of 598 hands. Clin Orthop 1972;83:29–40.
60. Phalen GS: Spontaneous compression of the median nerve at the wrist. JAMA 1951;145:1128–1133.
61. Onieal M-E: Essentials of musculoskeletal care. Rosemont, IL, AAOS, 1997.
62. Robert AW, Cynthia B, Thomas JA: Reverse Phalen's maneuver as an aid in diagnosing carpal tunnel syndrome. Arch Phys Med Rehab 1994;75:783–786.
63. Brain WR, Wright AD, Wilkinson M: Spontaneous compression of both median nerves in the carpal tunnel: six cases treated surgically. Lancet 1947;1:277–282.
64. Duck-Sun A: Hand elevation: a new test for carpal tunnel syndrome. Ann Plast Surg 2001;46:120–124.
65. Moberg E: Objective methods for determining the functional value of sensibility in the hand. J Bone Joint Surg 1958;40A:454–476.
66. Omer GE: Report of committee for evaluation of the clinical result in peripheral nerve injury. J Hand Surg 1983;8:754–759.
67. Finkelstein H: Stenosing tenovaginitis at the radial styloid process. J Bone Joint Surg 1930;12A:509.
68. Elson RA: Rupture of the central slip of the extensor hood of the finger: a test for early diagnosis. J Bone Joint Surg (Brit) 1986;68:229–231.
69. Preston D, Shapiro B: Electromyography and neuromuscular disorders. Clinical Electrophysiologic Correlations. Boston, MA, Butterworth-Heinemann, 1998.
70. Booher JM, Thibodeau GA: Athletic Injury Assessment. St Louis, MO, Mosby, 1989.
71. Guide to physical therapist practice. Phys Ther 2001;81:S13–S95.

10 | The Hip Joint

OVERVIEW

Due to its location, design, and function, the hip joint transmits truly impressive loads, both tensile and compressive. Loads of up to eight times body weight have been demonstrated in the hip joint during jogging, with potentially greater loads present during vigorous athletic competition.[1] Fortunately, under normal conditions, the structures about the hip are uniquely adapted to transfer such forces:

- *Acetabulum.* The acetabulum, which is actually made up of three bones, the ilium, ischium, and pubis, receives its name from the Latin term for the vinegar cup, which it resembles.
- *Labrum.* The acetabular labrum deepens the acetabulum and increases articular congruence.
- *Ligaments.* The major ligaments of the pelvis and hip are known to be the strongest in the body and are well adapted to the forces transferred between the spine and the lower extremities.
- *Muscles* (Table 10-1). The abdominal musculature and the erector muscles of the spine provide further stabilization of the hip region and must be considered in conditions that affect pelvic tilt and the hip joint. The balance of the muscles of the upper thigh, particularly the adductor muscles, with those of the lower abdomen requires further study.

In addition to providing stability, the hip joint permits a great deal of mobility. Thus, during activities involving the hip, a fine balance must be struck between mobility and stability. Any imbalance between these two variables can leave the hip joint and surrounding tissues prone to soft tissue injuries, impingement syndromes, and joint dysfunctions. Given that the hip region is also a common source of symptom referral from other regions, the examination of the hip rarely occurs in isolation, and almost always involves an assessment of the lumbar spine, pelvis, and knee joint complex.

EXAMINATION

History

The history should determine the patient's chief complaint and the mechanism of injury, if any. To aid the clinician as to the source of the symptoms, the patient should complete a pain diagram and a medical history questionnaire. The patient should also be encouraged to describe the location of pain (Table 10-2). Pain is a common presenting complaint in a local hip pathology (Table 10-3), but can also be present in more insidious conditions such as the inflammatory arthritides. Determining the location and type of pain (Table 10-3) can provide some clues as to the cause (Figures 10-1 and 10-2). The local sources of hip pain may include:

- Hip strains, tears, ruptures, and tendinitis (Table 10-4). The hip area is a common source of overuse injuries
- Bursitis (subtrochanteric and ischiogluteal)
- Contusions
- Snapping hip
- Loose body within the joint—associated with complaints of twinges of pain with hip motions

TABLE 10-1 Muscles Acting Across the Hip Joint

Muscle	Origin	Insertion	Innervation
Adductor brevis	External aspect of the body and inferior ramus of the pubis	By an aponeurosis to the line from the greater trochanter of the linea aspera of the femur	Obturator nerve, L3
Adductor longus	Pubic crest and symphysis	By an aponeurosis to the middle third of the linea aspera of the femur	Obturator nerve, L3
Adductor magnus	Inferior ramus of pubis, ramus of ischium, and the inferolateral aspect of the ischial tuberosity	By an aponeurosis to the linea aspera and adductor tubercle of the femur	Obturator nerve and tibial portion of the sciatic nerve, L2-4
Biceps femoris (long head)	Arises from the sacrotuberous ligament and posterior aspect of the ischial tuberosity	By way of a tendon, on the lateral aspect of the head of the fibula, the lateral condyle of the tibial tuberosity, the lateral collateral ligament, and the deep fascia of the leg	Tibial portion of the sciatic nerve, S1
Gemelli (superior and inferior)	Superior-dorsal surface of the spine of the ischium, inferior-upper part of the tuberosity of the ischium	Superior and inferior-medial surface of the greater trochanter	Sacral plexus, L5-S1
Gluteus maximus	Posterior gluteal line of the ilium, iliac crest, aponeurosis of the erector spinae, dorsal surface of the lower part of the sacrum, side of the coccyx, sacrotuberous ligament, and intermuscular fascia	Iliotibial tract of the fascia lata, gluteal tuberosity of the femur	Inferior gluteal nerve, S1-2
Gluteus medius	Outer surface of the ilium between the iliac crest and the posterior gluteal line, anterior gluteal line and fascia	Lateral surface of the greater trochanter	Superior gluteal nerve, L5
Gluteus minimus	Outer surface of the ilium between the anterior and inferior gluteal lines, and the margin of the greater sciatic notch	A ridge laterally situated on the anterior surface of the greater trochanter	Superior gluteal nerve, L5
Gracilis	The body and inferior ramus of the pubis	The anterior-medial aspect of the shaft of the proximal tibia, just proximal to the tendon of the semitendinosus	Obturator nerve, L2

Iliacus	Super two-thirds of the iliac fossa, upper surface of the lateral part of the sacrum	Fibers converge with tendon of the psoas major to lesser trochanter	Femoral nerve, L2
Obturator externus	Rami of the pubis, ramus of the ischium, medial two-thirds of the outer surface of the obturator membrane	Trochanteric fossa of the femur	Obturator nerve, L4
Obturator internus	Internal surface of the anterolateral wall of the pelvis, and obturator membrane	Medial surface of the greater trochanter	Sacral plexus, S1
Pectineus	Pecten pubis	Along a line leading from the lesser trochanter to the linea aspera	Femoral or obturator or accessory obturator nerves, L2
Piriformis	Front of the sacrum, gluteal surface of the ilium, capsule of the sacroiliac joint, and sacrotuberous ligament	Upper border of the greater trochanter of femur	Sacral plexus, S1
Psoas major	Transverse processes of all the lumbar vertebrae, bodies, and intervertebral disks of the lumbar vertebrae	Lesser trochanter of the femur	Lumbar plexus, L2-3
Quadratus femoris	Ischial body next to the ischial tuberosity	Quadrate tubercle on femur	Nerve to quadratus femoris
Rectus femoris	By two heads, from the anterior inferior iliac spine, and a reflected head from the groove above the acetabulum	Base of the patella	Femoral nerve, L3-4
Sartorius	Anterior superior iliac spine and notch below it	Upper part of the medial surface of the tibia in front of the gracilis	Femoral nerve, L2-3
Semimembranosus	Ischial tuberosity	The posterior-medial aspect of the medial condyle of the tibia	Tibial nerve, L5-S1
Semitendinosus	Ischial tuberosity	Upper part of the medial surface of the tibia behind the attachment of the sartorus and below that of the gracilis	Tibial nerve, L5-S1
Tensor of the fasciae latae	Outer lip of the iliac crest and the lateral surface of the anterior superior iliac spine	Iliotibial tract	Superior gluteal nerve, L4-5

TABLE 10-2 Differential Diagnosis for Pain in the Hip or Buttock Area[1]

Pain distribution	Potential cause
Groin area	Stress fractures of the pelvis and femur
	Crystal-induced synovitis (gout)
	An inguinal/femoral hernia
	Muscle calcification
	Hip adductor strain
	Iliopectineal bursitis
	Iliopsoas strain or avulsion fracture of the lesser trochanter
	Arthritis of the hip
	Hip arthrosis
	Femoral neck fracture
	Osteonecrosis of the femoral head
	Pubic symphysis dysfunction
	• Osteitis pubis
	• Osteomyelitis pubis
	• Pyogenic arthritis
	• Pubic fracture
	• Pubic osteolysis
	• Postpartum symphyseal pain
	Sacroiliac joint lesion
	Tumor
	Ureteral stone
	Hernia
	Inflammatory synovitis (e.g., rheumatoid arthritis, ankylosing spondylitis, systemic lupus)
	Subluxation
	Dislocation
	Transient synovitis
	Infection
	Loosened prosthesis
	Inflamed lymph nodes
	Lower abdominal
	Referred pain from viscera or spinal nerve
Pubic area	Sprain of pubic symphysis
	Osteitis pubis
	Abdominal muscle strain
	Bladder infection
Lateral buttock area	Trochanteric bursitis
	Tendinitis of abductors or external rotators
	Apophysitis of greater trochanter
	Referred pain from mid or lower lumbar spine
	Thrombosis of gluteal arteries
Anterior and lateral thigh	Strain of quadriceps
	Meralgia paresthetica
	Entrapment of femoral nerve
	Thrombosis of femoral artery or great saphenous vein
	Stress fracture of femur
	Referred pain from hip or mid lumbar spine
Medial thigh	Strain of adductor muscles
	Entrapment of obturator nerve
	Referred pain from hip or knee
ASIS	Apophysitis or sartorius or rectus femoris
Iliac crest	Strain of gluteal, oblique abdominals, tensor fasciae latae, quadratus lumborum
	Entrapment of iliohypogastric nerve
	Referred pain from upper lumbar spine

Source: Beattie P: The hip. In Malone TR, McPoil T, Nitz A (eds): Orthopaedic and Sports Physical Therapy, 3rd ed., p 506. St Louis, MO, Mosby, 1996.

TABLE 10-3 Clinical Findings, Differential Diagnosis, and Intervention Strategies of Some Hip Conditions

Diagnosis	History	Physical findings	Differential diagnosis
Legg-Calvé-Perthes disease	Insidious onset (1 to 3 months) of limp with hip or knee pain	Limited hip abduction, flexion, and internal rotation	Juvenile arthritis, other inflammatory conditions of the hip
Slipped capital femoral epiphysis	Acute (<1 month) or chronic (up to 6 months) presentation, pain may be referred to knee or anterior thigh	Pain and limited internal rotation, leg more comfortable in external rotation; chronic presentation may have leg length discrepancy	Muscle strain, avulsion fracture
Avulsion fracture	Sudden, violent muscle contraction; may hear or feel a "pop"	Pain on passive stretch and active contraction of involved muscle; pain on palpation of involved apophysis	Muscle strain, slipped capital femoral epiphysis
Hip pointer	Direct trauma to iliac crest	Tenderness over iliac crest, may have pain on ambulation and active abduction of hip	Contusion, fracture
Contusion	Direct trauma to soft tissue	Pain on palpation and motion, ecchymosis	Hip pointer, fracture, myositis ossificans
Myositis ossificans	Contusion with hematoma approximately 2 to 4 weeks earlier	Pain on palpation, firm mass may be palpable	Contusion, soft tissue tumors, callus formation from prior fracture
Femoral neck stress fracture	Persistent groin discomfort increasing with activity, history of endurance exercise, female athlete triad (eating disorder, amenorrhea, osteoporosis)	ROM may be painful, pain on palpation of greater trochanter	Trochanteric bursitis, osteoid osteoma, muscle strain
Osteoid osteoma	Vague hip pain present at night and increased with activities	Restricted motion, quadriceps atrophy	Femoral neck stress fracture, trochanteric bursitis
Illiotibial band syndrome	Lateral hip, thigh, or knee pain; snapping as iliotibial band passes over the greater trochanter	Positive Ober's test	Trochanteric bursitis

(Continued)

TABLE 10-3 Clinical Findings, Differential Diagnosis and Intervention Strategies of Some Hip Conditions (*Continued*)

Diagnosis	History	Physical findings	Differential diagnosis
Trochanteric bursitis	Pain over greater trochanter on palpation, pain during transitions from standing to lying down to standing	Pain on palpation of greater trochanter	Iliotibial band syndrome; femoral neck stress fracture
Avascular necrosis of the femoral head	Dull ache or throbbing pain in groin, lateral hip or buttock, history of prolonged steroid use, prior fracture, slipped femoral capital epiphysis	Pain on ambulation, abduction, internal and external rotation	Early degenerative joint disease
Piriformis syndrome	Dull posterior pain, may radiate down the leg mimicking radicular symptoms, history of track competition or prolonged sitting	Pain on active external rotation, passive internal rotation of hip and palpation of sciatic notch	Nerve root compression, stress fractures
Iliopsoas bursitis	Pain and snapping in medial groin or thigh	Reproduce symptoms with active and passive flexion/extension of hip	Avulsion fracture
Meralgia paresthetica	Pain or paresthesia of anterior or lateral groin and thigh	Abnormal distribution of lateral femoral cutaneous nerve on sensory examination	Other causes of peripheral neuropathy
Degenerative arthritis	Progressive pain and stiffness	Reduction in internal rotation early, in all motion later, pain on ambulation	Inflammatory arthritis
Legg-Calvé-Perthes disease	Normal CBC and ESR, plain films positive (early with changes in the epiphysis, later with flattening of the femoral head)	Maintain ROM, follow position of femoral head in relation to acetabulum radiographically	Orthopedic surgery if unresolved
Slipped capital femoral epiphysis	Plain films show widening of epiphysis early, later slippage of femur under epiphysis	Nonweight bearing, surgical pinning	Urgent orthopedic surgery with acute, large slips
Avulsion fracture	Plain films; if these are negative, CT or MRI	Rehabilitation program of progressive increase in ROM and strengthening	Orthopedic surgery if >2-centimeter displacement PT appropriate
Hip pointer	Plain films if suspect fracture	Rest, ice, NSAIDs, local steroid and anesthetic injection for severe pain, gradual return to activities with protection of site	

Condition	Diagnosis	Treatment	Recommendation
Contusion	Plain films negative	Rest, ice, compression, static stretch, NSAIDs	PT appropriate
Myositis ossificans	Radiograph or ultrasound examination reveals typical calcified, intramuscular hematoma	Ice, stretching of involved structure, NSAIDs; surgical resection after 1 year if conservative treatment fails	PT appropriate, orthopedic surgery if resection needed
Femoral neck stress fracture	Plain films may show cortical defects in femoral neck (superior or inferior surface); bone scan, MRI, CT may also be used if plain films are negative and diagnosis is suspected	Inferior surface fracture, no weight bearing until evidence of healing (usually 2 to 4 weeks) with gradual return to activities, superior surface fracture: ORIF	Orthopedic surgery for ORIF
Osteoid osteoma	Plain films, if these are negative and symptoms persist, MRI or CT	Surgical removal if unresponsive to medical therapy with aspirin or NSAIDs	Orthopedic surgery
Iliotibial band syndrome	Positive Ober's test	Modification of activity, footwear, stretching program, ice massage, NSAIDs	PT appropriate
Trochanteric bursitis	Plain films, bone scan, MRI negative for bony involvement	Ice, NSAIDs, stretching of iliotibial band, protection from direct trauma, steroid injection	PT appropriate
Avascular necrosis of the femoral head	Plain films, MRI	Protected weight bearing, exercises to maximize soft tissue function (strength and support), total hip replacement	PT trial appropriate, orthopedic surgery
Piriformis syndrome	EMG studies may be helpful, MRI of lumbar spine if nerve root compression is suspected	Stretching, NSAIDs, relative rest, correction of offending activity	PT appropriate
Iliopsoas bursitis	Plain films are negative	Iliopsoas stretching, steroid injection	PT appropriate
Meralgia paresthetica	Nerve conduction velocity testing may be helpful	Avoid external compression of nerve (clothing, equipment, pannus)	—
Degenerative arthritis	Plain films help with diagnosis and prognosis	Maximizing support and strength of soft tissues, ice, NSAIDs, modification of activities, cane, total hip replacement	PT trial appropriate, orthopaedic surgery

PPB = prepubescent; CBC = complete blood count; ESR = erythrocyte sedimentation rate; ROM = range of motion; CT = computed tomography; MRI = magnetic resonance imaging; NSAIDs = nonsteroidal anti-inflammatory drugs; PT = physical therapy; ORIF = open reduction internal fixation; EMG = electromyelography.

Source: Adkins SB, Figler RA: Hip pain in athletes. Am Fam Phys 2000;61:2109–2118.

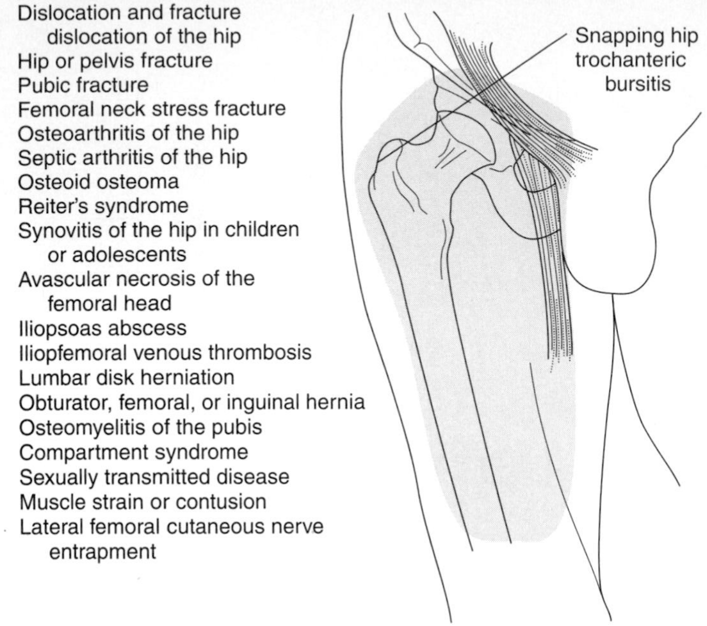

Dislocation and fracture
dislocation of the hip
Hip or pelvis fracture
Pubic fracture
Femoral neck stress fracture
Osteoarthritis of the hip
Septic arthritis of the hip
Osteoid osteoma
Reiter's syndrome
Synovitis of the hip in children
or adolescents
Avascular necrosis of the
femoral head
Iliopsoas abscess
Iliofemoral venous thrombosis
Lumbar disk herniation
Obturator, femoral, or inguinal hernia
Osteomyelitis of the pubis
Compartment syndrome
Sexually transmitted disease
Muscle strain or contusion
Lateral femoral cutaneous nerve
entrapment

Snapping hip
trochanteric
bursitis

FIG.10-1 Potential causes of anterior and lateral thigh pain. (*Reproduced with permission from Dutton M: Orthopaedic Examination, Evaluation, and Intervention, p 245 (Fig. 9-3). New York, McGraw-Hill, 2004.*)

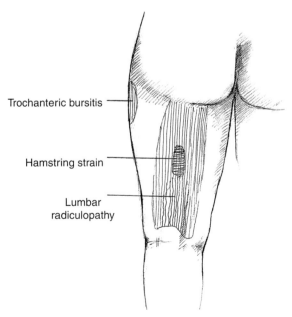

Trochanteric bursitis

Hamstring strain

Lumbar
radiculopathy

FIG.10-2 Potential causes of posterior thigh pain.

TABLE 10-4 Differentiation between Hip Strains and Tendinitis

Condition	Presentation	Examination findings	Imaging and diagnostic studies	Basis of diagnosis	Intervention
Muscle and tendon strains	Acute mechanism, localized pain occurring immediately	Local swelling and tenderness, ecchymosis, weakness	MRI or ultrasonography	Clinical findings with imaging if needed	Rest, ice, compression, progressive rehabilitation Address errors in training, technique, and mechanics
Tendinitis	Overuse, delayed onset, pain localized and worsening with activity	Local swelling and tenderness, crepitus "snapping," weakness	MRI or ultrasonography	Clinical findings with imaging if needed	Same as for strains

- Labral tears
- Stress fractures of the femoral neck
- Subluxations or dislocations of the hip

Osteoarthritis of the Hip Joint

It is important to correctly identify patients with symptomatic osteoarthritis (OA) and to exclude conditions that may be mistaken for or coexist with OA.[2,3] Periarticular pain that is not reproduced by passive motion and direct joint palpation suggests an alternate etiology such as bursitis, tendinitis, or periostitis. OA of the hip joint generally presents with fairly steady pain that becomes more severe as the disease advances. Progressively worsening pain with activity is common, and a painful, limping gait generally develops. Pain is worse initially with full internal rotation and extension of the hip, and hip range of motion is progressively lost. The distribution of painful joints is helpful to distinguish OA from other types of arthritis because metacarpophalangeal (MCP), wrist, elbow, ankle, and shoulder arthritis are unlikely locations for OA except after trauma.

Causes for symptom referral to the hip include:

- Occult hernia or nerve entrapment (Table 10-5)
- Tumors of the pelvis and lumbar spine (see *Systems Review*)
- *Inflammatory arthritides.* Inflammatory arthritides include seronegative spondyloarthropathies (ankylosing spondylitis, Reiter's syndrome, psoriatic arthropathy and enteropathic arthropathy), crystalline arthropathies (gout and pseudogout) and rheumatoid, and viral and septic arthritis. Symptoms including prolonged morning stiffness (greater than 1 hour) should raise suspicion for an inflammatory arthritis (Table 10-6). Typically, the pain with inflammatory arthritis is worse in the morning and improves with activity, although activity limitation may also occur. A careful history should be obtained to pinpoint other joint involvement, enthesopathy (tendinous pain and inflammation at the site of muscle insertion), associated skin disease, systemic symptoms, eye problems, sexually transmitted diseases, inflammatory bowel disease, and a family history of inflammatory disease.

The location of the symptoms can provide the clinician with some useful information. Anterior hip pain is a common complaint with many possible causes. The term "anterior hip pain" is applied to symptoms extending medially to the pubic symphysis, laterally to the anterior superior iliac spine (ASIS), superiorly to the lower abdomen and inferiorly to the proximal 5 to 10 centimeters of the anterior thigh. Anterior hip pain usually indicates pathology of the hip joint (i.e., degenerative arthritis), hip flexor muscle strains or tendinitis, and iliopsoas bursitis. However, OA of the hip may also cause pain behind the greater trochanter and knee due to the various nerves that crosses the hip.[4] In the adolescent, acute muscle contraction about the hip can result in avulsion of an apophysis (an ossification center at the attachment of tendon to bone). Whereas overuse is likely to result in tendinitis in an adult, it is more likely to cause apophysitis in the adolescent. Muscles with pelvic apophyseal attachments are listed in Table 10-7. Groin pain is a common complaint in this region and can result from local and referred sources (Table 10-8). The term "groin" refers to the inferomedial aspect of the anterior hip. One of the more common causes of groin pain in the older patient is OA of the hip. Lateral hip pain is usually associated with greater trochanteric pain syndrome, iliotibial band (ITB) syndrome, or meralgia

TABLE 10-5 Differentiation between Occult Hernia and Nerve Entrapment

Condition	Presentation	Examination findings	Imaging and diagnostic studies	Basis of diagnosis	Treatment
Sports hernia (occult hernia or tear of oblique aponeurosis)	Chronic groin pain (i.e., particularly common in soccer, and ice hockey); pain worse with "cutting" and sprinting	Tenderness at superficial inguinal ring	Herniography may identify occult hernia	Clinical findings	Herniorrhaphy Repair of aponeurosis
Obturator or ilioinguinal nerve entrapment	Same as for sports hernia but with adductor weakness or spasm	Adductor tenderness, decreased sensation	Electromyelography Obturator nerve block	Clinical findings and diagnostic tests	Surgical release of fascial entrapment of nerve

TABLE 10-6 Differentiation between osteoarthritis (OA) and rheumatoid arthritis (RA) of the Hip

Condition	Presentation	Examination findings	Imaging and diagnostic studies	Basis of diagnosis	Intervention
OA	Groin pain on activity, gradual worsening of pain, limp	Pain and decreased range of motion on internal rotation and extension	Radiographs: joint space narrowing, sclerosis, osteophytes	Clinical findings, confirmed with radiographs	Initially, oral analgesics and exercise Joint arthroplasty for end-stage disease
RA	Pain in the morning, activity limitation, systemic involvement	Generalized joint involvement, enthesopathy, skin or bowel symptoms	Elevated erythrocyte sedimentation rate and C-reactive protein level Arthrocentesis: white blood cell count in joint fluid of 2500 to 50,000 per mm^3 Radiographs: erosions, osteopenia	Clinical and laboratory findings Significant improvement with NSAIDs	NSAIDs and exercise, with disease progression, antirheumatic drugs

TABLE 10-7 Apophyseal Attachments of the Hip Muscles

Muscles	Apophyseal attachment
Internal and external obliques	Iliac crest
Sartorius	Anterior superior iliac spine
Rectus femoris	Anterior inferior iliac spine
Hamstrings	Ischium
Iliopsoas	Lesser trochanter

paresthetica (Table 10-9). Posterior hip pain is the least common pain pattern, and it usually suggests a source outside the hip joint. Posterior pain is typically referred from such disorders of the lumbar spine as degenerative disk disease, facet arthropathy, and spinal stenosis. Posterior hip pain is also caused by disorders of the sacroiliac joint, hip extensor and external rotator muscles, or, rarely, aortoiliac vascular occlusive disease.

After identifying whether the pain is anterior, lateral, or posterior, the clinician should focus on other characteristics of the pain—sudden versus insidious onset, movements and positions that reproduce the pain, predisposing activities, and the effect of ambulation or weight-bearing activity on the pain. As the hip is a weight-bearing joint, it is very important to gather information concerning the role of weight bearing in pain activities, particularly whether the patient has pain at rest as well as during weight bearing, or whether specific weight-bearing activities (e.g., stair climbing and walking) are the cause of increased pain.[5]

Information must be gathered with regard to the activities or times of day that appear to change the pain for better or worse. With any adult who has acute hip pain, the clinician should be alert for "red flags" that may indicate a more serious medical condition as the source of pain (see *Systems Review*).

Systems Review

Pain may be referred to the hip region from a number of sources. These include the lumbar spine, peripheral nerve entrapments, the sacroiliac joint, and the abdominal viscera. Complaints associated with referred pain include:

- Anterior thigh pain and knee pain may be indicative of lumbar radiculopathy.
- Pain that is decreased with walking up stairs may indicate the patient has lumbar spine stenosis, especially if the pain is increased when walking on the level.
- Pain with sitting could indicate a lumbar disk lesion, or ischial bursitis (weaver's bottom).
- Night pain that is unaffected by movement or positional changes is strongly suggestive of cancer.

Fever, malaise, night sweats, weight loss, night pain, intravenous drug abuse, a history of cancer, or known immunocompromised state should prompt you to consider such conditions as tumor, infection (i.e., septic arthritis or osteomyelitis), or an inflammatory arthritis. Intense inflammation on examination suggests infectious or microcrystalline processes such as gout or pseudogout. Weight loss, fatigue, fever, and loss of appetite should be sought out because these are clues to a systemic illness such as polymyalgia rheumatica, rheumatoid arthritis, lupus, or sepsis.

TABLE 10-8 Differentiation of Hip Pathologies that have the Potential to Produce Groin Pain

Factor	Congenital hip dislocation	Septic arthritis	Legg-Calvé-Perthes	Transient synovitis	Slipped femoral capital epiphysis	Avascular necrosis	Degenerative joint disease	Fracture
Age	Birth	Less than 2 years, rare in adults	2–13 years	2–12 years	Males 10–17 years, females 8–15 years	30–50 years	>40 years	Older adults
Incidence Male:female	Female > male Left > right Blacks < Whites	—	Male > female Rare in blacks, 15% bilateral	Male > female Unilateral	Male > female Blacks > Whites	Male > female	Women > men	Women > men
Observation	Short limb, associated with torticollis	Irritable child, motionless hip, prominent greater trochanter, mild illness	Short limb, high greater trochanter, quad atrophy, adductor spasm	Decreased flexion, abduction, external rotation, thigh atrophy, muscle spasm	Short limb, obese, quadriceps atrophy, adductor spasm	—	Frequently obese, joint crepitus, atrophy of gluteal muscles	Ecchymosis, may be swelling, short limb
Position	Flexed and abducted	Flexed, abducted, externally rotated	—	—	Flexion, abduction, external rotation	—	—	External rotation
Pain	—	Mild pain with palpation and passive motion, often referred to knee	Gradual onset; aching in hip, thigh and knee; tenderness	Acute: severe pain in knee Moderate: pain in thigh and knee, tenderness over hip	Vague pain in knee, suprapatellar area, thigh and hip; also in extreme motion	50% sharp pain, 50% insidious and intermittent pain in extreme ends of range	Insidious onset, pain with fall in barometric pressure	Severe pain in groin area

302

History	May be breech birth	Steroid therapy Fever	20–25% familial, low birth weight, growth delay	Low-grade fever	May be trauma	—	May be prolonged trauma, faulty body mechanics	May be trauma, fall
Range of motion	Limited abduction	Decreased	Limited abduction, extension	Decreased flexion, limited extension, internal rotation	Limited internal rotation, abduction, flexion, increased external adductor spasm	Decreased range of motion	Decreased motion external, internal rotation, and extreme flexion	Limited
Special tests	Galeazzi's sign Ortolani's sign Barlow's sign Piston's sign	Joint aspiration	—	—	—	—	—	—
Gait	—	Refused to walk	Antalgic gait after activity	Refused to walk, antalgic limp	Acute: antalgic Chronic: Trendelenburg External rotation	Coxalgic limp	Limp	—
Radiologic findings	Upward and lateral displacement, delayed development of acetabulum	CT scan: localized abscess, increased separation of ossification center from the lateral pelvic tear drop margin	In stages: increased density, fragmentation, flattening of epiphysis	Normal at first, widened medial joint space	Displacement of upper femoral epiphysis, especially in frog position	Flattening followed by collapse of femoral head	Increased bone density, osteophytes, subarticular cysts; degenerated articular cartilage	Fracture line, possible displacement; short femoral neck

Source: Richardson JK, Iglarsh ZA: The hip and pelvis. In Richardson JK, Iglarsh ZA, (eds): Clinical Orthopaedic Physical Therapy, pp 367–368. Philadelphia, PA, WB Saunders, 1994.

TABLE 10-9 Differential Diagnosis of Pain in the Greater Trochanter Region

Pathology	Clinical examination
Gluteus maximus insertional tendopathy	Local tenderness over the posterior aspect of the greater trochanter. May have pain with resisted hip extension, external rotation, or abduction in severe cases.
Calcification at the insertion of the gluteus maximus	Same clinical findings as for gluteus maximus insertional tendopathy
Subtendinous trochanteric bursitis	Same clinical findings as for gluteus maximus insertional tendopathy. Often passive hip flexion, external rotation, and adduction are also painful. Positive FABER test Pain with combined motion of passive flexion, external rotation, and adduction
Intertendinous trochanteric bursitis	Same clinical findings as for subtendinous trochanteric bursitis
Gluteus medius insertional tendopathy	Same clinical findings as for gluteus maximus insertional tendopathy, although tender area is slightly more proximal on the posterior aspect of the greater trochanter
Snapping hip (coxa saltans)	Snapping occurs during flexion of the hip from a position of extension or in alternating internal and external rotation from a position of hip flexion. Usually no associated pain
Lateral compartment syndrome of the thigh	Pain and local swelling over the tensor fascia latae muscle in the area over the greater trochanter, pain with sitting and activities
Stress fracture of the greater trochanter	Local pain with percussion/ultrasound
Referred pain from L4 or L5	Positive findings in lower quarter scanning examination

Source: Winkel D, Matthijs O, Phelps V: Appendix D. In Winkel D, Matthijs O, Phelps V, (eds): Diagnosis and Treatment of the Lower Extremities, p 595. Gaithersburg, MD, Aspen, 1997.

Newborns are routinely examined for hip dysplasia (Figure 10-3). Pediatric patients presenting with hip pathology, manifested by an antalgic gait or limp (Table 10-10) need a thorough investigation as to the cause (Table 10-11). The age of the child can provide some information (Table 10-12).

By combining the findings from a thorough history with the results of the examination and any pertinent imaging studies (Table 10-13), the clinician should be able to determine the suitability of the patient for a physical therapy intervention. If the clinician is concerned with any signs or symptoms of a visceral, vascular, neurogenic, psychogenic, spondylogenic, or systemic disorder that are out of the scope of physical therapy, the patient should be referred back to his or her physician, or to an appropriate health care professional. Examples of these kinds of signs and symptoms in the hip examination include an insidious onset of symptoms, evidence of radiculopathy, bowel or bladder changes or both, night pain unrelated to movement, and severe pain. The Cyriax lower quarter scanning examination should be used to screen for the presence of upper motor neuron or lower motor neuron lesions or the referral of symptoms from the spine.

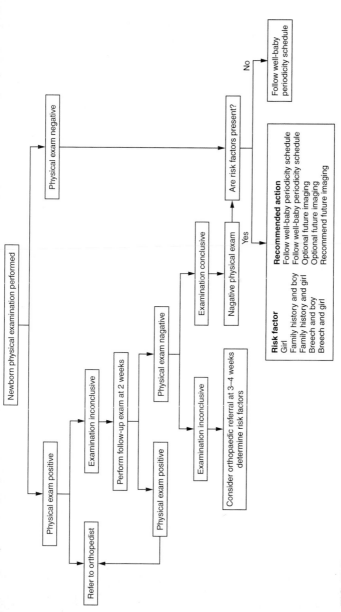

FIG.10-3 Hip dysplasia algorithm. *(Adapted from American Academy of pediatrics Committee on Quality Improvement. Clinical practice guideline: Early detection of developmental dysplasia of the hip. Pediatrics 2000;105:896–905.)*

TABLE 10-10 Differential Diagnosis of the Acutely Limping Child

Cause	Type
Trauma	Fracture
	Stress fracture
	Toddler's fracture (minimally displaced spiral fracture of the tibia)
	Soft tissue contusion
	Ankle sprain
Inflammatory	Juvenile rheumatoid arthritis
	Transient synovitis
	Systemic lupus erythematosus
Tumor	Spinal cord tumors
	Tumors of bone
	Benign: osteoid osteoma, osteoblastoma
	Malignant: osteosarcoma, Ewing's sarcoma
	Lymphoma
	Leukemia
Infection	Cellulitis
	Osteomyelitis
	Septic arthritis
	Lyme disease
	Tuberculosis of bone
	Gonorrhea
	Postinfectious reactive arthritis
Congenital	Developmental dysplasia of the hip
	Sickle cell
	Congenitally short femur
	Clubfoot
Neurologic	Cerebral palsy, especial mild hemiparesis
	Hereditary sensory motor neuropathies
Developmental	Legg-Calvé-Perthes disease
	Slipped capital femoral epiphysis
	Tarsal coalitions
	Osteochondritis dissecans (knee, talus)

Source: Leet AI, Skaggs DL: Evaluation of the acutely limping child. Am Fam Phys 2000;61:1011–1018.

Tests and Measures

Observation

The clinician observes the hip region noting any scars, bruising, swelling, and so forth. The patient is observed from the front, back, and sides for general alignment of the hip, pelvis, spine, and lower extremities (see *Orthopaedic Examination, Evaluation, and Intervention*, pp 686–687). The pelvic crossed syndrome demonstrates weakness and inhibition of the glutei muscles.[6] Atrophy of one buttock cheek compared with the other side may indicate superior or inferior gluteal nerve palsy. A balling-up of the gluteal muscle typically indicates a grade III tear of the gluteal muscles. Buttock swelling occurs with the sign of the buttock.[7] Swelling over the greater trochanter could indicate trochanteric bursitis. Adaptive shortening of the short hip adductors is indicated by a distinct bulk in the muscles of upper third of the thigh.[6] The bulk of the tensor of the fascia lata should not be distinct. A visible groove passing down the lateral aspect of the thigh may indicate that the tensor of the fascia latae (TFL) is overused, and both it and the ITB are adaptively shortened.[6]

The architecture and position of the hip joint and lower extremity is observed.

TABLE 10-11 Differentiation of Pediatric Hip Pathologies

	Congenital hip dislocation	Septic arthritis	Legg-Calvé-Perthes	Transient synovitis	Slipped femoral capital epiphysis
Age	Birth	Less than 2 years, rare in adults	2–13 years	2–12 years	Males 10–17 years Females 8–15 years
Incidence Male:female	Female > male Left > right Blacks < Whites	—	Male > female Rare in Blacks, 15% bilateral	Male > female Unilateral	Male > female Blacks > Whites
Observation	Short limb, associated with torticollis	Irritable child, motionless hip, prominent greater trochanter, mild illness	Short limb, high greater trochanter, quad atrophy, adductor spasm	Decreased flexion, abduction, external rotation, thigh atrophy, muscle spasm	Short limb; obese, quadriceps atrophy, adductor spasm
Position	Flexed and abducted	Flexed, abducted, externally rotated	—	—	Flexion, abduction, external rotation
Pain	—	Mild pain with palpation and passive motion, often referred to knee	Gradual onset; aching in hip, thigh, and knee; tenderness	Acute: severe pain in knee Moderate: pain in thigh and knee, tenderness over hip	Vague pain in knee, suprapatellar area, thigh and hip; also in extreme motion
History	May be breech birth	Steroid therapy Fever	20–25% familial, low birth weight, growth delay	Low-grade fever	May be trauma

(Continued)

307

TABLE 10-11 Differentiation of Pediatric Hip Pathologies (*Continued*)

	Congenital hip dislocation	Septic arthritis	Legg-Calvé-Perthes	Transient synovitis	Slipped femoral capital epiphysis
Range of motion	Limited abduction	Decreased	Limited abduction, extension	Decreased flexion, limited extension, internal rotation	Limited internal rotation, abduction, flexion, increased external adductor spasm
Special tests	Galeazzi's sign Ortolani's sign Barlow's sign	Joint aspiration	—	—	—
Gait	—	Refused to walk	Antalgic gait after activity	Refused to walk; antalgic limp	Acute: antalgic Chronic: Trendelenburg External rotation
Radiologic findings	Upward and lateral displacement, delayed development of acetabulum	CT scan: localized abscess, increased separation of ossification center from the lateral pelvic tear drop margin	In stages: increased density, fragmentation, flattening of epiphysis	Normal at first, widened medial joint space	Displacement of upper femoral epiphysis, especially in frog position

TABLE 10-12 Differential Diagnosis of the Acutely Limping Child by Age

Age group	Condition
All ages	Septic arthritis
	Osteomyelitis
	Cellulitis
	Stress fracture
	Neoplasm (including leukemia)
	Neuromuscular
Toddler (ages 1 to 3)	Septic hip
	Developmental dysplasia of the hip
	Occult fractures
	Leg-length discrepancy
Child (ages 4 to 10)	Legg-Calvé-Perthes disease
	Transient synovitis
	Juvenile rheumatoid arthritis
Adolescent (ages 11 to 16)	Slipped capital femoral epiphysis
	Avascular necrosis of femoral head
	Overuse syndromes
	Tarsal coalitions
	Gonococcal septic arthritis

Source: Leet AI, Skaggs DL: Evaluation of the acutely limping child. Am Fam Phys 2000;61:1011–1018.

Screening Tests

Screening tests for the hip joint include gait analysis and tests that load the joint.

Gait Analysis   Analysis of both the stance and swing phases of gait is essential to determine the problems that must be dealt with during the intervention (see *Orthopaedic Examination, Evaluation, and Intervention*, p 687). Determinants of stance-phase gait involve interaction between the pelvis and hip and distal limb joints (knee and ankle).[8,9]

Joint Loading Tests   Pain on weight bearing is a common complaint in some patients with hip joint pathology, including rheumatoid arthritis and OA.[10] Depending on the capability of the patient, the following weight bearing tests may produce pain.

- *High step.* The patient places one foot on a chair, and then leans onto it. The test is repeated on the other side. This test moves the hip joint through its full range of motion in the sagittal plane (flexion and extension). In addition, the pelvic innominates are also rotated in both directions (anterior and posterior).
- *Unilateral standing.* The patient stands on one leg. An inability to maintain the pelvis in a horizontal position during unilateral standing is called a positive Trendelenburg (see *Special Tests*).

Palpation

Palpation must be systematic and focus on specific anatomic structures. The optimal methods of palpating occur in regions where there is the least amount of overlying soft tissue.[11] The hip area should be palpated for warmth, tenderness, deformity, and crepitus. Palpation should include examination of the following structures.

TABLE 10-13 Correlating the History, Examination, and Diagnostic Studies

Category	History	Physical examination findings	Laboratory studies	Radiology
Traumatic	Fall	Localized pain, swelling, loss of motion	None unless infection is possible	Plain films, bone scan
Infectious	Fever, chills, erythema, pain	Rigid guarding, warmth, erythema	CBC, ESR, CRP, joint aspirate	Plain films, MRI, bone scan
Neoplastic	Night pain, pain unrelated to activity	Mass	CBC, ESR, CRP, alkaline phosphatase, calcium, electrolytes, joint aspirate	Plain films, MRI/CT, bone scan, staging work-up
Congenital	Problem since birth	Deformity, leg-length discrepancy, loss of ROM	None	Plain films
Neurologic	Ataxia, loss of balance, disorganized gait	High/low muscle tone, increased/decreased deep tendon reflexes, cavus foot or claw toes	Creatine kinase (if DMD is in differential diagnosis)	Plain films
Inflammatory	Pain >6 months, family history of rheumatoid arthritis	Warmth/erythema, one or more joints	CBC, ESR, CRP, joint aspiration	Plain films
Developmental	Painless limp (LCP disease) Knee pain (LCP disease, SCFE)	Loss of ROM in joints, asymmetric ROM, pain with ROM	None	Plain films

CBC = complete blood count; ESR = erythrocyte sedimentation rate; CRP = C-reactive protein; MRI = magnetic resonance imaging; CT = computed tomography; ROM = range of motion; DMD = Duchenne's muscular dystrophy; LCP = Legg-Calvé-Perthes; SCFE = slipped capital femoral epiphysis.
Source: Leet AI, Skaggs DL: Evaluation of the acutely limping child. Am Fam Phys 2000;61:1011–1018.

Anterior Aspect of Hip and Groin

Anterior Superior Iliac Spine   The anterior superior iliac spine serves as the origin for the sartorius muscle and the TFL.

Anterior Inferior Iliac Spine   The anterior inferior iliac spine (AIIS) can be palpated in the space formed by the sartorius and the TFL during passive flexion of the hip in the space known as the lateral femoral triangle. The lateral femoral cutaneous nerve passes through this triangle. Compression of this nerve produces a condition called meralgia paresthetica. The AIIS serves as the origin for the rectus femoris tendon.

Pubic Tubercle   Finding the groin crease and then traveling in an inferior-medial direction, or by following the tendon of the adductor longus proximally locate the pubic tubercle. Inguinal hernias are usually found cranial and medial to the tubercle, while femoral hernias are located lateral to the tubercle.

Adductor Magnus   The adductor magnus is palpable in a small triangle in the distal thigh, posterior to the gracilis muscle, and anterior to the semimembranosus.

Rectus Femoris   The rectus femoris has its origin at the AIIS, which is located just distal to the ASIS, between the TFL and sartorius.

Iliopsoas Bursa   To palpate this bursa the patient is positioned in supine with his or her hip positioned in approximately 40° flexion and external rotation, and resting on a pillow. At the proximal end of the femur, the clinician palpates the adductor tubercle and then moves to the ASIS. From there, the clinician proceeds to the inguinal ligament, under the fold of the external oblique (this area is more tender in men due to the proximity of the spermatic cord and tends to be the area for inguinal hernias in men), and into the femoral triangle. The psoas bursa is located under the floor of the triangle, close to the pubic ramus.

Femoral Triangle   The femoral artery lies superficial and medial to the iliopsoas muscle and is easily located by palpation of the pulse. The femoral nerve is the most lateral structure in the femoral triangle. To examine the femoral triangle, the patient is positioned in supine and, if it is possible for the patient to do this, the heel of the leg resting on the opposite knee. This places the patient in a position of flexion-abduction and external rotation.

Inguinal Ligament   The inguinal ligament is located in the fold of the groin, running from the ASIS to the pubic tubercle. It can be located by using transverse palpation.

Adductor Longus   Together with the gracilis, the adductor longus forms the medial border of the femoral triangle. The gracilis is located medial and posterior to the adductor longus. The adductor longus is best viewed during resisted adduction when it forms a cord like structure just distal to the pubic tubercle, before crossing under the sartorius.

Lateral Aspect of the Hip

The patient is positioned side lying.

Iliac Crest   The iliac crest is easy to locate (Figure 10-4). The cluneal nerves are superficial structures and can be located just superior to the crest.

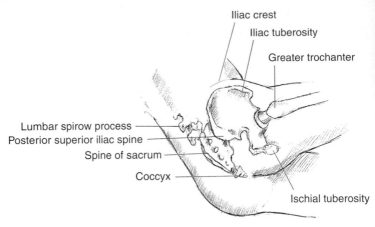

FIG.10-4   Bony landmarks—posterior and lateral view.

Greater Trochanter   The superior border of the greater trochanter represents the transverse axis of hip, and when the leg is abducted, an obvious depression appears above the greater trochanter. Palpation of the greater trochanter (Figure 10-4) is important because of the possibility of trochanteric bursitis. A number of muscles attach to the greater trochanter (Table 10-14). The gluteus medius inserts into the upper portion of the trochanter and can be palpated on the lateral aspect.[5]

Lesser Trochanter   The lesser trochanter, covered as it is with the iliopsoas and adductor magnus, is very difficult to palpate directly, but it can be located on the dorsal aspect if the hip is placed in extension and internal rotation, and the palpation is performed deeply lateral to the ischial tuberosity.

Piriformis Attachment   The origin of the piriformis can be found on the medial aspect of the superior point of the greater trochanter. Moving inferiorly from this point and the quadratus femoris, on the quadrate tubercle, the following tendon insertions can be palpated: superior gemelli, obturator internus, and inferior gemelli.

Psoas   The insertion for the psoas is located on the inferior aspect of the greater trochanter, and can be found by placing the patient's leg in maximum internal rotation of the hip. Once the superior aspect of the greater trochanter is located, the clinician moves in a posterior/medial/inferior direction to locate the inferior aspect of the greater trochanter.

TABLE 10-14 Muscles that Attach to the Greater Trochanter

Piriformis
Gluteus medius
Gluteus minimus
Obturator internus
Gemellus superior
Gemellus inferior

Posterior Aspect of the Hip

The patient is placed in side lying position.

Quadratus Lumborum   Palpation of the quadratus lumborum is best accomplished with the patient in side lying with the arm abducted overhead to open the space between the iliac crest and the 12th rib.

Ischial Tuberosity   The ischial tuberosity is best palpated in the side lying position with the hip flexed to 90° (see Figure 10-4). This position moves the gluteus maximus upward, so permitting direct palpation at the tuberosity. A number of structures have their attachments on the ischial tuberosity. These include the ischial bursa, the semimembranosus tendon, the long head of the biceps femoris and semitendinosus tendon, the sacrotuberous ligament, and the tendons of the quadratus femoris, adductor magnus, and inferior gemellus (Table 10-15). The *ischial bursa* is located on the inferior and medial aspect of the ischial tuberosity.

Sciatic Nerve   The sciatic nerve can be palpated at a point half way between the greater trochanter and the ischial tuberosity. Tenderness of this nerve can be produced by a piriformis muscle spasm, or by direct trauma.

Active, Passive, and Resistive Tests

During the examination of the range of motion, the clinician should note which portions of the range of motion are pain-free, and which portion causes the patient to feel pain. At the end of available active range of motion, passive overpressure is applied to determine the end-feel. The normal ranges and end-feels for the various hip motions are outlined in Table 10-16. Abnormal end-feels common in the hip are firm capsular end-feel before expected range, empty end-feel from severe pain, as in the Sign of the Buttock, and bony block in cases of advanced OA (Figure 10-5).[12] Horizontal abduction and adduction of the femur occur when the hip is in 90° of flexion. Because these actions require simultaneous, coordinated actions of several muscles, they can be used to assess the overall strength of the hip muscles.

Resisted testing is performed to provide the clinician with information about the integrity of the neuromuscular unit, and to highlight the presence of muscle strains (Table 10-17).[13]

If the history indicates that repetitive motions or sustained positions cause the symptoms, the clinician should have the patient reproduce these motions or positions.[14] In the child, pain and loss of range at the hip joint should always alert the clinician to the possibility of transient synovitis, Legg-Calvé-Perthes disease, or a slipped femoral capital epiphysis.

In addition to reports of pain and overall range of motion, the clinician also notes information about weakness, joint end-feel, palpation of the moving joint, and muscle tightness.

TABLE 10-15 Muscles that Attach to the Ischial Tuberosity

Semimembranosus
Semitendinosus
Long head of the biceps femoris
Adductor magnus
Quadratus femoris
Gemellus inferior

TABLE 10-16 Normal Ranges and End-Feels at the Hip

Motion	Range of motion (degrees)	End-feel
Flexion	110–120	Tissue approximation or tissue stretch
Extension	10–15	Tissue stretch
Abduction	30–50	Tissue stretch
Adduction	25–30	Tissue approximation or tissue stretch
External rotation	40–60	Tissue stretch
Internal rotation	30–40	Tissue stretch

Source: Beattie P: The hip. In Malone TR, McPoil T, Nitz A (eds): Orthopaedic and Sports Physical Therapy, 3rd ed., p 506. St Louis, MO, Mosby, 1996.

TABLE 10-17 Muscle Actions at the Hip

Hip flexion	Psoas
	Iliacus
	Rectus femoris
	Sartorius
	Pectineus
	Adductor longus
	Adductor brevis
	Gracilis
Hip extension	Biceps femoris
	Semimembranosus
	Semitendinosus
	Gluteus maximus
	Gluteus medius (posterior fibers)
	Adductor magnus (ischiocondylar portion)
Hip adduction	Adductor longus
	Adductor brevis
	Adductor magnus (ischiofemoral portion)
	Gracilis
	Pectineus
Hip abduction	Tensor of the fascia latae
	Gluteus medius
	Gluteus minimus
	Gluteus maximus
	Sartorius
Hip internal rotation	Adductor longus
	Adductor brevis
	Adductor magnus
	Gluteus medius (anterior fibers)
	Gluteus minimus (anterior fibers)
	Tensor of the fascia latae
	Pectineus
	Gracilis
Hip external rotation	Gluteus maximus
	Obturator internus
	Obturator externus
	Quadratus femoris
	Piriformis
	Gemellus superior
	Gemellus inferior
	Sartorius
	Gluteus medius (posterior fibers)

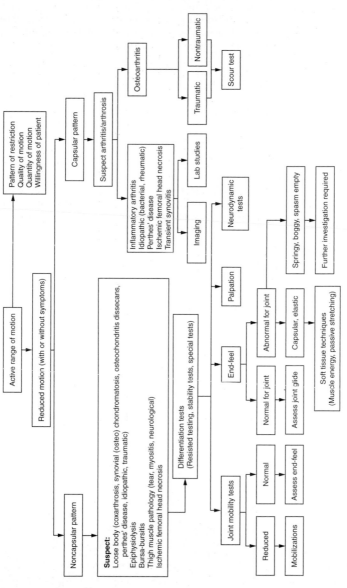

FIG. 10-5 Examination sequence in the presence of symptom-free or incomplete active range of motion at the hip.

315

Flexion

The six muscles primarily responsible for hip flexion are the iliacus, psoas major, pectineus, rectus femoris, sartorius, and TFL (see Table 10-17). The primary hip flexor is the iliopsoas muscle.

Hip flexion motion can be tested in sitting or supine first with the knee flexed (Figure 10-6), and then with the knee extended. With the hip flexed, the range of motion should be approximately 110°–120°. More hip flexion should be available with the knee flexed. Passive overpressure is applied.

Resisted tests are then performed.

To test the strength of the iliopsoas, the patient is supine with the thigh raised off the bed and the clinician applies resistance.

Asking the patient to bring the plantar aspect of the foot toward the opposite knee tests the action of the sartorius muscle, which flexes, abducts, and externally rotates the hip. The clinician applies resistance at the medial malleolus and at the lateral aspect of the thigh to resist flexion, abduction, and external rotation.

A painless weakness of hip flexion is rarely a good sign. Theoretically, it could indicate a disk protrusion at the L1 or L2 level. However, protrusions at these levels are not common. A more likely scenario is compression of the nerves by a neurofibroma or a metastatic invasion. Pain with the active motion or resisted tests, should prompt the clinician to examine the contractile tissues individually. Passive stretching can also produce pain in a contractile structure.

Extension

The primary hip extensor is the gluteus maximus. The hamstrings also serve as hip extensors. Hip extension also involves assistance from the adductor magnus, gluteus medius and minimus, and indirect assistance from the abdominals and the erector spinae.[15]

The patient is positioned prone or over the end of the table (Figure 10-7). As the clinician palpates the buttock mass, and stabilizes the sacrum to prevent

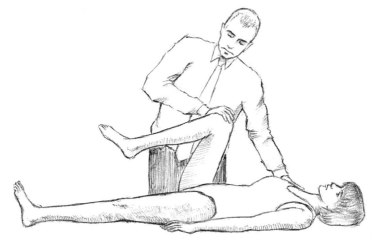

FIG.10-6 Active hip flexion with passive overpressure.

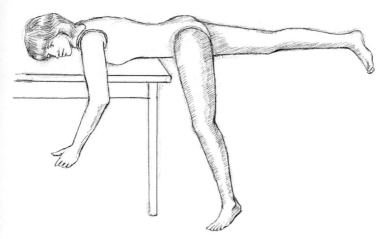

FIG.10-7   Position for testing hip extension range of motion and strength.

the lumbar spine from extending, the patient is asked to lift the thigh toward the ceiling.

The normal range of motion for hip extension is approximately 10–15°. Reduced hip extension can be the result of a number of reasons including adaptive shortening of the iliopsoas or a hip flexion contracture.

To test the strength of the gluteus maximus, the patient is positioned in prone, with his or her knee flexed. As before, the sacrum is stabilized and the patient is asked to raise the thigh off the table. The clinician then applies resistance. The hamstrings can be tested in supine with the knee extended. A strong and painful finding with resisted hip extension may indicate a grade I muscle strain of the gluteus maximus or hamstrings. It may also indicate a gluteal bursitis, or a lumbosacral strain.

Abduction/Adduction

Hip adduction and abduction range of motion can be tested while the patient is supine, making sure that both ASIS are level, and the legs are perpendicular to a line joining the ASIS (Figure 10-8).

Abduction   The patient is supine. The clinician monitors the ipsilateral ASIS, and the patient is asked to abduct the leg (Figure 10-8). The abduction motion is stopped when the ASIS is felt to move. The prime movers for this movement are the gluteus medius/minimus and the TFL. The quadratus lumborum functions as the stabilizer of the pelvis.

Adduction   Hip adduction is tested with the patient supine, and with the uninvolved leg adducted over the other leg, or held in flexion. As before, the ASIS is monitored for motion, indicating the end of range for adduction. The primary hip adductor is the adductor longus. Adaptive shortening of the hip adductors can theoretically result in inhibition of the gluteus medius, a decrease in frontal stability, ITB tendinitis, and anterior knee pain. Pain can be referred from the hip adductors into the anterior-lateral hip, groin, medial

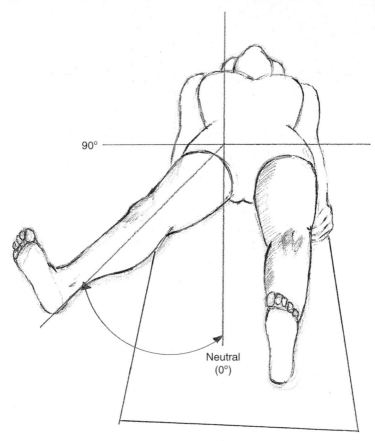

FIG.10-8   Active hip abduction.

thigh, the anterior knee, and medial tibia. Pain in these regions with passive abduction, or active adduction, may indicate a strain of one of the adductors. The cause of the pain can be differentiated between the two-joint gracilis and the other hip adductors (longus, brevis, and pectineus) in the following manner. The patient is positioned in side lying with the tested leg supported by the clinician. The clinician places the hip into the fully abducted position and the knee is flexed. If no pain is reproduced with this maneuver, the patient is asked to extend the knee, thereby bringing in the gracilis, and implicating it if the pain is now reproduced. This can be confirmed with resisted hip adduction and knee flexion. If the other adductors are implicated, this can be confirmed with resisted adduction (longus and brevis) or resisted hip adduction and hip flexion (pectineus).

The strength of the hip adductor muscle group is tested in side lying, by flexing the uninvolved leg over the tested leg, or by supporting the upper leg and then applying resistance. This position also stretches the hip abductors, and can be a source of pain in the case of an ITB syndrome.

The strength of the gluteus medius and minimus is tested with the patient in side lying. The patient is asked to perform hip abduction, without any flexion or external rotation occurring. The clinician applies resistance to the distal thigh.

A strong and painful finding with resisted adduction is usually the result of an adductor longus lesion, whereas a painless weakness with resisted abduction is often found in a palsy of the fifth lumbar root because of a disk herniation of the same level.

Internal and External Rotation

Although a number of muscles contribute to external rotation of the femur (see Table 10-17), six muscles function solely as external rotators.[16] These are the piriformis, gemellus superior, gemellus inferior, obturator internus, obturator externus, and quadratus femoris. Normal range of motion for hip external rotation is approximately 40°–60°. Excessive external rotation of the hip may indicate hip retroversion.

The major internal rotator of the femur is the gluteus minimus, assisted by the gluteus medius, TFL, semitendinosus, and semimembranosus. The internal rotators of the femur are estimated to be only approximately one-third the strength of the external rotators.[17] Normal range of motion for hip internal rotation is approximately 30°–40°. Excessive internal rotation of the hip may indicate hip anteversion.

To assess the range of motion of the hip rotators, the patient is positioned in supine with the leg in 90° of hip flexion, and 90° of knee flexion. Alternatively, the patient can be positioned prone, with the knee flexed to 90° and the hip in neutral.

Functional Assessment

Table 10-18 outlines a functional assessment tool for the hip.[18] An assessment of the patient's functional status can also be made through observation or through use of a self-report measure, which allows a patient to rate his or her capacity to perform.

Passive Accessory Movements

Due to the extreme congruency of the joint partners at the hip joint, this is a difficult area to assess with any degree of accuracy, especially as the glides that occur are very slight. Thus, only one accessory motion, lateral distraction, is examined.

The patient is positioned supine with the hip and knee flexed to 90°, with the knee placed on the clinician's shoulder (Figure 10-9). The clinician places one hand over the greater trochanter and the other close to the superior aspect of the medial thigh (Figure 10-9). A distraction force and then a compression force are applied in line with the femoral neck. The test is positive if excessive movement is detected.

Special Tests

Special tests are merely confirmatory tests and should not be used alone to form a diagnosis. The results from these tests are used in conjunction with the other clinical findings to help guide the clinician. To assure accuracy with these tests, both sides should be tested for comparison.

TABLE 10-18 Functional Test of the Hip

Starting position	Action	Functional test	
Standing	Hip flexion—lift foot onto an 8-inch or 20-centimeter step and return	5–6 repetitions 3–4 repetitions 1–2 repetitions 0 repetitions	Functional Functionally fair Functionally poor Nonfunctional
Standing	Hip extension—sit in a chair and return to standing	5–6 repetitions 3–4 repetitions 1–2 repetitions 0 repetitions	Functional Functionally fair Functionally poor Nonfunctional
Standing	Hip abductors—lift leg to balance on one leg while keeping pelvis level	Hold 1–1.5 minutes Hold 30–59 seconds Hold 1–29 seconds Cannot hold	Functional Functionally fair Functionally poor Nonfunctional
Standing	Hip adductors—walk sideways 6 meters	6–8 meters one way 3–6 meters one way 1–3 meters one way 0 meter	Functional Functionally fair Functionally poor Nonfunctional
Standing	Hip internal rotation—test leg off floor (holding on to object for balance if necessary) internally rotate non-weight bearing hip	10–12 repetitions 5–9 repetitions 1–4 repetitions 0 repetitions	Functional Functionally fair Functionally poor Nonfunctional
Standing, facing closed door	Hip external rotation—test leg off floor (holding on to object for balance if necessary) externally rotate non-weight-bearing hip	10–12 repetitions 5–9 repetitions 1–4 repetitions 0 repetitions	Functional Functionally fair Functionally poor Nonfunctional

Source: Palmer ML, Epler M: Clinical Assessment Procedures in Physical Therapy. Philadelphia, PA, JB Lippincott, 1990.

Quadrant (Scour) Test

The quadrant or scour test is a dynamic test of the inner quadrant and outer quadrant of the hip joint surface.[19]

The patient is positioned in supine, close to the edge of the bed, with his or her hip flexed and foot resting on the bed. The clinician interlocks the fingers of both hands and places them over the top of the patient's knee. The patient's hip is placed in 90° of flexion with the knee allowed to flex comfortably. From this point, the clinician adducts the hip to the point when the patient's pelvis begins to lift on the bed to assess the inner quadrant (Figure 10-10). At the end

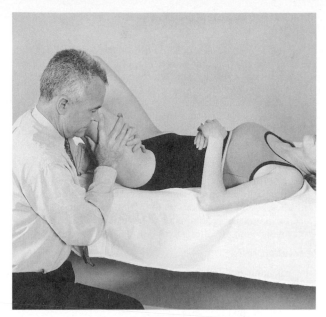

FIG.10-9 Hip distraction. (*Reproduced with permission from Dutton M: Orthopaedic Examination, Evaluation, and Intervention, p 695 (Fig. 17-20). New York, McGraw-Hill, 2004.*)

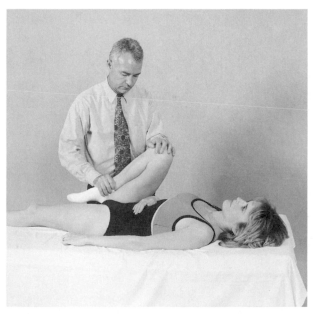

FIG.10-10 Scour test. (*Reproduced with permission from Dutton M: Orthopaedic Examination, Evaluation, and Intervention, p 695 (Fig. 17-21). New York, McGraw-Hill, 2004.*)

range of flexion and adduction, a compression force is applied at the knee along the longitudinal axis of the femur. From this point, the clinician moves the hip into a position of flexion and abduction to examine the outer quadrant. Throughout the entire movement, the femur is held midway between internal and external rotation, and the movement at the hip joint should follow the smooth arc of a circle. An abnormal finding is resistance felt anywhere during the arc. The resistance may be caused by capsular tightness, an adhesion, a myofascial restriction, or a loss of joint congruity.

FABER (Flexion, Abduction, External Rotation) or Patrick's Test

The FABER test (flexion, abduction, and external rotation) test is a screening test for hip, lumbar or sacroiliac joint dysfunction, or an iliopsoas spasm.

A positive test results in pain or loss of motion as compared with the uninvolved side or both. Having the patient demonstrate where the pain is with this test may assist with the interpretation of this test.

SI Provocation Tests

Unless the patient history or the physical examination highlights the presence of a sacroiliac dysfunction, the clinician relies on two simple stress tests to rule out sacroiliac pathology, the anterior gapping (Figure 10-11) and posterior gapping (Figure 10-12) tests.

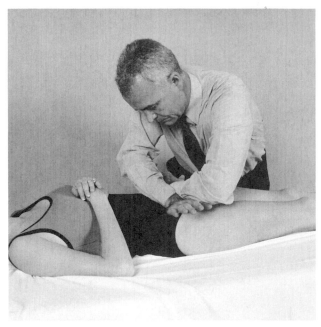

FIG.10-11 Anterior gapping of the SI joint. (*Reproduced with permission from Dutton M: Orthopaedic Examination, Evaluation, and Intervention, p 696 (Fig. 17-23). New York, McGraw-Hill, 2004.*)

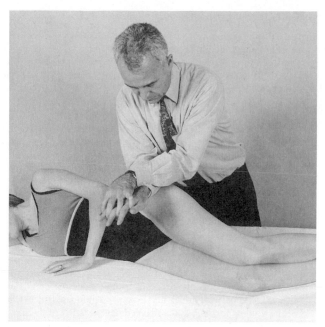

FIG.10-12 Posterior gapping of the SI joint. (*Reproduced with permission from Dutton M: Orthopaedic Examination, Evaluation, and Intervention, p 696 (Fig. 17-24). New York, McGraw-Hill, 2004.*)

In addition to the provocative tests, the passive motions of the hip can be examined with the innominate stabilized. The hip motions and their respective innominate motions, in parenthesis, are outlined in Table 10-19.

Craig Test

The Craig test is used to assess femoral anteversion/retroversion. The patient is positioned in prone with the knee flexed to 90°. The clinician rotates the hip through the full ranges of hip internal and external rotation while palpating the greater trochanter and determining the point in the range at which the greater trochanter is the most prominent laterally. If the angle is greater than 8°–15° in the direction of internal rotation when measured from the vertical and long axis of the tibia, the femur is considered to be in anteversion.[20–23]

TABLE 10-19 Hip Motions and Their Associated Innominate Motions

Flexion (posterior rotation)
Extension (anterior rotation)
Abduction (upward)
Adduction (downward)
Internal rotation (IR)
External rotation (ER)

Flexion-Adduction Test

This test is used as a screening test for early hip pathology.[24] The patient is positioned in supine and the hip is passively flexed to 90° and in neutral rotation. From this position, the clinician stabilizes the pelvis and the hip is passively adducted. The resultant end-feel, restriction, discomfort, or pain is noted and compared with the normal side.

Trendelenburg Sign

The Trendelenburg sign indicates weakness of the gluteus medius muscle during unilateral weight bearing. This position produces a strong contraction of the gluteus medius, which is powerfully assisted by the gluteus minimus and TFL, to keep the pelvis horizontal. For example, when the right foot supports the body weight, the right hip abductors contract isometrically, and eccentrically, to prevent the left side of the pelvis from being pulled downward.

The clinician crouches or kneels behind the patient with his or her eyes level with the patient's pelvis, and ensures that the patient does not lean to one side during the testing. The patient is asked to stand on one limb for approximately 30 seconds and the clinician notes whether the pelvis remains level. If the hip remains level, the test is negative. A positive Trendelenburg sign is indicated when, during unilateral weight bearing, the pelvis drops toward the unsupported limb. A number of dysfunctions can produce the Trendelenburg sign. These include superior gluteal nerve palsy, a lumbar disk herniation, weakness of the gluteus medius, and advanced degeneration of the hip.

Pelvic Drop Test[25]

The patient is asked to place one foot on a 20-centimeter (8-inch) stool or step and to stand up straight. The patient then lowers the non-weight-bearing leg to the floor. On lowering the leg, there should be no arm abduction, anterior or pelvic motion, or trunk flexion. Nor should there be any hip adduction or internal rotation of the weight-bearing hip. These compensations are indications of an unstable hip or weak external rotators.

Sign of the Buttock

To test for the presence of this syndrome, the patient is positioned in supine. The clinician performs a passive unilateral straight leg raise. If there is a unilateral restriction, the clinician flexes the knee and notes whether the hip flexion increases. If the restriction was a result of the lumbar spine or hamstrings, hip flexion increases. If the hip flexion does not increase when the knee is flexed, it is a positive sign of the buttock test. If the sign of the buttock is encountered, the patient must be immediately returned to the physician for further investigation.

Muscle Length Tests

Thomas Test and Modified Thomas Test　The original Thomas test was designed to test the flexibility of the iliopsoas complex, but has since been modified and expanded to assess a number of other soft tissue structures.

The original test involved positioning the patient in supine, with one knee held to the chest at the point when the lumbar spine begins to flex (Figure 10-13). The clinician assesses whether the thigh of the extended leg maintains full contact with the surface of the bed. If the thigh is raised off the surface of the treatment table, the test is positive (Figure 10-13). A positive test indicates a decrease in flexibility in the rectus femoris or iliopsoas muscles or both.

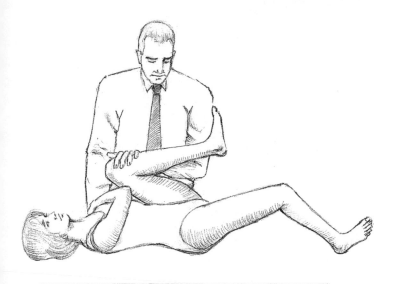

FIG.10-13   Thomas test.

A modified version to this test is commonly used. For the modified version, the patient is positioned in sitting at the end of the bed (Figure 10-14). From this position, the patient is asked to lie down, while bringing both knees against the chest. Once in this position, the patient is asked to perform a posterior pelvic tilt. While the contralateral hip is held in maximum hip flexion with the arms, the tested limb is lowered over the end of the bed, toward the floor. In this position, the thigh should be parallel with the bed, in neutral rotation, and neither abducted nor adducted, with the lower leg perpendicular to the thigh and in neutral rotation. A knee flexion of 100°–110° should be present with the thigh in full contact with the table.

Ely's Test   This is a test to assess the flexibility of the rectus femoris. The patient is positioned in prone lying and the knee is flexed. If the rectus is tight, the pelvis is observed to anteriorly rotate early in the range of knee flexion, and the hip flexes.

Ober's Test   The Ober test is used to evaluate tightness of the iliotibial band and tensor fascia lata (see *Thomas Test* also).[26] The patient is placed in the side lying position, and, with the hip extended and abducted, and the knee flexed, the proximal part of the leg is allowed to drop passively onto the contralateral limb (Figure 10-15). The test is considered positive when the leg fails to lower. There have been some doubts expressed as to the reliability of the Ober test as a measure for ITB tightness.[27]

Straight Leg Raise Test for Hamstring Length   The patient is positioned in supine with the legs together and extended. The clinician stands on the side of the leg to be tested and grasps the patient's ankle with one hand, while using the other hand to stabilize the opposite thigh. With the patient's knee extended, the clinician lifts the patient's leg, flexing the hip, until motion is seen to occur

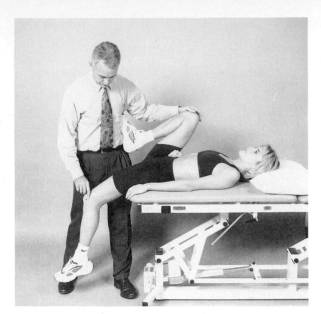

FIG.10-14 Modified Thomas test. (*Reproduced with permission from Dutton M: Orthopaedic Examination, Evaluation, and Intervention, p 698 (Fig. 17-27). New York, McGraw-Hill, 2004.*)

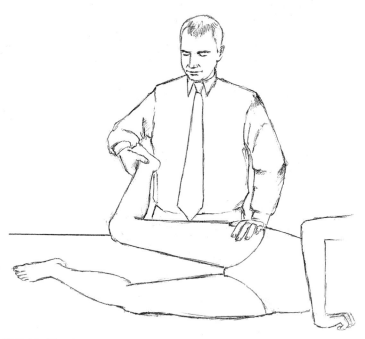

FIG.10-15 Ober test.

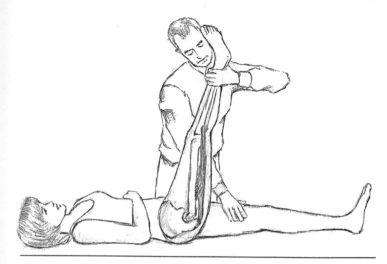

FIG.10-16   Hamstring length.

at the opposite ASIS (Figure 10-16). The angle of flexion from the treatment table is measured. The clinician returns the leg to the table and repeats the maneuver from the other side of the table with the other leg. The hamstrings are considered shortened if a straight leg cannot be raised to an angle of 80° from the horizontal, while the other leg is straight.[6] Any limitation of flexion is interpreted as being caused by contracted hamstring muscles.

This straight leg raise test may also be used as a screen for adverse neural tension, particularly of the sciatic nerve.

90-90 Straight Leg Raise   The hamstring length can also be assessed with the patient positioned in supine and the tested leg flexed at the hip and knee to 90°. From this position, the patient is asked to extend the knee of the involved side without extending the hip. The measurement is taken at the first resistance barrier.

Piriformis   The patient is positioned in supine. The clinician flexes the involved hip to 60°. After stabilizing the patient's pelvis, the clinician applies a downward pressure through the femur, and maximally adducts the involved hip. From this position, the hip is moved into internal rotation and then external rotation. Internal rotation stresses the superior fibers, while external rotation stresses the inferior fibers. Normal range of motion should be 45° into either rotation.

Hip Adductors   The patient is positioned supine with the leg to be tested close to the edge of the mat table. The leg not to be tested is 15°–25° abducted at the hip joint with the heel over the end of the mat table. Maintaining the tested knee in extension, the clinician passively abducts the tested leg. The normal range is 40°. When the full range is reached, the knee of the tested leg is passively flexed and the leg abducted further. If the maximum range does not increase when the knee is flexed, the one-joint adductors (pectineus, adductor magnus, adductor longus, and adductor brevis) are shortened. If the range does increase with the knee passively flexed, the two-joint adductors (gracilis, biceps femoris, semimembranosus, and semitendinosus) are shortened.

Leg Length Discrepancy

The test for a leg length discrepancy is best performed radiographically. However, the following clinical test can be used to highlight the more significant discrepancies.

The patient is positioned in supine and the clinician palpates the ASIS. From this point, the clinician slides distally into the depression and then measures from this point to the tip of the malleolus making sure that the course of the tape follows the same route for both legs.

Fulcrum Test

The fulcrum test[28] is used to test for the presence of a stress fracture of the femoral shaft. The patient is positioned in sitting with his or her knees bent over the edge of the bed, and feet dangling. A firm towel roll is placed under the involved thigh, and is moved proximal to distal as gentle pressure is applied to the dorsum of the knee with the clinician's hand. A positive test is when the patient reports sharp pain or expresses apprehension when the fulcrum arm is placed under the fracture site.

Pediatric Screening Tests for Congenital or Developmental Dysplasia of the Hip

The value of the neonatal hip screening examination remains controversial.[29] At present, the Ortolani and Barlow tests are currently used to examine the infant. Both tests are designed to detect motion between the femoral head and the acetabulum.[29] The reproducibility of these tests is dependent on ligamentous or capsular laxity, which usually disappears by 10 to 12 weeks of age.[29]

In addition to the special tests, the clinician looks for asymmetry between the lower extremities. Asymmetric thigh folds, a short leg appearance, or a prominent greater trochanter may be significant findings.[29]

In addition to the clinical tests, both congenital hip dysplasia (CHD) and developmental dysplasia of hip (DDH) can be detected with radiographs or ultrasound.

Neurovascular Assessment

Manual muscle testing and sensation testing may be used to assess the integrity of the neurologic structures. In addition, neurodynamic mobility tests including the straight leg raise and the prone knee bending tests may be used (see *Orthopaedic Examination, Evaluation, and Intervention*, Chapter 12). In order to gain the most from these tests, the clinician should be aware of the dermatomal pattern as well as the areas supplied by the peripheral nerves (inferior femoral cutaneous, lateral femoral cutaneous, and posterior femoral cutaneous nerves). It is very important to remember, that reports of paresthesia in the "saddle" region is indicative of cauda equina compression and constitutes a medical emergency.

Imaging Studies

Imaging studies continue to be developed and refined to help clinicians diagnose more accurately, and these often provide prognostic information. These imaging studies are most effective when selected on the basis of a thorough history and physical examination.

Radiographs

Pain in the hips is often difficult to assess with plain radiographs. Plain anteroposterior radiographs of the pelvis will clearly show a hip dislocation in most patients but lateral views may be required to confirm the diagnosis and to show the direction if the signs are subtle. Anteroposterior (AP) and lateral views are also used to demonstrate most fractures. For patients in whom femoral neck fracture is strongly suspected but standard x-ray findings are negative, an AP view with hip internally rotated provides a better view of the femoral neck.

Early avascular necrosis in patients of any age and fractures in patients with osteopenia are especially problematic. Avascular necrosis may not show significant radiographic changes until it has advanced.

In cases of pigmented villonodular synovitis, radiographs of the hip may show erosions in the head and neck of the femur and acetabulum.

Magnetic Resonance Imaging

When plain radiographs show no apparent fracture in an elderly patient who has osteoarthritic as well as osteoporotic changes in the hips, but the physical examination findings strongly suggest one, magnetic resonance imaging (MRI) can more accurately assess these subtle occult fractures because it is very sensitive to marrow edema.

MRI is highly sensitive and specific for the diagnosis of pigmented villonodular synovitis of the hip.[30] Characteristic MRI findings include hip joint effusion, lifting of the joint capsule, low signal intensity on both T_1- and T_2-weighted images (because of hemosiderin deposition), hyperplastic synovium (that appears as a lobulated synovial mass), bony erosions, and preservation of bone density.[30]

In addition, MRI is superior to radiographs in the early detection of avascular necrosis, enabling institution of appropriate intervention. MRI can also be used to assess for abdominal aortic dissection, aneurysms, vascular anomalies, and coarctation.

In the athletic population, there is increasing use of MRI to diagnose pelvic and hip fractures, muscle contusion and strain, tendon injuries, acetabular labral tears, bursitis, and osteitis pubis and chronic symphyseal injury.[31]

Computed Tomography

A computed tomography (CT) scan may be required to confirm the diagnosis of a hip dislocation if the signs are subtle. Associated acetabular wall fractures and femoral head fractures also may be identified by CT scans. CT is also more sensitive in detecting osteochondral fragments.

Because MRI is susceptible to artifacts due to patient motion, dissection and aneurysms are still usually evaluated with rapid helical CT.

Ultrasonography

Ultrasonography provides visualization of the cartilage, hip stability, and features of the acetabulum, and has been identified as the technique of choice for clarifying a physical finding suggestive of developmental dysplasia of the hip (DDH), both for assessing a high-risk infant and for monitoring the condition.

EXAMINATION CONCLUSIONS—THE EVALUATION

Following the examination, and once the clinical findings have been recorded, the clinician must determine a specific diagnosis or a working hypothesis, based on a summary of all the findings. This diagnosis can be structure related (medical diagnosis) (Table 10-20), or a diagnosis based on the preferred practice patterns as described in the *Guide to Physical Therapist Practice*.[32]

TABLE 10-20 Differential Diagnosis for Common Causes of Hip Pain

Condition	Patient age	Mechanism of injury or onset	Area of symptoms	Symptoms aggravated by	Observation	AROM	PROM	Resisted	Tenderness with palpation
Trochanteric bursitis	15–45	Direct trauma Microtrauma	Lateral aspect of hip or thigh	Lying on involved side	Unremarkable	Painful hip abduction with rotation	Pain at end range hip ER Pain with hip ER with abduction	Pain with resisted hip abduction Pain with resisted hip IR	Lateral thigh over greater trochanter
Groin strain	20–40	Sudden overload	Anteromedial thigh Medial thigh	Running	Possible bruising around medial thigh	Hip extension only limited movement Hip ER limited and painful	Pain at end range hip extension Pain at end range hip abduction	Pain with resisted hip adduction	Proximal medial thigh
Hamstring muscle tear	15–45	Sudden overload	Buttock and posterior thigh	Running	Possible bruising around posterior thigh	SLR limited and painful	Pain at end range hip flexion Pain at end range hip extension Pain with passive SLR	Pain with resisted hip extension Pain with resisted knee flexion	Posterior thigh
Piriformis syndrome	25–55	Gradual	Buttock and posterior thigh Back of leg	Prolonged sitting	Unremarkable	SLR limited and painful	Pain at end range hip ER Pain with passive SLR	Pain with resisted hip ER	Buttock

Condition	Age	Onset	Location of pain	Aggravating factors	Observation	Active movement	Passive movement	Resisted tests	Palpation
Hip OA	50+	Gradual	Anterior thigh Anteromedial thigh	Weight bearing	Possible atrophy of thigh muscles Altered gait	Limited hip IR and extension Painful hip IR Painful hip extension	Pain at end range hip IR All movements feel stiff	Weak hip abduction General weakness of hip muscles	Anterior hip
Iliotibial band syndrome	25–55	Overuse	Lateral aspect of thigh Lateral aspect of knee	—	Unremarkable	Pain on moving from knee extension to flexion	Pain at end range hip ER with abduction	All resistive tests negative	Lateral epicondyle of femur Lateral aspect of knee
Psoas bursitis	20–40	Overuse	Anteromedial thigh	—	Unremarkable	Hip extension only limited movement	Pain at end range hip extension	Pain with resisted hip flexion	Anterior hip
Lumbar or thoracic disk pathology	20–50	Gradual Sudden overload	Varies according to spinal nerve root involved but occurs in dermatomal distribution	Lumbar or thoracic flexion (bending or sitting) Activities that increase intrathecal pressure	May have associated deviation of trunk	Increased symptoms with trunk flexion Increased symptoms with hip flexion with knee extended (SLR)	Symptoms invariably increased with passive SLR	Fatigable weakness of associated myotome	Possible tenderness over involved spinal segment

SLR = straight leg raire

REFERENCES

1. Crowninshield RD, et al.: A biomechanical investigation of the human hip. J Biomech 1978;11:75–85.
2. Spiera H: Osteoarthritis as a misdiagnosis in elderly patients. Geriatrics 1987;37–42.
3. Schon L, Zuckerman JD: Hip pain the elderly: evaluation and diagnosis. Geriatrics 1988;43:48–62.
4. Wroblewski BM: Pain in osteoarthrosis of the hip. Practitioner 1978;1315:140–141.
5. Echternach JL: Evaluation of the hip. In Echternach JL (ed): Physical Therapy of the Hip, pp 17–32. New York, Churchill Livingstone, 1990.
6. Jull GA, Janda V: Muscle and Motor control in low back pain. In Twomey LT, Taylor JR (eds): Physical Therapy of the Low Back: Clinics in Physical Therapy, p 258. New York, Churchill Livingstone, 1987.
7. Cyriax J: Textbook of Orthopaedic Medicine, Diagnosis of Soft Tissue Lesions, 8th ed. London, Bailliere Tindall, 1982.
8. Inman VT, Ralston HJ, Todd F: Human Walking. Baltimore, MD, Williams & Wilkins, 1981.
9. Lehmkuhl LD, Smith LK: Brunnstrom's Clinical Kinesiology. Philadelphia, PA, FA Davis, 1983.
10. Yoder E: Physical therapy management of nonsurgical hip problems in adults. In Echternach JL (ed): Physical Therapy of the Hip, pp 103–137. New York, Churchill Livingstone, 1990.
11. Mattingly GE, Mackarey PJ: Optimal methods for shoulder tendon palpation: a cadaver study. Phys Ther 1996;76:166–174.
12. Fagerson TL: Hip. In Wadsworth C (ed): Current Concepts of Orthopedic Physical Therapy—Home Study Course, Orthopaedic Section. La Crosse, WI, APTA, 2001.
13. Hoppenfeld S: Physical examination of the hip and pelvis. In Physical Examination of the Spine and Extremities, p 143. East Norwalk, CT, Appleton-Century-Crofts, 1976.
14. McKenzie R, May S: History. In McKenzie R, May S (eds): The Human Extremities: Mechanical Diagnosis and Therapy, pp 89–103. Waikanae, New Zealand, Spinal Publications, 2000.
15. Janda V: Muscle Function Testing, pp 163–167. London, Butterworths, 1983.
16. Hall SJ: The biomechanics of the human lower extremity. In Basic Biomechanics, pp 234–281. New York, McGraw-Hill, 1999.
17. Johnston RC: Mechanical considerations of the hip joint. Arch Surg 1973;107:411.
18. Palmer ML, Epler M: Clinical Assessment Procedures in Physical Therapy, pp 68–73. Philadelphia, PA, JB Lippincott, 1990.
19. Maitland GD: The Peripheral Joints: Examination and Recording Guide. Adelaide, Australia, Virgo Press, 1973.
20. Gelberman RH., et al.: Femoral anteversion. J Bone Joint Surg 1987;69B:75.
21. Pizzutillo PT, MacEwen GD, Shands AR: Anteversion of the femur. In Tonzo RG (ed): Surgery of the Hip Joint. New York, Springer-Verlag, 1984.
22. Reikeras O, Bjerkreim I, Kolbenstvedt A: Anteversion of the acetabulum and femoral neck in normals and in patients with osteoarthritis of the hip. Acta Orthop Scan 1983;54:18–23.
23. Ruwe PA, et al.: Clinical determination of femoral anteversion: a comparison with established techniques. J Bone Joint Surg 1992;74:820.
24. Woods D, Macnicol M: The flexion-adduction test: an early sign of hip disease. J Pediatr Orthop 2001;10:180–185.
25. Zimney NJ: Clinical reasoning in the evaluation and management of undiagnosed chronic hip pain in young adult. Phys Ther 1998;78:62–73.
26. Grelsamer RP, McConnell J: The Patella: A Team Approach. Gaithersburg, MD, Aspen, 1998.
27. Melchione WE, Sullivan MS: Reliability of measurements obtained by the use of an instrument designed to indirectly measure ilio-tibial band length. J Orthop Sports Phys Ther 1993;18:511–515.
28. Johnson AW, Weiss CB, Wheeler DL: Stress fractures of the femoral shaft in athletes—more common than expected: a new clinical test. Am J Sports Med 1994;22:248–256.

29. Aronsson DD, et al.: Developmental dysplasia of the hip. Pediatrics 1994;94 (2 Pt 1): 201–208.
30. Dorwart RH, et al.: Pigmented villonodular synovitis of synovial joints: clinical, pathologic, and radiologic features. AJR Am J Roentgenol 1984;143:877–885.
31. Kneeland JB: MR imaging of sports injuries of the hip. Magn Reson Imaging Clin N Am 1999;7:105–115.
32. Guide to physical therapist practice. Phys Ther 2001;81:S13–S95.

11 | The Knee Joint Complex

OVERVIEW

The knee is the largest and most complex joint in the body. It is considered a "physiologic" joint because it requires the normal functioning of all its parts (e.g., bony, ligamentous, and muscular) to simultaneously provide smooth motion, stability in stance, and protection against deterioration over time.[1,2] The knee joint complex includes three articulating surfaces, which form two distinct joints contained within a single joint capsule: the patellofemoral and tibiofemoral joint. Despite its proximity to the tibiofemoral joint, the patellofemoral joint can be considered as its own entity, in much the same way as the craniovertebral joints are when compared to the rest of the cervical spine.

TIBIOFEMORAL JOINT

The tibiofemoral joint, or knee joint, is a ginglymoid, or modified hinge joint, which has six degrees of freedom (see *Orthopaedic Examination, Evaluation, and Intervention*, p 735). The bony configuration of the knee joint complex is geometrically incongruous and lends little inherent stability to the joint. Joint stability is therefore dependent on the static restraints of the joint capsule, ligaments, and menisci, and the dynamic restraints of the quadriceps, hamstrings, and gastrocnemius.[3,4]

PATELLOFEMORAL JOINT

The patella is a passive component of the knee extensor mechanism, where the static and dynamic relationships of the underlying tibia and femur determine the patellar-tracking pattern. To assist in the control of the forces around the patellofemoral joint, there are a number of static and dynamic restraints (see *Orthopaedic Examination, Evaluation, and Intervention*, p 753).

One of the problems facing the knee joint complex is the fact that it was not originally designed for bipedal motion.[5] Evolutionary modifications in femoral rotation, distal femoral physeal obliquity, and the development of an osseous patella have allowed the knee to adapt to the major changes placed on it during functional demands.[2] Despite these adaptations, however, the knee is one of the most commonly injured joints in the body.

Knee injuries generally result from acute trauma or overuse. Broadly speaking, acute injuries fall into one of five categories: (1) contusions, (2) fractures or physeal injuries, (3) ligamentous injuries, (4) meniscal tears, and (5) patellar subluxation or dislocation.[6]

Whatever the underlying injury to the knee joint complex, the foundation of the intervention is a timely diagnosis. Accurate diagnosis requires knowledge of knee anatomy, common pain patterns in knee injuries, frequently encountered causes of knee pain, as well as specific physical examination skills.[5]

EXAMINATION

The examination of the knee joint complex should include a thorough and detailed history, a careful inspection and palpation of the knee for point tenderness, assessment of joint effusion, range-of-motion and strength testing, an evaluation of the ligaments for injury or laxity, an assessment of patella motion, and assessment of the integrity of the menisci (see *Orthopaedic Examination, Evaluation, and Intervention*, pp 757–782). The examination of the knee joint complex rarely occurs in isolation, and almost always involves an assessment of the lumbar spine, pelvis, hip, foot, and ankle.

HISTORY

With the larger number of specific tests available for the knee joint complex, it is tempting to overlook the important role of the history. The complete history should include information about how and when the injury occurred (onset), how the patient characterizes the symptoms, and whether the patient has had any previous knee disorders.[7] In addition, the clinician should ask questions about the location (anterior, medial, lateral, or posterior knee) (Table 11-1 and Figures 11-1 through 11-4), quality (e.g., dull, sharp, achy), severity, and duration of the patient's symptoms; the presence or absence of mechanical symptoms (locking, popping, giving way); joint effusion (timing, amount, recurrence); and the degree of dysfunction and disability.[8] A history of locking episodes suggests a meniscal tear. A sensation of popping at the time of injury suggests ligamentous injury, probably a complete rupture of a ligament (third-degree tear) (Table 11-2). The anterior cruciate ligament (ACL) and the medial collateral ligament (MCL) are the most commonly injured knee ligaments. The lateral collateral ligament (LCL) and the posterior cruciate ligament (PCL) are rarely injured. Episodes of giving way are consistent with some degree of knee instability and may indicate patellar subluxation or ligamentous rupture.

The patient's age can provide some initial clues (Table 11-3). For example, teenage girls and young women are more likely to have patellar tracking problems such as patellar subluxation and patellofemoral pain syndrome, whereas teenage boys are more likely to have knee extensor mechanism problems such as tibial apophysitis (Osgood-Schlatter lesion) and patellar tendinitis. Osteoarthritis of the knee joint is common in older adults.

Information about the patient's activity level can provide the clinician with useful clues. For example, active patients are more likely to have acute ligamentous sprains and overuse injuries such as pes anserine bursitis and medial plica syndrome (see *Orthopaedic Examination, Evaluation, and Intervention*, p 797).

TABLE 11-1 Differential Diagnosis of Knee Pain by Anatomic Site

Anterior knee pain	Medial knee pain	Lateral knee pain	Posterior knee pain
Patellar subluxation or dislocation	Medial collateral ligament sprain	Lateral collateral ligament sprain	Popliteal cyst (Baker's cyst)
Tibial apophysitis (Osgood-Schlatter lesion)	Medial meniscal tear	Lateral meniscal tear	Posterior cruciate ligament injury
Jumper's knee (patellar tendinitis)	Pes anserine bursitis	Iliotibial band tendinitis	
Patellofemoral pain syndrome (chondromalacia patellae)	Medial plica syndrome		

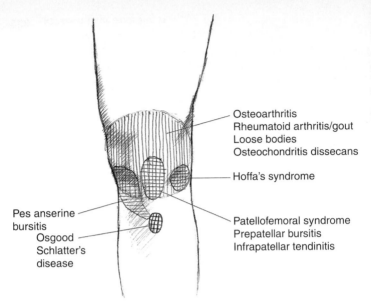

FIG. 11-1   Anterior knee pain and the possible causes.

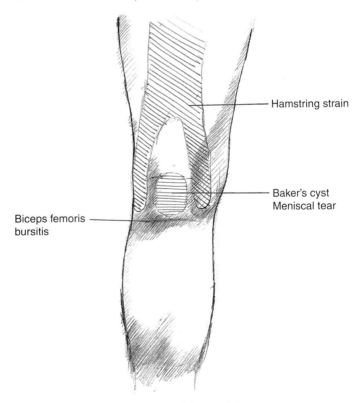

FIG. 11-2   Posterior knee pain and the possible causes.

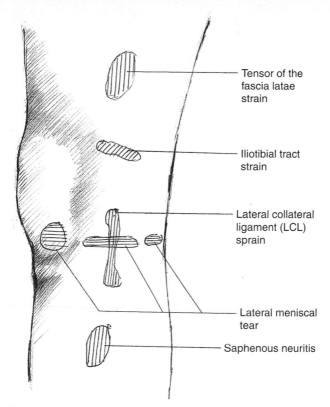

FIG. 11-3 Lateral knee pain and the possible causes.

TABLE 11-2 Common Ligamentous and Meniscal Injuries

Structure	Mechanism of injury	Subjective complaints
MCL	Most commonly involves valgus (contact) stress or external rotational force with leg firmly planted. Often associated with ACL injury	Reports of swelling developing within 12 hours of injury, localized swelling and tenderness over injured area
ACL	Most commonly injured with noncontact pivoting/twisting mechanism while foot is planted, noncontact hyperextension, sudden deceleration, forced internal rotation, sudden valgus impact	Reports of being immediately disabled/unable to continue activity, extreme pain at time of injury, hearing "pop" in the knee, experiencing tearing sensation, acute knee swelling (within 1–2 hours of injury), episodes of "giving way"
Meniscus	Usually caused by noncontact injury, rotational force applied to partly or completely flexed knee as occurs with squatting then rapidly rotating while coming to a standing position	Reports being able to continue/complete with activity. Reports of swelling developing within 12 hours of injury, localized swelling and tenderness over injured area. History of popping or clicking with knee motions

Source: Austermuehle PD: Common knee injuries in primary care. Nurse Pract 2001;26:32–45;quiz 46–47.

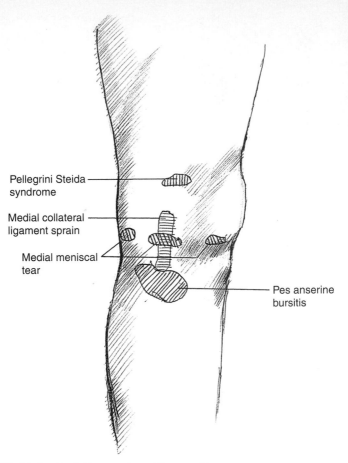

FIG. 11-4 Medial knee pain and the possible causes.

TABLE 11-3 Common Causes of Knee Pain by Age Group

Children and adolescents	Young adults (20–45 years)	Older adults (50+ years)
Patellar subluxation	Patellofemoral pain syndrome (chondromalacia patellae)	Osteoarthritis
Tibial apophysitis (Osgood-Schlatter lesion)	Medial plica syndrome	Crystal-induced inflammatory arthropathy: gout, pseudogout
Jumper's knee (patellar tendinitis)	Pes anserine bursitis	Popliteal cyst (Baker's cyst)
Referred pain: slipped capital femoral epiphysis, others	Trauma: ligamentous sprains (anterior cruciate, medial collateral, lateral collateral), meniscal tear	
Osteochondritis dissecans	Inflammatory arthropathy: rheumatoid arthritis, Reiter's syndrome	
	Septic arthritis	

Aggravating and alleviating factors, drugs, or interventions used, and the injury's relationship to a specific activity also need to be identified.[9]

The timing and amount of joint effusion are important clues to the diagnosis. Rapid onset (within 2 hours) of a large, tense effusion suggests rupture of the ACL or fracture of the tibial plateau with resultant hemarthrosis, whereas slower onset (24 to 36 hours) of a mild to moderate effusion is consistent with meniscal injury or ligamentous sprain. Recurrent knee effusion after activity is consistent with meniscal injury.

The primary mechanisms of injury in the knee are direct trauma, a varus or valgus force (with or without rotation), hyperextension, flexion with posterior translation, a twisting force, rapid deceleration, and overuse (see Table 11-2).[10] For example, hyperextension with an audible pop and immediate onset of swelling raises the suspicion of an ACL tear.[6] A direct blow to the lateral aspect of the knee commonly results in injury to the MCL depending on the amount of valgus stress. Similarly, a blow to the medial aspect of the knee can stress the LCL. A direct blow to the anterior aspect of the knee can disrupt the PCL. The position of the joint at the time of the traumatic force dictates which anatomic structures are at risk for injury; hence, an important aspect of obtaining the patient's history for acute injuries is to allow him or her to describe the position of the knee and direction of forces at the time it was injured.[11] Twisting injuries are somewhat less specific in terms of determining the injured structure as they can be associated with ACL tears, meniscal tears, or patellar subluxation or dislocation.[6]

Anterior knee pain is most commonly associated with patellofemoral dysfunction, which is a frequent source of impairment.[12] The differential diagnosis of anterior knee pain should include tears of the menisci, medial synovial plica syndrome, inflammatory or degenerative arthritis, tumors of the joint, ligament injuries that mimic patellar instability, osteochondritis dissecans of the medial femoral condyle, prepatellar bursitis, patellar tendinitis, inflammation of the patellar fat pad, and Sinding-Larsen-Johansson syndrome.[13–17]

Patients with overuse injuries often describe a precipitating event and gradual onset of symptoms. Overuse injuries can be caused by both extrinsic factors, such as poor training techniques or inadequate footwear, and intrinsic factors, such as poor flexibility or structural abnormalities.[8]

Pain that is not alleviated with rest could indicate a nonmechanical source of pain, or a chemically induced source, such as an inflammatory reaction. A hot and swollen joint without a history of trauma should provoke suspicions about hemophilia, rheumatoid arthritis, an infection, or gout (Table 11-4).

TABLE 11-4 Synovial Fluid Findings

Findings	Normal	Noninflammatory	Inflammatory	Septic
Color	Clear	Yellow	Yellow to green	Yellow
Clarity	Transparent	Transparent	Opaque	Opaque
Viscosity	High	High	Low	Variable
WBC per mm^3	<200	200–2000	2000 to 150,000	15,000 to 200,000
PMNs	<25%	<25%	>50%	>75%
Mucin clot	Good	Good	Good to poor	Poor

WBC = white blood cells; PMNs = polymorphonuclear cells.
Source: McGahan JP, Shoji H: Knee effusions. J Fam Pract 1977;4:141–144.

Septic arthritis may develop in patients of any age, but crystal-induced inflammatory arthropathy is more likely in adults.

Finally, the patient should be asked about previous episodes and interventions for his or her knee symptoms, including the use of medications, supporting devices, and physical therapy.

SYSTEMS REVIEW

Knee pain can be referred to the knee from the lumbosacral region (L3 to S2 segments) and the hip. Referred pain from the hip occurs with hip joint pathology, such as slipped capital femoral epiphysis. The peripheral nerves are also capable of referring pain to this area. Medial knee pain, with a burning quality could indicate saphenous nerve neuritis (Figure 11-3). Pain that is constant and burning in nature should alert the clinician to the possibility of reflex sympathetic dystrophy, gout, or radicular pain. Intermittent pain usually indicates a mechanical problem (meniscus). The more common causes of referred knee pain and those causes of a more serious nature are described in Chapter 9 of the *Orthopaedic Examination, Evaluation, and Intervention*.

TESTS AND MEASURES

Observation

The observation component of the examination begins as the clinician meets the patient and ends as the patient is leaving. This informal observation should occur at every visit. The patient should be observed while he or she walks, stands, sits, and in nonweight bearing.[8] When possible the clinician should compare the involved knee with the asymptomatic knee. During gait, the clinician should observe for antalgia, step length, pelvic tilt, and cadence.[5] The major motion at the knee during the gait cycle occurs in the sagittal plane, including an arc of motion from full extension to approximately 60° of flexion, and is characterized by two flexion waves (see *Orthopaedic Examination, Evaluation, and Intervention*, Chapter 13).[2] The stance phase knee flexion wave peaks early in stance, which allows the quadriceps muscle to function as a shock absorber, whereas the swing phase knee flexion wave facilitates foot clearance and limb advancement.[2]

With the patient standing, the clinician observes whether the pelvis is level, the knees symmetrical and the leg lengths equal.[18] This includes inspecting the injured knee for bruising erythema, discoloration, and swelling. The presence of bruising or erythema is an important piece of information regarding the nature and severity of the injury.[5] Swelling above the patella is most likely a joint effusion; below the patella, prepatellar bursitis; and behind the knee, a popliteal cyst.[2] With the patient supine, large knee effusions fill in the normal recesses on either side of the patella.[6] This can be confirmed using the *ballottement sign* (see *Orthopaedic Examination, Evaluation, and Intervention*, pp 757–758).

Morphology is important to function and should be recorded. The clinician should observe the knees in standing in both the coronal (bowlegs, genu varum; knock knees, genu valgum) and sagittal planes (flexion or hyperextension, genu recurvatum). Normally, when a patient stands with his or her feet together, the medial aspects of both knees and ankles are also in contact.[6] Knees with more than 15° of misalignment in any plane (varus, valgus, recurvatum) do not do well if subject to ligamentous disruption.[19] In addition, assessing the hip and ankle joints is important as problems in these joints can exacerbate knee injuries or cause referred knee pain:

- Increased anteversion (internal rotation) of the femur often occurs in combination with external torsion (external rotation) of the tibia.[6] This pattern of misalignment predisposes the patient to patellofemoral problems.
- Pronation of the foot or pes planus (flatfoot) can cause internal rotation of the femur, which also predisposes the patient to patellofemoral joint dysfunction.

The musculature above and below the knee should be symmetric bilaterally. In particular, the vastus medialis obliquus of the quadriceps should be evaluated to determine if it appears normal or shows signs of atrophy. Thigh atrophy can have significant detrimental effects on both patellar tracking and knee performance.[6] A well-defined gastrocnemius is usually indicative of an active lifestyle.[19]

Palpation

For the palpation to be reliable, the clinician must have a sound knowledge of surface anatomy and the clinician should employ a logical sequence. The results from the palpation examination should be correlated with other findings. The knee can be positioned in 30° or 90° of flexion. The former position allows the cruciate ligaments to be relaxed and allows for better palpation of the anterior half of the menisci.[19] The latter position brings the menisci more anteriorly, and the collateral ligaments more posteriorly.[19] The knee is palpated and assessed for pain, warmth, and effusion. Point tenderness should be sought, particularly at the patella (all four poles), tibial tubercle, anterolateral (Figure 11-5) and anteromedial (Figure 11-6) joint line, medial joint line, and lateral joint line. Specific

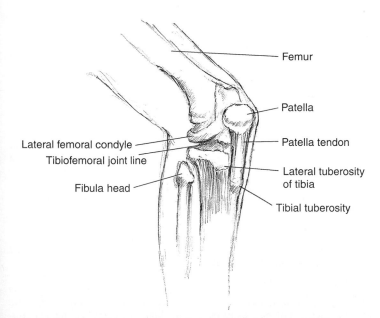

Femur

Patella

Patella tendon

Lateral femoral condyle

Tibiofemoral joint line

Fibula head

Lateral tuberosity of tibia

Tibial tuberosity

FIG. 11-5 Palpable structures on the anterolateral aspect of the knee.

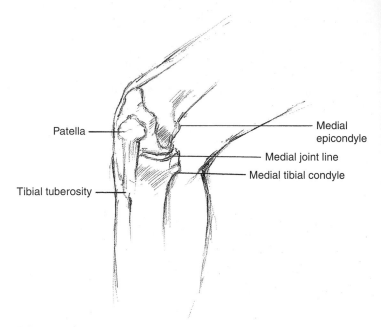

FIG. 11-6 Palpable structures on the anteromedial aspect of the knee.

structures to be palpated include the quadriceps muscle, patella, patella tendon, iliotibial band, LCL, MCL, medial hamstrings, lateral hamstrings, and the pes anserinus. Tenderness and/or differences in temperature between these structures when compared to the uninvolved knee suggest inflammation. The popliteal fossa, through which the principal neurovascular structures of the knee (popliteal artery and vein, tibial nerve, common fibular nerve) pass, should also be palpated.

Active Range of Motion, Passive Range of Motion, and Then Passive Overpressure

Range of motion testing for the tibiofemoral joint should include assessment of knee flexion and extension, tibial internal and external rotation. Normal knee motion (Figure 11-7 and Table 11-5) has been described as 0° of extension to 140° of flexion, although hyperextension is frequently present to varying degrees.[20] The range of motion testing can often be diagnostic and provides the clinician with some clues as to the cause of the problem (Figure 11-8). It is important to examine the uninvolved knee first to allay any patient fears and to determine what the normal range of motion is. In addition, observation of the uninvolved knee can afford the clinician information about the patellofemoral joint and the tracking of the patella.[5]

Patella Motion Tests

Probably the most important part of the patellofemoral examination is the observation of the dynamics of patellar tracking in weight bearing and non-weight bearing. Excessive lateral tracking of the patella as the patient nears

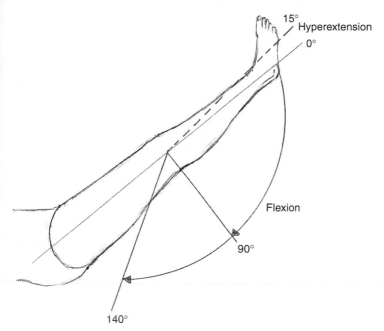

FIG. 11-7 Normal knee motion.

full extension ("J" sign) is a common finding with patellofemoral dysfunction.[6] The various contact areas of the patella are engaged at different parts of the range of motion (Table 11-6). Pain elicited in some but not all of the range provides the clinician with valuable information about the diagnosis and the ranges to avoid during the intervention.

Ankle Motions

Ankle motions are tested because a number of structures share a common relationship with the foot and ankle and the knee joint complex.

Hip Motions

A number of muscles cross both the hip and the knee. These include the rectus femoris, the gracilis, the sartorius, and the hamstrings. Adaptive shortening of

TABLE 11-5 Normal Ranges and End-Feels at the Knee

Motion	Range of motion (degrees)	End-feel
Flexion	0–140	Tissue approximation or tissue stretch
Extension	0–15	Tissue stretch
External rotation of the tibia on the femur	30–40	Tissue stretch
Internal rotation of the tibia on the femur	20–30	Tissue stretch

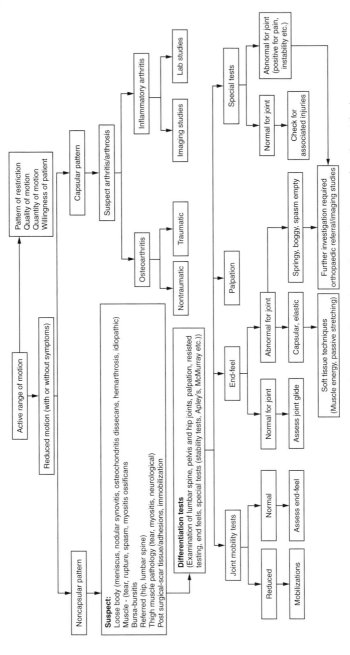

FIG. 11-8 Examination sequence in the presence of symptom-free or incomplete active range of motion at the knee.

TABLE 11-6 Patella Contact during Ranges

Knee range of flexion	Facet contact
0	No contact
15–20	Inferior pole
45	Middle pole
90	All facets
Full flexion (135)	Odd facet and lateral aspect

Sources: Goodfellow JW, Hungerford DS, Woods C:
Patellofemoral joint mechanics and pathology: I and II. J Bone
Joint Surg 1976;58B:287–299.
Aglietti P, et al.: A new patella prosthesis. Clin Orthop 1975;107:
175–187.

any of these structures may cause alterations in postural mechanics and gait.
The hip rotators can also influence other aspects of the lower kinetic chain.

Strength Testing

Gross muscle testing is useful in checking for deficits in the lower extremities
(Table 11-7). Strength testing involves the performance of resisted isometric
tests (see *Orthopaedic Examination, Evaluation, and Intervention*, pp 763–764).
The primary extensor of the knee is the quadriceps (femoral nerve, L2, 3, 4),
and the primary flexors are the hamstring muscles (tibial portion of the sciatic
nerve, L5, S1). For each of the tests, the joint is placed as close to its open
packed position as possible to minimize any joint compression forces. Strength
testing of the hip, foot, and ankle muscles should also be included.

TABLE 11-7 Muscles of the Knee: Their Actions, Nerve Supply, and Nerve
Root Derivation

Action	Muscles acting	Nerve supply	Nerve root derivation
Flexion of Knee	Biceps femoris	Sciatic	L5, S1-2
	Semimembranosus	Sciatic	L5, S1-2
	Semitendinosus	Sciatic	L5, S1-2
	Gracilis	Obturator	L2-3
	Sartorius	Femoral	L2-3
	Popliteus	Tibial	L4-5, S1
	Gastrocnemius	Tibial	S1-2
	Tensor fascia latae	Superior gluteal	L4-5
Extension of Knee	Rectus femoris	Femoral	L2-4
	Vastus medialis	Femoral	L2-4
	Vastus intermedisus	Femoral	L2-4
	Vastus lateralis	Femoral	L2-4
	Tensor fascia latae	Superior gluteal	L4-5
Internal rotation of flexed leg (nonweight bearing)	Popliteus	Tibial	L4-5
	Semimembranosus	Sciatic	L5, S1-2
	Semitendinosus	Sciatic	L5, S1-2
	Sartorius	Femoral	L2-3
	Gracilis	Obturator	L2-3
External rotation of flexed leg (nonweight bearing)	Biceps femoris	Sciatic	L5, S1-2

Functional Tests

Functional outcome following knee injury must consider the patient's perspective, and not just objective measurements of instability. Functional motion requirements of the knee vary according to the specific task. In normal level ground walking, 60°–70° of knee flexion is required. This requirement increases to 80°–85° with stair climbing, and to 120°–140° for running.[21] Approximately 120° of knee flexion is necessary for activities such as squatting to tie a shoelace or to don a sock.[22] Table 11-8 outlines the amounts of knee range of motion that must be available for common activities of daily living.

Special Tests

Special tests for the knee joint complex are dependent on the clinician's needs, the structure of each joint and the subjective complaints (Table 11-9). These tests are only performed if there is some indication that they would be helpful in arriving at a diagnosis. The special tests help confirm or implicate a particular structure and may also provide information as to the degree of tissue damage.

Stress Testing

The stress tests are used to determine the integrity of the joint, ligaments, and the menisci. A complete history and physical examination can diagnose approximately 90% of ligamentous injuries. The primary stabilizers of the knee joint complex are the ACL, which is responsible for restricting anterior translation of the tibia; the PCL, which is responsible for restricting posterior translation of the tibia; the MCL, which restricts medial translation (valgus stress); and the LCL, which restricts lateral translation (varus stress) (Table 11-10).

The goal of the stress tests is to identify the degree of separation and the quality, or end-feel of the separation. Intact ligaments have an abrupt and firm end-feel, whereas sprained ligaments have a soft or indistinct end-feel depending on the degree of injury. A comparison should always be made with the uninvolved knee before a determination is made. It is important to remember that both pain and swelling can hamper the sensitivity of these tests.[8] Serious

TABLE 11-8 Approximate Range of Motion Required for Common Activities of Daily Living

Activity	Required flexion range of motion (degrees)
Running	120–140
Squatting	120
Tying shoelace	120
Donning a sock	120
Climbing downstairs	110
Sitting and rising	85
Climbing upstairs	80
Swing phase of gait	70
Stance phase of gait	20

Source: Laubenthal KN, Smidt GL, Kettelkamp DB: A quantitative analysis of knee motion for activities of daily living. Phys Ther 1972;52:34–42.

TABLE 11-9 Subjective Complaint, Potential Diagnosis and Confirmatory Test

Subjective complaint	Potential diagnosis	Confirmatory test(s)
My knee hurts when I get up from a chair or go up steps	Patellofemoral dysfunction	Patellofemoral grind test
My knee gives out when I step down from the curb	Subluxation/dislocation of the patella	Patella apprehension test
My knee locks	1. Torn medial meniscus 2. Loose body within the knee joint	McMurray test and Apley grinding and distraction tests
My knee feels swollen and tight	Fluid within the knee	Patellar effusion tests
My knee buckles; it gives out	1. Unstable knee joint (torn collateral or cruciate ligament) 2. Torn medial meniscus	Valgus and varus stress tests, anterior drawer, Lachman, posterior sag, strength testing (neuro screen), meniscus tests
I can't straighten my knee out	1. Fluid in the knee 2. Torn meniscus	Meniscus tests, patellar ballottement test, bounce home test
I have pain on the inside of my leg	1. Torn medial collateral ligament 2. Bursitis, pes anserinus bursa	Valgus stress test Palpation of the pes anserinus bursa
I made a quick turn wile playing sports while my foot was planted, and my leg suddenly collapsed and the knee became swollen	Torn medial meniscus	Apley test and McMurray test
I have bow legs and they hurt	1. Osteoarthritis 2. Ligamentous instability	Range of motion (capsular) Patellofemoral grinding test Ligament stability tests
I have swelling in the back of my knee	Popliteal cyst	Palpation of popliteal fossa
I landed heavily on the front of my knee and it hurts	1. Patellar fracture 2. Chondromalacia 3. Fat pad syndrome 4. Prepatellar bursitis 5. Infrapatellar bursitis	Radiograph Palpation
I can't move my knee in any direction without pain	Infected knee joint	Joint aspiration

Source: Hoppenfeld S: Physical examination of the knee joint by complaint. Ortho Clin N Am 1979;10:3–20.

TABLE 11-10 Primary and Secondary Restraints of the Knee

Tibial motion	Primary restraints	Secondary restraints
Anterior translation	ACL	MCL, LCL: middle third of mediolateral capsule, popliteus corner, semimembranosus corner, iliotibial band
Posterior translation	PCL	MCL, LCL: posterior third of mediolateral capsule, popliteus tendon, anterior and posterior meniscofemoral ligaments
Valgus rotation	MCL	ACL, PCL: posterior capsule when knee fully extended, semimembranosus corner
Varus rotation	LCL	ACL, PCL: posterior capsule when knee fully extended, popliteus corner
Lateral rotation	MCL, LCL	Popliteus corner
Medial rotation	ACL, PCL	Anteroposterior meniscofemoral ligaments, semimembranosus corner

ACL = anterior cruciate ligament; LCL = lateral collateral ligament; MCL = medial collateral ligament; PCL = posterior cruciate ligament.
Source: Irrgang JJ, Safran MC, Fu FH: The knee: ligamentous and meniscal injuries. In Zachazewski JE, Magee DJ, Quillen WS (eds): Athletic Injuries and Rehabilitation, pp 623–692. Philadelphia, PA, WB Saunders, 1996.

functional instability of the knee appears to occur unpredictably. The reasons for such discrepancies are unknown, but they may be due to:[4]

- Varying definitions of instability
- Varying degrees of damage of the ACL[23,24]
- Different combinations of injuries[25]
- Different mechanisms of compensation for the loss of the ACL
- Differences in rehabilitation
- The diverse physical demands and expectations of different populations

One-Plane Medial Instability

Abduction Valgus Stress   The clinician applies a strong valgus force, with a counter force applied at the lateral femoral condyle (see Figure 11-9). Normally, there is little or no valgus movement in the knee, and, if present, should be less than the amount of varus motion. Under normal conditions, the end-feel is firm. With degeneration of the medial or lateral compartments, varus and valgus motions may be increased, while the end-feels will be normal.

With the knee tested in full extension, any demonstrable instability is usually very significant. Pain with this maneuver is caused by an increase in tension of the medial collateral structures, or the connection of these structures with the medial meniscus. If pain or an excessive amount of motion is detected compared with the other extremity, a hypermobility or instability should be suspected. The following structures may be implicated:

- Superficial and deep fibers of the MCL
- Posterior oblique ligament
- Posterior-medial capsule
- Medial capsular ligament
- Anterior cruciate ligament
- Posterior cruciate ligament

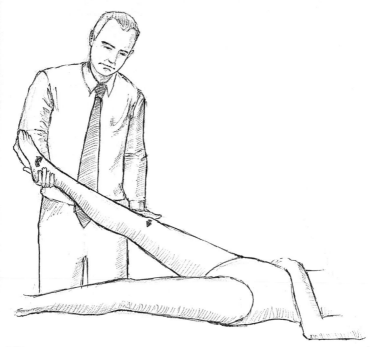

FIG. 11-9   Valgus test of the knee.

The test is then repeated at 10°–30° of flexion to further assess the MCL, the posterior oblique ligament, and the PCL. MCL injuries are classified into three grades. In grade I injuries, the MCL is tender and swollen but does not exhibit increased laxity with valgus testing. Increased laxity of the valgus test, but with a firm end-feel, while the knee is positioned in 30° of flexion usually denotes a tearing, of at least a grade II tearing of the middle third of the capsular ligament and the parallel fibers of the MCL. An indefinite end-feel characterizes a grade III tear with the valgus test.

The posterior fibers of the MCL can be isolated, by placing the knee in 90° of flexion with full external rotation of the tibia.[26] The femur is prevented from rotating by the clinician's shoulder. The clinician places one hand on the dorsum of the foot and the other on the heel, and an external rotation force is applied using the foot as a lever.

One-Plane Lateral Instability

The clinician applies a strong varus force, with a counter force applied at the medial femoral condyle. To be able to assess the amount of varus movement, the clinician should repeat the maneuver several times, applying slight overpressure at the end of the range of motion. Under normal conditions, the end-feel is firm, after slight movement.

If this test is positive for pain or excessive motion as compared with the other extremity, the following structures may be implicated:

• Lateral collateral ligament
• Lateral capsular ligament
• Arcuate-popliteus complex
• Anterior cruciate ligament
• Posterior cruciate ligament

If the instability is gross, one or both cruciate ligaments may be involved, as well as, occasionally, the biceps femoris tendon and the iliotibial band, leading to a rotary instability, if not in the short term, certainly over a period of time.[27]

The test is then repeated at 10°–30° of flexion and the tibia in full external rotation to further assess the LCL, the posterior-lateral capsule and the arcuate-popliteus complex.

One-Plane Anterior Instability

A number of tests have been advocated for testing the integrity of the ACL. Two of the more commonly used ones are the Lachman, and the anterior drawer test.

The Lachman Test   The Lachman test is one of the easiest and most accurate diagnostic measures used to assess ACL injuries.[28] The knee is held in 30° of flexion, while the tibia is anteriorly translated with respect to the femur. A number of factors can influence the results of the Lachman test. These include:

• An inability of the patient to relax
• The degree of knee flexion
• The size of the clinician's hand
• The stabilization (and thus relaxation) of the patient's thigh

According to Weiss et al.,[29] these factors can be minimized by the use of the modified Lachman test. In this test, the patient is positioned supine with his or her feet resting firmly on the end of the table and his or her knees flexed from 10° to 15°. The clinician stabilizes the distal end of patient's femur using his or her thigh rather than his or her hand as in the Lachman test, and then attempts to displace patient's tibia anteriorly (Figure 11-10). If the tibia moves forward, and the concavity of the patellar tendon/ligament becomes convex, the test is considered positive.

The grading of knee instability is as follows:[30–32]

1+ (mild): 5 millimeter or less
2+ (moderate): 5–10 millimeter
3+ (serious): more than 10 millimeter

False negatives with this test can occur. A significant hemarthrosis, protective hamstring spasm, or a tear of the posterior horn of the medial meniscus may cause false negatives with this test.[33]

Anterior Drawer Test   The aforementioned Lachman test is a modification of the anterior drawer test, of which there are a number of variations, all of which involve positioning the patient in supine:[26]

Anterior drawer test in 80° of flexion without rotation.[26] The clinician grasps the lower leg of the patient just distal to the joint space of the knee. The patient's knee is flexed 80°, and the lower leg is not rotated. The clinician fixates the patient's leg by sitting on the foot (Figure 11-11). The clinician can place the thumbs, either in the joint space, or just distal to it, to assess mobility.

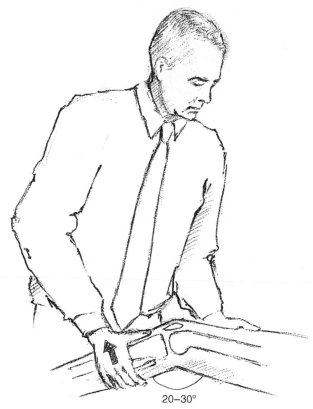

20–30°

FIG. 11-10   Lachman test.

The clinician tests the tension in the musculature. It is important that all muscles around the knee be relaxed to allow any translatory movement to occur. With both hands, the clinician now abruptly pulls the lower leg forward. This test is positive when an abnormal anterior movement of the tibia occurs compared with the other extremity.

Anterior drawer test in 80° of flexion and maximal external rotation.[26] The initial positions of the patient and clinician are the same as in the test *Anterior Drawer Test in 80° of flexion without rotation* above, with the exception that the lower leg is positioned in maximum external rotation. For the performance, refer to the *Anterior Drawer Test in 80° flexion without rotation*. The ACL and the medial and posterior-medial capsuloligamentous structures are tested in this position. If this test is positive, there is likely to be an anterior-medial rotatory instability. The specific medial and posterior-medial structures that are affected can be further differentiated by the valgus tests previously described.

Anterior drawer test in 80° of flexion and 50% internal rotation.[26] The initial positions of the patient and clinician are the same as in test *Anterior Drawer Test in 80° of flexion without rotation*, with the exception that the lower leg is placed in 50% internal rotation. For the performance, refer to test

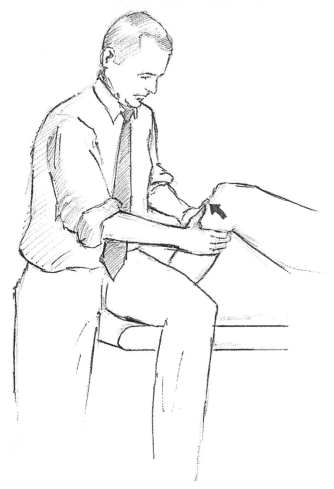

FIG. 11-11 Anterior drawer.

Anterior Drawer Test in 80° of flexion without rotation. The ACL and the posterior-lateral capsuloligamentous structures are tested in this position. If this test is positive, there is likely to be an anterior-lateral rotatory instability. The varus tests (*Passive Varus Test in Slight Knee Flexion* and *Passive Varus Test in Knee Extension*) allow for further determination as to which of the lateral and posterior-lateral structures are affected.

Anterior drawer test in 80° of flexion and maximal internal rotation.[26] The initial positions of the patient and clinician are the same as in test: *Anterior Drawer Test in 80° of flexion without rotation*, with the exception that the lower leg is now maximally internally rotated. Performance of this test is the same as described for the *Anterior Drawer Test in 80° of flexion without rotation*. When in maximal internal rotation, the PCL can completely restrict anterior translation of the tibia. Thus for this test to demonstrate excessive anterior translation, the PCL, the ACL, and the lateral or posterior-lateral capsuloligamentous structures have to be affected.

The anterior drawer test has been found to be 40.9% sensitive and 96.8% specific.[34] False-negatives may occur with this test for the same reasons as those in the Lachman test.

One-Plane Posterior Instability

The PCL is very strong and is rarely completely torn. It is typically injured in a dashboard injury, or in knee flexion activities (kneeling on the patella). A number of tests have been advocated to test the integrity of the PCL:[26]

- *Gravity (Godfrey) sign.* The patient is positioned in supine with the knee flexed to about 90°. The clinician assesses the contour of the tibial tuberosity. If there is a rupture (partial) of the PCL, the tibial tuberosity on the involved side will be less visible than on the noninvolved side.[35] This is caused by an abnormal posterior translation, resulting from a rupture of the PCL. In cases of doubt, the patient can be asked to contract the hamstrings slightly by pushing his or her heels into the clinician's hands. This will usually result in an increase in the posterior translation of the tibia. This maneuver is often performed as a quick test for integrity of the PCL.
- *Posterior drawer.* The patient is positioned in supine with the knee flexed to 90°. The clinician attempts a posterior displacement of the tibia on the femur.

Rotary Instabilities

Rotary or complex instabilities occur when the abnormal or pathologic movement is present in two or more planes. The ligamentous laxities, present at the knee joint in these situations, allow motion to take place around the sagittal, coronal, and the horizontal axis.

Posterior-Lateral Instability   This type of instability is relatively rare, as it requires complete posterior cruciate laxity. It occurs when the lateral tibial plateau subluxes posteriorly on the femur, with the axis shifting posteriorly and medially to the medial joint area. With a hyperextension test, this posterior displacement is obvious and has been labeled the external rotation recurvatum sign.

Active Posterolateral Drawer Test[36]   The patient sits with the foot on the floor in neutral rotation and the knee flexed to 80°–90°. The patient is asked to isometrically contract the hamstrings, while the clinician stabilizes the foot. A positive result for the test is a posterior subluxation of the lateral tibial plateau.

Hughston's Posteriorolateral Drawer Test[31,32]   The patient is positioned supine with the involved leg flexed at the hip to 45°, the knee flexed to 80°–90°, and the lower leg in slight external rotation.[37] The clinician pushes the lower leg posteriorly. If the tibia rotates posteriorly during the test, the test is positive for posteriolateral instability, and indicates that the following structures may have been injured:

- Posterior cruciate ligament
- Arcuate-popliteus complex
- Lateral collateral ligament
- Posterior-lateral capsule

The one-plane medial and lateral stability tests can be used to help differentiate further which lateral and posteriolateral structures are affected.

Hughston's External Rotational Recurvatum Test[31,32] This test is used to detect an abnormal relationship between the femur and tibia in knee extension. The patient is positioned supine with his or her legs straight, and the clinician positioned at the foot of the table. The clinician gently grasps the great toes of both feet at the same time, and lifts the feet from the table, while focusing on the tibial tuberosity of both legs. The patient must be completely relaxed. In the presence of a posteriolateral rotary instability, the knee moves into relative hyperextension at the lateral side of the knee, and the tibia externally rotates.[37]

Posterior-Medial Rotary Instability

Hughston's Posterior-Medial Drawer Test The patient is positioned supine with the involved leg flexed at the hip to 45°, the knee flexed to 80°–90°, and the lower leg in slight internal rotation.[37] The clinician pushes the lower leg posteriorly. If the tibia rotates posteriorly during the test, the test is positive for posterior-medial instability, and indicates that the following structures may have been injured:

- Posterior cruciate ligament
- Posterior oblique ligament
- Medial collateral ligament
- Posterior-medial capsule
- Anterior cruciate ligament

The one-plane medial and lateral stability tests can be used to help differentiate further which medial and posterior-medial structures are affected.

Anterior-Lateral Rotary Instability

The pathology for this condition almost certainly involves the PCL and, clinically, the instability allows the medial tibial condyle to sublux posteriorly, as the axis of motion has moved to the lateral joint compartment.[27]

The diagnosis of anterior-lateral instability is based on the demonstration of a forward subluxation of the lateral tibial plateau as the knee approaches extension and the spontaneous reduction of the subluxation during flexion, in the lateral pivot shift test.[27] This form of instability usually occurs when the individual is either decelerating or changing direction, and the sudden shift of the lateral compartment is experienced as a "giving way" phenomenon, often associated with pain.[27]

Pivot-Shift Test Since the majority of patients with an ACL rupture complain of a "giving-way" sensation, the pivot shift test is regarded in current literature as capable of identifying rotational instability.[38–40]

There are two main types of clinical tests to determine the presence of the pivot shift, the reduction test and the subluxation test.

In the reduction test, the knee is flexed from full extension under a valgus moment.[41] A sudden reduction of the anteriorly subluxed lateral tibial plateau is seen as the pivot shift.[42]

The subluxation test is effectively the reverse of the reduction test.[32] However, only 35% to 75% of patients whose knees pivot while the patient is under anesthesia will experience such pivot when awake.[43–46] The test begins with patients' knees extended. The clinician internally rotates the patient's tibia with one hand and applies a valgus stress to the patient's knee joint with the other (Figure 11-12). As the clinician gradually flexes the patient's ACL-deficient knee joint, the patient's subluxed anterior tibia snaps back into normal alignment at 20° to 40° of flexion.[38]

There is little agreement in the literature with regard to the sensitivity of the pivot shift test, which varies between 0 and 98%.[45,47,48]

The pivot shift can be positive with an isolated ACL injury,[45,49] or a tear or stretching of the lateral capsule,[50,51] although an injury to the MCL reduces the likelihood of a pivot shift even with ACL injury.[45,52]

MacIntosh (True Pivot-Shift)   The MacIntosh test[53] is the most frequently used test to detect anterior-lateral instability, although Hughston,[32] Slocum, and Losee[51] have all described variations, with the latter author having received credit for describing the instability simultaneously, and independently, from MacIntosh.

The clinician picks up the relaxed leg by grasping the ankle, and flexes the leg by placing the heel of the other hand over the lateral head of the gastrocnemius. The knee is then extended and a slight valgus stress is applied to its lateral aspect to support the tibia. Under the influence of gravity, the femur falls backward and, as the knee approaches extension, the tibial plateau subluxes forward. This subluxation can be accentuated by gently internally rotating the tibia with the hand that is cradling the foot and ankle. At this point, a strong valgus force is placed on the knee by the upper hand, thereby impinging the subluxed tibial plateau against the lateral femoral condyle, by jamming the two joint surfaces together. This will prevent easy reduction as the tibia is then flexed on the femur. At approximately 30°–40° of flexion, the displaced tibial plateau will suddenly reduce, often in a dramatic fashion.

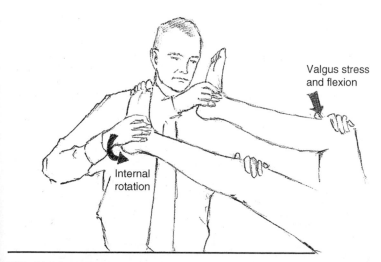

Valgus stress and flexion

Internal rotation

FIG. 11-12   Pivot shift test.

Anterior-Medial Instability

Patients who demonstrate excessive anterior medial tibial condylar displacement during the anterior drawer test are exhibiting anterior-medial instability, as the axis of motion has moved to the lateral joint compartment.[27] The pathology involves the ACL, the MCL, and the posterior medial capsule.[27]

Slocum Test The Slocum test is designed to assess for both rotary and anterior instabilities.[54] The patient is positioned in supine and his or her knee is flexed to 80°–90°, with the hip flexed to 45°. The foot of the involved leg is first placed in 30° of internal rotation. Excessive internal rotation results in a tightening of the remaining structures and can lead to false negatives. The clinician sits on the foot to maintain its position, and pulls the tibia forward (Figure 11-13). A positive test results from movement occurring primarily on the lateral side of the knee, and indicates a lesion to one or more of the following structures:

- Anterior cruciate ligament
- Posterior-lateral capsule
- Arcuate popliteus complex
- Lateral collateral ligament
- Posterior cruciate ligament

If this test is positive, the second part of the test, which assesses anterior-medial rotary instability, is less reliable.[55]

The second half of the test is similar to the first, except that the patient's foot is placed in about 15° of external rotation. Again, by placing the foot in too much external rotation, the clinician runs the risk of false negatives during testing. Movement occurring primarily on the medial side of the knee during testing is a positive result, and indicates a lesion to one or more of the following structures:

- Medial collateral ligament
- Posterior oblique ligament
- Posterior-medial capsule
- Anterior cruciate ligament

Patellar Stability Tests

Patellar stability is assessed by gently pushing the patella medially and laterally while the knee is relaxed in a position of 90° of flexion. This position is

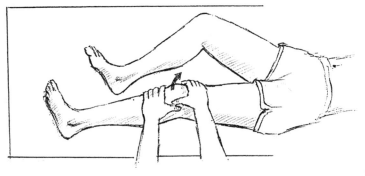

FIG. 11-13   Slocum test.

used because this is the position when all the retinacula are on stretch. If this test is positive for laxity, further testing is needed. The further testing involves application of medial, and lateral, patellar glides, tilts, and rotations, with the knee in relaxed extension, and noting any limitations of motion, or excessive excursion.[56]

The apprehension test may also be used if patella instability is suspected. The patient lies supine and the knee is positioned in 30° of flexion. In this position, the patella is at a point where, in most patients, it is about to engage in the femoral groove. The clinician slowly pushes the patella in a lateral direction. Patients who anticipate patellar dislocation will demonstrate visible apprehension or involuntary contraction of the quadriceps with this maneuver.

Meniscal Lesion Tests

McMurray Test[26]

The McMurray test was originally developed to diagnose posterior horn lesions of the medial meniscus.

The patient is positioned in supine and the clinician maximally flexes the hip and knee. This is performed by grasping the dorsum of the patient's foot in such a way that the thumb is lateral, the index and middle fingers are medial, and the ring and little fingers hold the medial edge of the foot (Figure 11-14). One hand is placed against the lateral aspect of the patient's knee (Figure 11-14). By rotating the patient's lower leg several times, the clinician can assess whether the

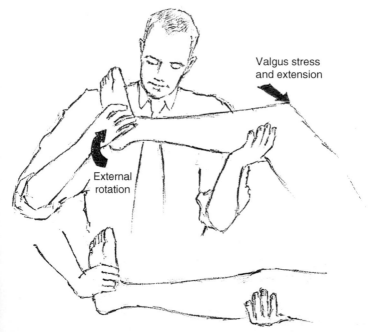

Valgus stress
and extension

External
rotation

FIG. 11-14   McMurray's test.

patient is fully relaxed. While the lower leg is slightly externally rotated, the ipsi-lateral hand moves the patient's foot in a varus direction. The knee is flexed as far as comfortable, after which the foot is brought into a valgus direction with simultaneous internal rotation of the lower leg. The clinician then gently extends the knee to about 120°, and at the same time exerts valgus pressure on the knee with the hand (see Figure 11-14). This test is positive when a palpable click, or audible thump, is elicited that is also painful. It is thought that pain with passive external rotation implicates lesions of the posterior horn of the lateral meniscus, while pain with passive internal rotation implicates a lesion of the posterior horn of the medial meniscus, although false-positives are common.

By modifying this test, it is possible to diagnose other meniscus lesions as well.

Apley's Test[57]

The patient is positioned in the prone position with his or her knee flexed to 90°. The patient's thigh is stabilized by the clinician's knee (Figure 11-15).

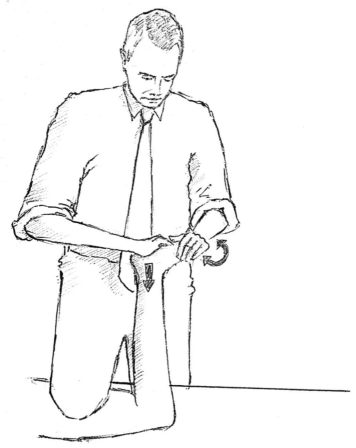

FIG. 11-15 Apley's grind test.

The clinician applies internal and external rotation with compression to the lower leg, noting any pain, and the quality of motion. Pain with this maneuver may indicate a meniscal lesion.

Steinmann's Tenderness Displacement Test[26]

Steinmann's test can be used to diagnose meniscus lesions as theoretically tenderness moves posteriorly when the knee is flexed and anteriorly when the knee is extended with such lesions. If the most painful site is found in the joint space at the level of the MCL, the test is less reliable, because both the medial meniscus and the ligament move posteriorly during flexion.

Special Tests for Specific Diagnoses

Plical Irritation

Plical irritation has a characteristic pattern of presentation. The anterior pain in the knee is episodic and associated with painful clicking, giving-way, and the feeling of something catching in the knee. Careful palpation of the patellar retinaculum and fat pad, with the knee extended and then flexed, can be used to detect tender plicae, and for the differentiation of tenderness within the fat pad, from tenderness over the anterior horn of the menisci.

Patellar Mobility and Retinaculum Tests

Patella glides can be used to examine for retinacular mobility. The patella should be able to translate at least 33% of its width both medially and laterally (Figure 11-16). Inability to do this indicates tightness of the retinacula. Hypermobility of the patella is demonstrated if the patella can be translated 100% of its width medially or laterally (Figure 11-16).

Hamstring Flexibility

The popliteal angle is the most popular method reported in the literature for assessing hamstring tightness, especially in the presence of a knee flexion contracture.[58] Hamstring flexibility can also be assessed with a passive straight leg raise, while ensuring that the lumbar spine is flattened on the treatment table and the pelvis is stabilized. However, this method may be used only if there is full extension at the knee of the leg being examined. Normal hamstring length should allow 80° to 85° of hip flexion, when the knee is extended and the lumbar spine is flattened.[56]

ITB Flexibility

The cardinal sign for iliotibial contracture is that in the supine patient an abduction contracture is present when the hip and knee are extended, but is eliminated by flexion of the hip and knee.[59]

Quadriceps Flexibility

Placing the patient prone and passively flexing the knee, bringing the heel toward the buttocks, examine quadriceps flexibility. The lumbar spine is monitored and stabilized if necessary to prevent motion. The heel should touch the buttocks.

Neurovascular Status

The neurovascular assessment should include pulse, sensation, and reflex testing. A working knowledge of the dermatomes and myotomes around the

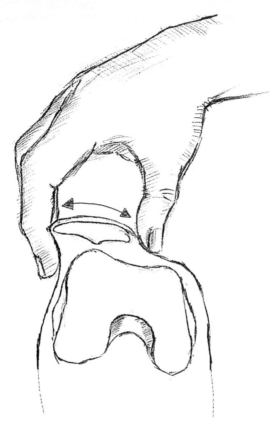

FIG. 11-16   Patellar mobility testing.

knee is essential. The L3 dermatome (femoral nerve) supplies the anterior thigh just above the knee, L4 the anteromedial portion of the knee and the leg (saphenous nerve), and L5 the lateromedial portion of the knee and leg (sural and peroneal nerves).[5] The skin over the posterior aspect of the knee is mostly innervated by the S2 dermatome.[5]

Laboratory Tests

The presence of warmth, exquisite tenderness, painful effusion, and marked pain with even slight range of motion of the knee joint is consistent with septic arthritis or acute inflammatory arthropathy. Arthrocentesis can be used as a diagnostic tool and therapeutic procedure.[60] Although not all knee effusions require aspiration, arthrocentesis is recommended in patients with knee effusion without a history of trauma and with a clinical suspicion of infectious etiology.[60] Synovial fluid obtained by arthrocentesis is sent for analysis (see Table 11-4). In addition to obtaining the results from a complete blood count with differential and an erythrocyte sedimentation rate (ESR), the results of any arthrocentesis should be obtained to help differentiate simple effusion from hemarthrosis or occult osteochondral fracture.

Diagnostic Imaging[2,8]

Plain Radiography

Plain film radiographs can be important tools in the evaluation of acute knee injuries. The Ottawa Knee Rules provide guidelines when radiographs of the knee are necessary.[61] These rules aim to identify patients with clinically significant knee fractures, defined as a bone fragment at least 5 millimeter in breadth or an avulsion fracture associated with complete disruption of tendons or ligaments. With a sensitivity of 100%, the Ottawa guidelines recommend knee radiographs when one or more of the following are present: age 55 or older, tenderness at the head of the fibula, no bone tenderness of the knee other than the patella, inability to flex the knee to 90°, and the inability to bear weight or walk more than four steps immediately after injury. When radiographs are indicated, anteroposterior and lateral views are usually supplemented with five additional views. The anteroposterior view is helpful for evaluating the distal femoral physis, the proximal tibial physis, the tibial intercondylar eminence, and the patella. The lateral view is useful for evaluating the position of the patella and the tibial tubercle. Two oblique views may be ordered secondarily to better appreciate minimally displaced fractures about the knee. Varus and valgus stress views may reveal physeal fractures and collateral ligament injury or laxity. The tunnel or notch view is an anteroposterior radiograph with the knee flexed 20°. This view shows the articular surfaces of the distal femoral condyles and is used when osteochondritis dissecans is suspected. The sunrise or sulcus view is used to assess the congruity of the patellofemoral articulation. The alignment view, a standing anteroposterior view of the entire lower extremity (including the hip, knee, and ankle joints), allows for assessment of anatomic, mechanical, and weight-bearing axes, and compartment space narrowing.

Magnetic Resonance Imaging

Magnetic resonance imaging (MRI) is used to highlight both soft tissue and bone. The soft tissues include the menisci, cruciate and collateral ligaments, and synovial lining of the joint space. Osseous structures defined uniquely by MRI include articular cartilage, physeal cartilage, subchondral bone, periosteum, and marrow elements. MRI is most often used to confirm or clarify a diagnosis or to plan arthroscopy or surgery.[9]

Plain tomograms or computed tomographic (CT) scans may be helpful in diagnosing tibial plateau fractures and osteochondral fractures.[6]

EXAMINATION CONCLUSIONS—THE EVALUATION

Following the examination, and once the clinical findings have been recorded, the clinician must determine a specific diagnosis or a working hypothesis, based on a summary of all the findings. This diagnosis can be structure related (medical diagnosis) (Table 11-11), or a diagnosis based on the preferred practice patterns as described in the *Guide to Physical Therapist Practice*.[62]

TABLE 11-11 Differential Diagnosis of Common Causes of Knee Pain

Condition	Patient age	Mechanism of injury	Area of Symptoms	Symptoms aggravated by	Observation	AROM	PROM	End-feel	Resisted	Tenderness with palpation
Patellofemoral syndrome	20–50	Gradual Macrotrauma Microtrauma	Anterior knee	Prolonged sitting Stairs Kneeling	Possible soft tissue thickening/swelling at anterior knee	Usually no limited ranges	Pain at end range knee flexion	Usually unremarkable	Usually no pain with resisted tests	Anterior knee especially with patella compression
Patellar tendinitis	15–50	Gradual (repeated eccentric overloading during deceleration activities)	Anterior knee	Squatting, jumping	Usually unremarkable	Usually unremarkable	Pain at end range knee flexion	Usually unremarkable	May have pain with resisted knee extension	Over the patellar tendon, inferior or superior to the patellar
Quadriceps muscle tear	20–40	Sudden overload	Anterior thigh	Squatting	Possible bruising over anterior thigh/knee Possible swelling over anterior thigh/knee	Limited knee flexion	Pain with combined hip extension and knee flexion	Spasm/empty depending on extent of injury	Pain with resisted hip flexion Pain with resisted knee extension	Anterior thigh
Knee osteoarthritis	50+	Gradual due to microtrauma Macrotrauma (traumatic arthritis)	Generalized knee	Weight bearing	Possible soft tissue thickening/swelling around knee	Loss of motion in a capsular pattern	Pain at end range knee flexion and extension	Unremarkable	Generalized weakness	Typically posterior knee if present at all

Anterior cruciate ligament sprain/tear	15–45	Trauma to knee (sudden deceleration, an abrupt change of direction, valgus force, rotary force) while foot is fixed	Varies according to number of associated structures involved Typically associated with immediate swelling of knee (acute hemarthrosis)	Weight bearing	Knee swelling	Loss of some knee flexion and extension (depending on extent of swelling)	Pain at end ranges	Loss of firm end-feel with Lachman/anterior drawer	Pain with resisted knee rotation	Depends on associated injuries
Collateral ligament injury	Varies	Trauma to contralateral aspect of knee (valgus or varus)	Distal femur on medial or lateral aspect depending on whether MCL or LCL is involved	Varus stress (LCL) Valgus stress (MCL)	Swelling may be present depending on extent of trauma	Depends on extent of trauma	Possible pain at end range of tibial rotation	Depends on extent of injury	Usually negative	Distal medial femur to medial joint line (MCL) Distal lateral femur to lateral joint line (LCL)
Prepatellar bursitis	15–50	Direct trauma to anterior aspect of knee History of prolonged kneeling	Anterior knee	Kneeling	Local swelling, fluctuation	Unremarkable	Sometimes passive flexion is painful	Usually unremarkable	Usually unremarkable	Anterior aspect of knee

(Continued)

TABLE 11-11 Differential Diagnosis of Common Causes of Knee Pain (*Continued*)

Condition	Patient age	Mechanism of injury	Area of Symptoms	Symptoms aggravated by	Observation	AROM	PROM	End-feel	Resisted	Tenderness with palpation
Patellar subluxation/ dislocation	Varies	Twisting injury with the femur internally rotating on a fixed foot, although there may be no history of trauma	Varies according to tissues involved	Weight bearing	Dependent on the degree of trauma	Dependent on extent of trauma	Dependent on extent of trauma, apprehension usually present	Spasm/empty	Usually unable to perform secondary to pain	Lateral femoral condyle, retinacular, patellar facet
Lumbar disk pathology	20–50	Gradual Sudden overload of lumbar spine	L3 dermatome	Trunk flexion Bearing down	May have associated trunk deviation	Usually pain with trunk flexion	Unremarkable	May have painful SLR	Fatigable weakness in associated myotome	May have tenderness over involved spinal segment

REFERENCES

1. Dye SF: An evolutionary perspective of the knee. J Bone Joint Surg 1987; 69A:976–983.
2. Davids JR: Pediatric knee. Clinical assessment and common disorders. Ped Clin N Am 1996;43:1067–1090.
3. Wojtys EM, Huston LJ: Neuromuscular performance in normal and anterior cruciate ligament-deficient lower extremities. Am J Sports Med 1994;22:89–104.
4. Frank CB, Jackson DW: The science of reconstruction of the anterior cruciate ligament. J Bone Joint Surg 1997;79(10):1556–1576.
5. Mendelsohn CL, Paiement GD: Physical examination of the knee. Primary Care 1996;23:321–328.
6. Rothenberg MH, Graf BK: Evaluation of acute knee injuries. Postgrad Med 1993;93:75–82, 85–86.
7. Clancy WG: Evaluation of acute knee injuries. In Finerman G (ed): American Association of Orthopaedic Surgeons, Symposium on Sports medicine: The Knee, pp 185–193. St Louis, MO, Mosby, 1985.
8. Austermuehle PD: Common knee injuries in primary care. Nurse Pract 2001;26:32–45, quiz 46–47.
9. Bergfeld JA, Ireland ML, Wojtys EM: Pinpointing the cause of acute knee pain. Patient Care Arch 1997;31:100–117.
10. Tria AJ: Ligaments of the knee. New York, Churchill Livingstone, 1995.
11. Solomon DH, et al.: The rational clinical examination. Does this patient have a torn meniscus or ligament of the knee? Value of the physical examination. JAMA 2001;286:1610–1620.
12. Sisk TD: Knee injuries. In Crenshaw AH (ed): Campbell's Operative Orthopaedics, pp 2283–2496. St Louis, MO, Mosby, 1987.
13. Tria AJ, Palumbo RC, Alicia JA: Conservative care for patellofemoral pain. Orthop Clin North Am 1992;23:545–554.
14. Bentley G, Dowd G: Current concepts of etiology and treatment of chondromalacia patella. Clin Orthop 1984;189:209.
15. Insall JN: Patella pain syndromes and chondromalacia patellae. Inst Course Lect 1981;30:342–356.
16. Kummel B: The treatment of patellofemoral problems. Primary Care 1980;7:217–229.
17. Reider B, et al.: The anterior aspect of the knee joint: an anatomical study. J Bone and Joint Surg [Am] 1981;63A:351–356.
18. Brinker MR, Miller MD: In Brinker MR, Miller MD (eds): Fundamentals of orthopedics, pp 294–321. Philadelphia, PA, WB Saunders, 1999.
19. Feagin JA, Jr.: The office diagnosis and documentation of common knee problems. Clin Sports Med 1989;8:453–459.
20. Barber-Westin SD, Noyes FR, Andrews M: A rigorous comparison between the sexes of results and complications after anterior cruciate ligament reconstruction. Am J Sports Med 1997;25:514–526.
21. Reinking MF: Knee anatomy and biomechanics. In Wadsworth C (ed): Disorders of the Knee—Home Study Course. La Crosse, WI, Orthpaedic Section, APTA, 2001.
22. Laubenthal KN, Smidt GL, Kettelkamp DB: A quantitative analysis of knee motion for activities of daily living. Phys Ther 1972;52:34–42.
23. Rauch G, et al.: Is conservative treatment of partial or complete anterior cruciate ligament rupture still justified? An analysis of the recent literature and a recommendation for arriving at a decision. Zeitschr Orthop 1991;129:438–446.
24. Sommerlath K, Odensten M, Lysholm J: The late course of acute partial anterior cruciate ligament tears. A nine to 15-year follow-up evaluation. Clin Ortho Relat Res 1992;281:152–158.
25. Terry GC, et al.: How iliotibial tract injuries of the knee combine with acute anterior cruciate ligament tears to influence abnormal anterior tibial displacement. Am J Sports Med 1993;21:55–60.

26. Winkel D, Matthijs O, Phelps V: Examination of the knee. Diagnosis and Treatment of the Lower Extremities, pp 166–197. Maryland, MD, Aspen, 1997.

27. Reid DC: Knee ligament injuries, anatomy, classification, and examination. In Reid DC (ed): Sports Injury Assessment and Rehabilitation, pp 437–493. New York, Churchill Livingstone, 1992.

28. Liu SH, et al.: The diagnosis of acute complete tears of the anterior cruciate ligament. J Bone Joint Surg 1995;77(6):586.

29. Weiss JR, et al.: A functional assessment of anterior cruciate ligament deficiency in an acute and clinical setting. J Orthop Sports Phys Ther 1990;11:372–373.

30. Hanten WP, Pace MB: Reliability of measuring anterior laxity of the knee joint using a knee ligament arthrometer. Phys Ther 1987;67:357–359.

31. Hughston JC, et al.: Classification of knee ligament instabilities. Part 2. J Bone Joint Surg 1976;58A:173–179.

32. Hughston JC, et al.: Classification of knee ligament instabilities. Part 1. J Bone Joint Surg 1976;58A:159–172.

33. Torg JS, Conrad W, Kalen V: Clinical diagnosis of anterior cruciate ligament instability in the athlete. Am J Sports Med 1976;4(2):84–93.

34. Katz JW, Fingeroth RJ: The diagnostic accuracy of ruptures of the anterior cruciate ligament comparing the Lachman's test, the anterior drawer sign, and the pivot-shift test in acute and chronic knee injuries. Am J Sports Med 1986;14:88–91.

35. Strobel M, Stedtfeld HW: Diagnostic Evaluation of the Knee. Berlin, Springer-Verlag, 1990.

36. Shino K, Horibe S, Ono K: The voluntary evoked posterolateral drawer sign in the knee with posterolateral instability. Clin Orthop 1987;215:179–186.

37. Hughston JC, Norwood LA: The posterolateral drawer test and external rotation recurvatum test for posterolateral rotary instability of the knee. Clin Orthop 1980;147:82–87.

38. Jensen K: Manual laxity tests for anterior cruciate ligament injuries. J Orthop Sports Phys Ther 1990;11:474–481.

39. Jakob RP, St Ñubli HU, Deland JT: Grading the pivot shift. J Bone Joint Surg 1987;69B:294–299.

40. Noyes FR, et al.: An analysis of the pivot shift phenomenon. Am J Sports Med 1991;19:148–155.

41. Bull AM, et al.: Incidence and mechanism of the pivot shift. An in vitro study. Clin Ortho Rel Res 1999;363:219–231.

42. Galway HR, Beaupre A, MacIntosh DL: Pivot shift: a clinical sign of symptomatic anterior cruciate deficiency. J Bone Joint Surg 1972;54B:763–764.

43. Bach BR Jr, et al.: Arthroscopy-assisted anterior cruciate ligament reconstruction using patellar tendon substitution. Two- to four-year follow-up results. Am J Sports Med 1994;22:758–767.

44. Daniel DM, Stone ML, Riehl B: Ligament surgery: the evaluation of results. In Daniel DM, Akeson WH, O'Connor JJ (eds): Knee Ligaments, Structure, Function and Repair, pp 521–534. New York, Raven, 1990.

45. Donaldson WF, Warren RF, Wickiewicz TL: A comparison of acute anterior cruciate ligament examinations. Am J Sports Med 1985;13:5–10.

46. Norwood LA, et al.: Acute anterolateral rotatory instability of the knee. J Bone Joint Surg 1979;61A:704–709.

47. DeHaven KE: Diagnosis of acute knee injuries with hemarthrosis. Am J Sports Med 1980;8:9–14.

48. Otter C, Aufdemkampe G, Lezeman H: Diagnostiek van knieletsel en relatie tussen de aanwezigheid van knieklachten en de resultaten van functionele testen en Biodex-test. In Jaarboek 1994 Fysiotherapie Kinesitherapie, pp 195–228. Houten, Bohn, Stafleu, van Loghum, 1994.

49. Harilainen A, et al.: Prospective preoperative evaluation of anterior cruciate ligament instability of the knee joint and results of reconstruction with patellar ligament. Clin Orthop 1993;297:17–22.

50. Losee RE: Concepts of the pivot shift. Clin Orthop 1983;172:45–51.

51. Losee RE, Johnson TR, Southwick WO: Anterior subluxation of the lateral tibial plateau. A diagnostic test and operative repair. J Bone Joint Surg 1978;60A: 1015–1030.

52. Gerber C, Matter P: Biomechanical analysis of the knee after rupture of the anterior cruciate ligament and its primary repair. An instant-centre analysis of function. J Bone Joint Surg 1983;65B:391–399.

53. MacIntosh DL, Galway RD: The lateral pivot shift. A symptomatic and clinical sign of anterior cruciate insufficiency. In 85th Annual Meeting of American Orthopaedic Association. Tucker's Town, Bermuda, 1972.

54. Slocum DB, Larson RL: Rotary instability of the knee. J Bone Joint Surg 1968;50A:211–225.

55. Slocum, DB, et al.: A clinical test for anterolateral rotary instability of the knee. Clin Orthop 1976;118:63–69.

56. Grelsamer RP, McConnell J: Examination of the patellofemoral joint. In The Patella: A Team Approach, pp 109–118. Maryland, MD, Aspen, 1998.

57. Apley AG: The diagnosis of meniscus injuries: some new clinical methods. J Bone Joint Surg 1947;29B:78–84.

58. Kuo L, et al.: The hamstring index. J Pediatr Orthop 1997;17:78–88.

59. Gautam VK, Anand S: A new test for estimating iliotibial band contracture. J Bone Joint Surg 1998;80B:474–475.

60. Johnson MW: Acute knee effusions: a systematic approach to diagnosis. Am Fam Phys 2000;61:2391–2400.

61. Steill IG, et al.: Implementation of the Ottawa Knee Rule for the use of radiography in acute knee injuries. JAMA 1997;278:2075–2079.

62. Guide to physical therapist practice. Phys Ther 2001;81:S13–S95.

12 | The Ankle and Foot

OVERVIEW

Despite the fact that the ankle complex is endowed with multiple structural supports, it is the most commonly injured part in the body.[1] The majority of the support provided to the ankle and foot joints (Table 12-1) come by way of the arrangement of the ankle mortise and by the numerous ligaments found here (Table 12-2). Further stabilization is afforded by an abundant number of tendons that cross this joint complex (Tables 12-3, 12-4). These tendons are also involved in producing foot and ankle movements and are held in place by retinaculae.

Even with this remarkable level of protection, the foot and ankle complex is at the mercy of truly impressive forces that act on it during normal and athletic activities. As elsewhere, injuries to this area can be either microtraumatic or macrotraumatic. However, because of the sophisticated musculoskeletal arrangement of the ankle and foot complex, determining the exact diagnosis can be difficult. Obtaining an accurate diagnosis necessitates a thorough knowledge of anatomy and biomechanics (see *Orthopaedic Examination, Evaluation, and Intervention*, pp 833–857) combined with the findings of a detailed history and physical examination.

EXAMINATION

The exact form of the examination of the foot and ankle complex is very dependent on the acuteness of the condition (see *Orthopaedic Examination, Evaluation, and Intervention*, p 878). An inability to bear weight, severe pain, and rapid swelling indicate a serious injury such as a capsular tear, fracture, or grade III ligament sprain.[2–5] In such cases the patient should be referred for further medical examination.

History

The clinician must determine whether the onset was the result of an injury or whether the symptoms occurred gradually. Information about the mechanism should include, when, where, and how the injury occurred. Details about the mechanism of injury allow the clinician to infer the pathologic status and structures involved, although it must be remembered that the patient's recollection of the mechanism frequently does not correspond to the structures damaged.[6,7] Where possible, the position of the foot and ankle at the time of the injury should also be determined. Most ankle sprains occur when the foot is plantar flexed, inverted, and adducted (Table 12-5, Figure 12-1). However, this same mechanism can also lead to more serious conditions such as a malleolar or talar dome fracture (Table 12-6). A dorsiflexion injury with associated snapping and pain on the lateral aspect of the ankle that rapidly diminishes may indicate a tear of the peroneal retinaculum.[8]

Information about the time of injury, the time of the onset of swelling, and its location are important. Most often the patient can point to the location of the initial pain. The patient may note hearing a "snap," "crack," or "pop" at the time of injury, which could indicate a ligamentous injury or a fracture. It is worth remembering that the clinical presentation of subtle fractures can be similar to that of ankle sprains, and these fractures are frequently missed on the initial examination.

TABLE 12-1 The Joints of the Foot and Ankle: Their Open Pack, Close Pack Positions, and Capsular Patterns

Joints of the hind foot	Open pack position	Close pack position	Capsular pattern
Tibiofibular joint	Plantar flexion	Maximum dorsiflexion	Pain on stress
Talocrural joint	10° plantar flexion and midway between inversion and eversion	Maximum dorsiflexion	Plantar flexion, dorsiflexion
Subtalar joint	Midway between extremes of range of motion	Supination	Varus, valgus
Joints of the midfoot			
Midtarsal Joints	Midway between extremes of range of motion	Supination	Dorsiflexion, plantar flexion, adduction, medial rotation
Joints of the forefoot			
Tarsometatarsal joints	Midway between extremes of range of motion	Supination	None
Metatar-sophalangeal joints	10° extension	Full extension	Great toe: Extension, flexion Second–fifth toes: Variable
Interphalangeal joints	Slight flexion	Full extension	Flexion, extension

Determining the location of the pain can provide some clues as to the cause (Figure 12-2). The site and severity of the pain can be measured using a body diagram and visual analogue scale respectively. A stress fracture, or tendinitis, typically has a localized site of pain, whereas diffuse pain is often associated with compartment syndromes. The distribution of pain is important and the clinician should rule out whether the pattern is dermatomal, from a peripheral nerve, or referred from a distal structure (refer to *Systems Review*).[9]

Information should be gleaned about activities that aggravate the symptoms. For example, pain with forced dorsiflexion and eversion, and with squatting activities, may suggest ankle instability. Pain after activity suggests an overuse, or chronic injury. Pain during an activity suggests stress on the injured structure.

If there is no traumatic event, the clinician must determine if there has been a change in exercise or activity intensity (increased mileage with runners), training surface, or changes in body weight or shoe wear (causal agents).[6,7] Pain that is related to a time of day may indicate an activity-related problem. Increased symptoms associated with an increase in exercise or activity intensity likely indicates an overuse injury. Achilles tendinitis is an overuse injury associated with an insidious onset of posterior calcaneal pain. Complaints of cramping may accompany muscular fatigue or intermittent claudication from arterial insufficiency. Increased symptoms when walking or running on uneven terrain as compared with an even terrain may suggest ankle instability. Increased symptoms when walking or running on hard surfaces as compared to a stiffer surface may suggest a lack of shock absorbency of the foot or shoe.

TABLE 12-2 Ankle and Foot Joints and Associated Ligaments

Joint	Associated ligament	Fiber direction	Motions limited
Distal tibiofibular	Anterior tibiofibular	Distolateral	Distal glide of fibula
	Posterior tibiofibular Interosseous	Distolateral	Plantar flexion Distal glide of fibular
	Interosseous group Interosseous III		Plantar flexion Separation of tibia and fibula
Ankle	Deltoid (medial collateral)		
	Superficial	Plantar-anterior	Plantar flexion, abduction
	Tibionavicular	Plantar, plantar-posterior	Eversion, abduction
	Tibiocalcaneal		Dorsiflexion, abduction
	Posterior tibiotalar	Plantar-posterior	Eversion, abduction, plantar flexion
	Deep Anterior tibiotalar	Anterior	Plantar flexion Inversion
	Lateral or fibular collateral		Anterior displacement of foot
	Anterior talofibular Calcaneofibular	Anterior-medial	Inversion Dorsiflexion
	Posterior talofibular Lateral talocalcaneal	Posterior-medial Horizontal (lateral)	Dorsiflexion Posterior displacement of foot
	Anterior capsule Posterior capsule	Posterior-medial	Inversion Dorsiflexion Plantar flexion Dorsiflexion
Subtalar	Interosseous talocalcaneal		
	Anterior band	Proximal-anterior-lateral	Inversion
	Posterior band	Proximal-posterior-lateral	Joint separation
	Lateral talocalcaneal	(See ankle)	Inversion
	Deltoid	(See ankle)	Joint separation
	Lateral collateral	(See ankle)	Dorsiflexion
	Posterior talocalcaneal	Vertical	Eversion
	Medial talocalcaneal	Plantar-anterior	Inversion
	Anterior talocalcaneal (cervical ligaments)	Plantar-posterior-lateral	
Main ligamentous support of longitudinal arches	Long plantar	Anterior, slightly medial	Eversion
	Short plantar	Anterior	Eversion
	Plantar calcaneonavicular	Dorsal-anterior-medial	Eversion
	Plantar aponeurosis	Anterior	Eversion

(Continued)

TABLE 12-2 Ankle and Foot Joints and Associated Ligaments (*Continued*)

Joint	Associated ligament	Fiber direction	Motions limited
Midtarsal or transverse	Bifurcated		Joint separation
	Medial band	Longitudinal	Plantar flexion
	Lateral band	Horizontal	Inversion
	Dorsal talonavicular	Longitudinal	Plantar flexion of talus on navicular
	Dorsal calcaneocuboid	Longitudinal	Inversion, plantar flexion
	Ligaments supporting the arches		
Intertarsal	Numerous ligaments named by two interconnected bones (dorsal and plantar ligaments)		Joint motion in direction causing ligament tightness
	Interosseous ligaments connecting cuneiforms, cuboid, and navicular		Flattening of transverse arch
	Ligaments supporting arches		
Tarsometatarsal	Dorsal, plantar, and interosseous		Joint separation
Intermetatarsal	Dorsal, plantar, and interosseous		Joint separation
	Deep transverse metatarsal		Joint separation
			Flattening of transverse arch
Metatarsophalangeals	Fibrous capsule	Plantar-anterior	Flexion
	Dorsally, thin—separated from extensor tendons by bursae		Extension
	Inseparable from deep surface of plantar and collateral ligaments		Flexion, abduction, or adduction in flexion
	Collateral		Extension
	Plantar, grooved for flexor tendons		
Interphalangeal	Collateral		Flexion, abduction, or adduction in flexion
	Plantar		Extension
	Extensor hood replaces dorsal ligaments		Flexion

Plantar fasciitis is a condition associated with a lack of shock absorbency and typically associated with an insidious onset of heel pain and pain felt when first weight bearing in the morning.

Additionally, questions regarding past medical history, previous ankle injury, goals of the patient regarding the functional results, and level and intensity of sports involvement are important in order to individualize the intervention.

TABLE 12-3 Intrinsic Muscles of the Foot

Muscle	Proximal	Distal	Innervation
Extensor digitorum brevis	Distal superior surface of calcaneus	Dorsal surface of second through fourth toes, base of proximal phalanx	Deep peroneal S1 and S2
Abductor hallucis	Tuberosity of calcaneus and plantar aponeurosis	Base of proximal phalanx, medial side	Medial plantar L5 and S1 (L4)
Adductor hallucis	Base of second, third, and fourth metatarsals, and deep plantar ligaments	Proximal phalanx of first digit lateral side	Medial and lateral plantar S1 and S2
Lumbricals	Medial and adjacent sides of flexor digitorum longus tendon to each lateral digit	Medial side of proximal phalanx and extensor hood	Medial and lateral plantar L5, S1, and S2 (L4)
Plantar interossei			
First	Base and medial side of third metatarsal	Base of proximal phalanx and extensor hood of third digit	Medial and lateral plantar S1 and S2
Second	Base and medial side of fourth metatarsal	Base of proximal phalanx and extensor hood of fourth digit	
Third	Base and medial side of fifth metatarsal	Base of proximal phalanx and extensor hood of fifth digit	
Dorsal interossei			
First	First and second metatarsal bones	Proximal phalanx and extensor hood of second digit medially	Medial and lateral plantar S1 and S2
Second	Second and third metatarsal bones	Proximal phalanx and extensor hood of second digit laterally	
Third	Third and fourth metatarsal bones	Proximal phalanx and extensor hood of third digit laterally	
Fourth	Fourth and fifth metatarsal bones	Proximal phalanx and extensor hood of fourth digit laterally	
Abductor digiti minimi	Lateral side of fifth metatarsal bone	Proximal phalanx of fifth digit	Lateral plantar S1 and S2

TABLE 12-4 Extrinsic Muscle Attachments and Innervation

Muscle	Proximal	Distal	Innervation
Gastrocnemius	Medial and lateral condyle of femur	Posterior surface of calcaneus through Achilles tendon	Tibial S2 (S1)
Plantaris	Lateral supracondylar line of femur	Posterior surface of calcaneus through Achilles tendon	Tibial S2 (S1)
Soleus	Head of fibula, proximal third of shaft, soleal line and midshaft of posterior tibia	Posterior surface of calcaneus through Achilles tendon	Tibial S2 (S1)
Tibialis anterior	Distal to lateral tibial condyle, proximal half of lateral tibial shaft, and interosseous membrane	First cuneiform bone, medial and plantar surfaces and base of first metatarsal	Deep fibular (peroneal) L4 (L5)
Tibialis posterior	Posterior surface of tibia, proximal two-thirds posterior of fibula, and interosseous membrane	Tuberosity of navicular bone, tendinous expansion to other tarsals and metatarsals	Tibial L4 and L5
Fibularis (Peroneus) longus	Lateral condyle of tibia, head and proximal two-thirds of fibula	Base of first metatarsal and first cuneiform, lateral side	Superficial fibular (peroneal) L5 and S1 (S2)
Fibularis (Peroneus) brevis	Distal two-thirds of lateral fibular shaft	Tuberosity of fifth metatarsal	Superficial fibular (peroneal) L5 and S1 (S2)
Fibularis (Peroneus) tertius	Lateral slip from extensor digitorum longus	Tuberosity of fifth metatarsal	Deep fibular (peroneal) L5 and S1
Flexor hallucis brevis	Plantar surface of cuboid and third cuneiform bones	Base of proximal phalanx of great toe	Medial plantar S3 (S2)

(Continued)

373

TABLE 12-4 Extrinsic Muscle Attachments and Innervation (*Continued*)

Muscle	Proximal	Distal	Innervation
Flexor hallucis longus	Posterior distal two-thirds fibula	Base of distal phalanx of great toe	Tibial S2 (S3)
Flexor digitorum brevis	Tuberosity of calcaneus	One tendon slip into base of middle phalanx of each of the lateral four toes	Medial and lateral plantar S3 (S2)
Flexor digitorum longus	Middle three-fifths of posterior tibia	Base of distal phalanx of lateral four toes	Tibial S2 (S3)
Extensor hallucis longus	Middle half of anterior shaft of fibula	Base of distal phalanx of great toe	Deep fibular (peroneal) L5 and S1
Extensor hallucis brevis	Distal superior and lateral surfaces of calcaneus	Dorsal surface of proximal phalanx	Deep fibular (peroneal) S1 and S2
Extensor digitorum longus	Lateral condyle of tibia proximal anterior surface of shaft of fibula	One tendon to each lateral four toes, to middle phalanx and extending to distal phalanges	Deep fibular (peroneal) L5 and S1

TABLE 12-5 Physical Findings in Lateral Ankle Sprains by Grade

Sign/symptom	Grade I	Grade II	Grade III
Loss of functional ability	Minima	Some	Great
Pain	Minimal	Moderate	Severe
Swelling	Minimal	Moderate	Severe
Ecchymosis	Usually not	Frequently	Yes
Difficulty bearing weight	No	Usually	Almost always

Systems Review

As symptoms can be referred distally to the foot and ankle from a host of other joints and conditions, the clinician must be able to differentially diagnose from the presenting signs and symptoms. The cause of the referred symptoms may be neurologic or systemic in origin. If a disorder involving a specific nerve root (L4, L5, S1, or S2) is suspected, the necessary sensory, motor, and reflex testing should be performed. Peripheral nerve entrapments, although not common, may also occur in this region, and often go unrecognized. These include Morton's neuroma, and entrapment of the tibial nerve or its branches—the deep fibular (peroneal) nerve, superficial fibular (peroneal) nerve, sural, and saphenous nerves.[10]

Systemic problems that may involve the leg, foot, and ankle include diabetes mellitus (peripheral neuropathy), osteomyelitis, gout and pseudogout, sickle cell disease, complex regional pain syndrome, peripheral vascular disease, and rheumatoid arthritis. A systemic problem, such as rheumatoid arthritis may be associated with other signs and symptoms, including other joint pain, although the other joint pain may also be the result of overcompensation in the rest of the kinetic chain.

Warning signs at the ankle and foot, which should alert the clinician to a more insidious condition include:

- Immediate and continuous inability to bear weight, which may indicate a fracture (see Table 12-6)
- Nocturnal pain—unrelated to movement, which may indicate a malignancy, hemarthrosis, fracture, or infection
- Gross pain during valgus motions of the ankle, which may indicate compression of a fractured fibular malleolus
- Pain and weakness during resisted eversion, which may indicate fracture of the fifth metatarsal bases
- Calf pain with or without tenderness, swelling with pitting edema, increased skin temperature, superficial venous dilatation, or cyanosis may indicate the presence of a deep vein thrombosis, which requires immediate medical attention (see *Orthopaedic Examination, Evaluation, and Intervention*, p 261)
- Gross tenderness during pressure on the distal fibula, which may indicate a fibular fracture
- Feelings of warmth or coldness in the foot. An abnormally warm foot can indicate local inflammation but can also originate from a tumor in the pelvis or lumbar region.[11] An abnormally cold foot usually indicates a vascular problem.[11]

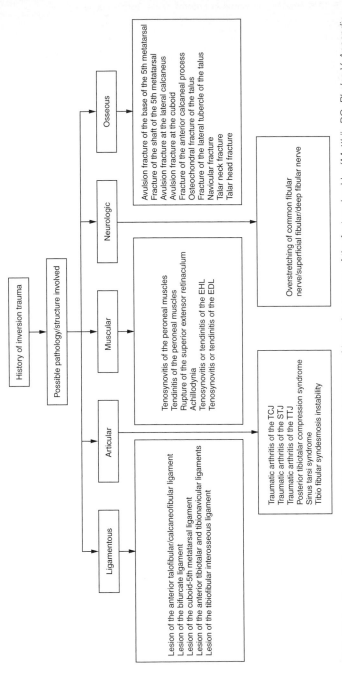

FIG. 12-1 Examination sequence in the presence of a history of inversion trauma of the foot and ankle. (*Matthijs DO, Phelps V, Appendix F. In Winkel D, Matthijs O, Phelps V, (eds): Diagnosis and Treatment of the Lower Extremities, pp 645–646. Maryland, MD, Aspen, 1997.*)

TABLE 12-6 Summary and Comparison of Common Foot and Ankle Fractures

Fracture type	Mechanism of injury	Important physical examination findings[a]	Radiograph[b]
Talar dome (lateral)	Inversion with dorsiflexion	Tenderness anterior to the lateral malleolus, along the anterior border of the talus	Mortise view: shallow, wafer-shaped lesion
Talar dome (medial)	Inversion with plantar flexion or atraumatic	Tenderness posterior to the medial malleolus, along the posterior border of the talus	AP view: deep, cup-shaped lesion; initial radiograph can be normal because changes in subchondral bone may not develop for weeks.
Lateral talar process	Rapid inversion with dorsiflexion	Point tenderness over the lateral process (anterior and inferior to the lateral malleolus)	Mortise view: lateral view may show subtalar effusion
Posterior talar process (lateral tubercle)	Hyperplantar flexion or forced inversion	Tenderness to deep palpation anterior to the Achilles tendon over posterolateral talus Plantar flexion may reproduce pain.	Lateral radiograph (an accessory ossicle, the os trigonum, may be present)
Posterior talar process (medial tubercle)	Dorsiflexion with pronation	Tenderness to deep palpation between the medial malleolus and the Achilles tendon	Difficult with standard views; an oblique ankle radiograph taken with the foot placed in 40° of external rotation has been successful.
Anterior process of the calcaneus	Inversion with plantar flexion can lead to an avulsion fracture. Forced dorsiflexion can cause a compression fracture.	Point tenderness over the calcaneal cuboid joint (approximately 1 centimeter inferior and 3 to 4 centimeters anterior to the lateral malleolus)	Lateral radiograph (an accessory ossicle, the calcaneus secondarium, may be present)

AP = anteroposterior.
[a] Acutely, most fractures will have symptoms very similar to those of ankle sprains: swelling, ecchymosis, ligamentous laxity, tenderness, and decreased range of motion.
[b] All these fractures can have subtle findings on plain radiograph, and computed tomography or magnetic resonance imaging may be required to accurately confirm or characterize a fracture.
Source: Judd DB, Kim DH: Foot fractures frequently misdiagnosed as ankle sprains. Am Fam Phys 2002;66:785–794.

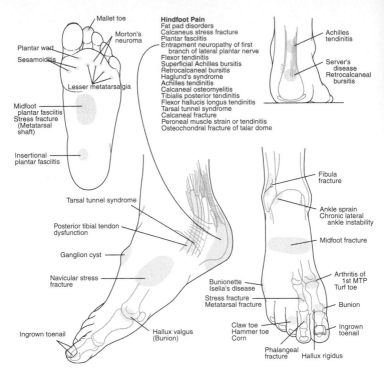

FIG. 12-2   Pain location and possible diagnoses. (*Reproduced with permission from Dutton M: Orthopaedic Examination, Evaluation, and Intervention, p 262 (Fig. 9-7). New York, McGraw-Hill 2004.*)

Tests and Measures

Observation

The observation of the foot and ankle complex can provide the clinician with a wealth of information, including clues about static and dynamic, structural or mechanical foot abnormalities. It is extremely important to observe the entire kinetic chain when assessing the foot and ankle. Weight-bearing and non-weight-bearing alignment and postures of the lower extremity are compared where possible. An important part of the examination of the foot and ankle is the gait assessment (see *Orthopaedic Examination, Evaluation, and Intervention,* Chapter 13). If an antalgic gait is present, the clinician must determine why to help rule out weight-bearing pain from other structures within the kinetic chain.

In addition to evaluating alignment, the leg, foot, and ankle are observed for the presence of bruising, cyanosis, erythema, pallor, skin breakdown, swelling, or unusual angulation. Cyanosis and pallor indicate problems with vascular supply.[12] The appearance of bluish-black plaques on the posterior and posterior-lateral aspect of one or both heels in a young distance runner is found in a condition called *black-dot heel*, which results from a shearing stress or a pinching of the heel between the counter and the sole of the shoe at heel strike during running. Retromalleolar swelling could suggest a tear of the fibularis (peroneus) brevis tendon. Swelling and pain on the posterior aspect of the distal fibula may indicate a traumatic fibularis (peroneal) tendon subluxation.[13] Swelling only on the antero-lateral aspect of the ankle joint can indicate an anterolateral ankle impingement. This can be confirmed if pain is elicited with passive forced ankle dorsiflexion, and extreme ankle eversion and inversion.[14]

Callus formation on the sole of the foot is an indicator of dysfunction. Calluses provide the clinician with an index to the degree of shear stresses applied to the foot, and clearly outline abnormal weight-bearing areas.[15] In adequate amounts, calluses provide protection, but in excess, may cause pain. Callus formation under the second and third metatarsal heads could indicate excessive pronation in a flexible foot, or Morton's neuroma if just under the former. A callus under the fifth, and sometimes the fourth metatarsal head may indicate an abnormally rigid foot.

The weight bearing and wear patterns of the shoes should be noted. The greatest amount of wear on the sole of the shoe should occur beneath the ball of the foot, in the area corresponding to the first, second, and third metatar-sophalangeal (MTP) joints and slight wear to the lateral side of the heel. Old running shoes belonging to patients who excessively pronate tend to display overcompression of the medial arch of the midsole and extensive wear of the lateral regions of the heel counter and medial forefoot. The upper portion of the shoe should demonstrate a transverse crease at the level of the MTP joints. A stiff first MTP joint can produce a crease line that runs obliquely, from forward and medial to backward and lateral.[16] The cup, at the rear of the shoe, which is formed by the heel counter, should be vertical and symmetrical with respect to the shoe, and should be of a durable enough material to hold the heel in place.[17] A medial inclination of the cup, with bulging of the lateral lip of the counter, indicates a pronated foot.[16] A lateral bulge of the heel counter indicates a supinated foot. Scuffing of the shoe might indicate tibialis anterior weakness.[18]

The non weight-bearing component of the examination is initiated by having the patient seated on the edge of the bed, feet dangling. In this position, the feet should adopt an inverted and plantar flexed pose. A mobile on nonstructural flat foot will take on a more normal configuration in nonweight bearing, whereas a fixed or structural flat foot will maintain its planus state. By placing one hand on the patella, and the other hand on the tips of the malleoli, the clinician should note approximately 20°–30° of external rotation of the ankle in relation to the knee.[19]

Palpation

Careful palpation should be performed of the involved and uninvolved leg, foot, and ankle to differentiate tenderness of specific structures (Figure 12-3). Areas of localized swelling and ecchymosis over the ligaments on the medial or lateral aspects of the foot and ankle should be noted. In addition, the clinician should note the borders of ecchymosis, the temperature and tautness of the shin, as well as the suppleness of the soft tissues.[12] Inflamed tendons are often characterized by swollen tendon sheaths, pain with direct palpation, and pain with both active movement and passive stretching of the tendon.[12] Partial rupture of tendons may present with an enlarged, bulbous thickening of the tendon at the rupture site.[12]

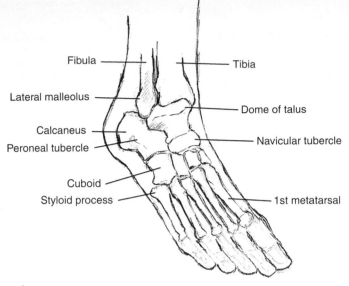

A

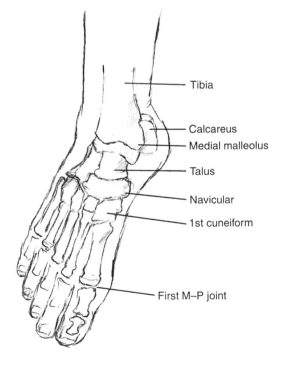

B

FIG. 12-3 Palpation points.

Posterior Aspect of Foot and Ankle

- *Achilles tendon.* The Achilles tendon is inspected for contour changes such as swelling, erythema, and thickening. Any gaps or nodules in the tendon and specific sites of pain should be carefully examined. Palpable gaps in the tendon, accompanied by an inability to rise up on the toes could indicate a rupture of the tendon. The most common site of Achilles tendon rupture is 2 to 6 centimeters proximal to the insertion of the Achilles tendon into the calcaneus.[12]

- *Calcaneus.* At the distal end of the Achilles tendon is the calcaneal tuberosity. The posterior aspect of the calcaneus and surrounding soft tissue is palpated for evidence of exostosis ("pump bump" or Haglund's deformity) and associated swelling (retrocalcaneal bursitis). The inferior medial process of the calcaneus, just distal to the weight-bearing portion serves as the attachment of the plantar fascia and is often tender with plantar fasciitis.

Anterior and Anterior-Medial Aspect of Foot and Ankle

While reading the next section, the reader may find it helpful to remove a shoe and sock, and self-palpate.

- *Great toe and the phalanges.* Beginning medially, the clinician locates and palpates the great toe and its two phalanges. The first metatarsal bone is more proximal, the head of which should be palpated for tenderness on the lateral aspect (bunion) and inferior aspect (sesamoiditis).

  Moving laterally from the phalanges of the great toe, the clinician palpates the phalanges and metatarsal heads of the other four toes. Tenderness of the second metatarsal head could indicate the presence of Freiberg's disease, an osteochondritis of the second metatarsal head. A callus under the second and third metatarsal head may indicate a fallen metatarsal arch. Palpable tenderness in the region of the third and fourth metatarsal heads could indicate a Morton's neuroma, especially if walking barefoot relieves the characteristic sharp pain between the toes of this condition. Tenderness on the lateral aspect of the fifth metatarsal head could indicate the presence of a tailor's bunion.

- *Cuneiform.* The first cuneiform is located at the proximal end of the first metatarsal, and is palpated for tenderness.

- *Navicular.* The navicular is the most prominent bone on the medial aspect of the foot. The navicular tuberosity can be located by moving proximally from the medial aspect of the first cuneiform. The talonavicular joint line lies directly proximal to the navicular tuberosity. In addition, the posterior tibialis, which can be made more prominent with resisted plantarflexion, adduction, and supination, can be used as a reference as it inserts on the plantar surface of the navicular (see later). Tenderness of the navicular could indicate the presence of a fracture, or osteochondritis of the navicular (Köhler's disease).

- *Second and third cuneiforms.* These two bones can be palpated by moving laterally from the first cuneiform. Tenderness of these bones may indicate a cuneiform fracture.

- *Dorsal pedis pulse.* The pulse of the dorsal pedis artery, a branch of the anterior tibial artery, can be palpated over the cuneiform bones, between the first and second cuneiform, or between the first and second metatarsal bones.

- *Medial malleolus.* The medial malleolus is palpated for swelling or tenderness. Moving proximally from the anterior aspect of the medial malleolus, the distal aspect of the tibia is palpated. Distal to that is the talus bone. Moving distal from the tibia, the clinician palpates the long extensor tendons, the tibialis anterior, and the extensor retinaculum. The tendon of the tibialis anterior is visible at the level of the medial cuneiform and the base of the first metatarsal bone, especially if the foot is positioned in dorsiflexion and supination. Tenderness along the posterior and inferior aspect of the medial malleolus, which can radiate distally to the medial arch, could indicate the presence of flexor hallucis longus tendinitis.[12]

- *Tarsal tunnel.* The tarsal tunnel is a fibro-osseous tunnel located just posterior to the medial malleolus on the inside of the ankle. The roof of the tarsal tunnel is formed by the deep fascia of the leg and the deep transverse fascia. The proximal and inferior borders of the tunnel are formed by inferior and superior margins of the flexor retinaculum. The superior aspect of the calcaneus, the medial wall of the talus, and the distal-medial aspect of the tibia form the floor of the tunnel. The tendons of the flexor hallucis longus muscle, flexor digitorum longus muscle, tibialis posterior muscle, the posterior tibial nerve and the posterior tibial artery pass through the tarsal tunnel. Irritation of the posterior tibial nerve can be detected by applying gentle localized percussion over the area of the nerve entrapment (Tinel's sign). A positive test is the reproduction of a tingling sensation in the distribution of the posterior tibial nerve (see *Special Tests*).

- *Talus.* The talus can be located by moving from the distal aspect of the medial malleolus along a line joining the navicular tuberosity. Its location can be made easier by everting and inverting the foot. Eversion causes the talar head to become more prominent while inversion causes the head to be less visible.

- *Sustentaculum tali.* Distal and inferior to the medial malleolus, a shelf-like bony prominence of the calcaneus (the sustentaculum tali) can be palpated. At the dorsal aspect of the sustentaculum tali, the talocalcaneal joint line can be palpated.

- *Posterior tibialis tendon.* This tendon is palpable at the level of the medial malleolus especially with the foot held in plantarflexion and supination. Distal and medial to this tendon, the crossing of the flexor digitorum longus and flexor hallucis tendons can be felt. Palpation of the posterior tibialis tendon along its course will often identify specific areas of pain in the region of synovitis or partial tendon rupture.[12]

- *Posterior tibial artery.* The posterior tibial artery can be located posterior to the medial malleolus, and anterior to the Achilles tendon.

- *Medial (deltoid) ligaments.* The medial (deltoid) ligaments are divided into superficial and deep ligaments. The palpable, although difficult to differentiate superficial ligaments include the tibionavicular, calcaneotibial, and the superficial posterior talotibial ligament. These ligaments are usually palpated as a group on the medial aspect of the ankle. It is worth remembering that isolated injury to these ligaments is rare. It is difficult to diagnose these injuries by physical examination alone—often stress radiographs in external rotation[20] and valgus talar tilt[21] are needed to confirm suspicion.[12]

Anterior and Anterior-Lateral Aspect of the Foot and Ankle

- *Tibial crest.* The tibial crest is palpated for tenderness, which may indicate the presence of shin splints. Swelling in this area may indicate the presence of anterior compartment syndrome. The muscles of the lateral compartment (fibularis (peronei)) and anterior compartment (tibialis anterior and the long extensors) are palpated here for swelling or tenderness. Swelling or tenderness of these structures usually indicates inflammation.

- *Lateral malleolus.* The lateral malleolus is located at the distal aspect of the fibula. Distal to the lateral malleolus is the calcaneus.
- *Fibularis (peroneus) longus.* The tendon of the fibularis (peroneus) longus runs superficially behind the lateral malleolus. Resisted pronation and plantarflexion of the foot makes the tendon more prominent. Tenderness along the lateral calcaneal wall to the cuboid may indicate tendinitis of the fibularis (peroneus) longus.[12] Pain with resisted plantarflexion and pronation over the tendon will help implicate the fibularis (peroneus) longus tendon.[13]
- *Fibularis (peroneus) brevis.* The origin for the fibularis (peroneus) brevis is more distal to the fibularis (peroneus) longus and lies deeper. It becomes superficial on the lateral aspect of the foot at its insertion at the tuberosity of the fifth metatarsal. Tenderness over the posterior and distal aspect of the lateral malleolus may indicate tendinitis of the fibularis (peroneus) brevis.[12] Pain with resisted plantarflexion and abduction over the tendon will help implicate the fibularis (peroneus) brevis tendon.[13]
- *Anterior talofibular ligament.* The anterior talofibular ligament (ATFL) can be palpated two to three fingerbreadths anterior-inferior to the lateral malleolus.[2] This is usually the area of most extreme tenderness following an inversion sprain. The anterior aspect of the distal tibiofibular syndesmosis may also be tender following this type of sprain.
- *Calcaneofibular ligament.* The calcaneofibular ligament (CFL) can be palpated one to two fingerbreadths inferior to the lateral malleolus.[2]
- *Posterior talofibular ligament.* The posterior talofibular ligament (PTFL) can be palpated posterior-inferior to the posterior edge of the lateral malleolus.[2]
- *Sinus tarsi.* The sinus tarsi is visible as a concave space between the lateral tendon of the extensor digitorum longus muscle and the anterior aspect of the lateral malleolus. The origin of the extensor digitorum brevis is at the level of this tunnel.
- *Cuboid.* The cuboid bone can be palpated by moving distally about one-finger width from the sinus tarsi.

Active and Passive Range of Motion

Range of motion testing is divided into active range of motion (AROM) (Figure 12-4), and passive range of motion (PROM) with overpressure to assess the end-feel. AROM tests are used to assess the patient's willingness to move and the presence of movement restriction patterns such as a capsular on noncapsular pattern. The end-feel may provide the clinician with information as to the cause of a motion restriction. The normal ranges of motion, end-feels, for the lower leg, ankle, and foot are outlined in Table 12-7. The open- and closed-pack positions and capsular patterns are outlined in Table 12-1. General AROM of the foot and ankle in the non-weight-bearing position is assessed first, with painful movements being performed last. Weight bearing tests are then performed. In addition to the foot and ankle tests, the clinician should also assess hip and knee range of motion.

If the symptoms are experienced in the hind foot during the general tests, then passive, active, and resisted inversion and eversion of the heel must be tested. If these and the weight-bearing tests are negative, there is probably no immediate need to proceed with a more detailed examination although this may have to be done if no other region can be inculpated. However, a more detailed articular

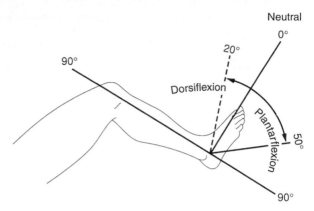

FIG. 12-4   Range of motion of the foot and ankle. (*Reproduced with permission from Luttgens K, Hamilton N: Kinesiology, 9th ed. p 623 (Fig. C-10). New York, McGraw-Hill 1997.*)

scanning examination is required if the symptoms increase or the range of motion decreases or both, or an abnormal end-feel is detected.

Distal Tibiofibular Joint   Specific motion at this joint cannot be produced voluntarily. However, the function of this joint can be assessed indirectly by asking the patient to twist around both feet in each direction while weight bearing, or with weight-bearing dorsiflexion.

Dorsiflexion   The patient is positioned in supine, with the knee slightly flexed and supported by a pillow, while the clinician stands at the foot at the table, facing the patient.

TABLE 12-7 Normal Ranges of Motion and End-Feels for the Lower Leg, Ankle, and Foot

Motion	Normal range (degrees)	End-feel
Plantar flexion	30–50°	Tissue stretch
Dorsiflexion	20°	Tissue stretch
Hind foot inversion (supination)	20°	Tissue stretch
Hind foot eversion (pronation)	10°	Tissue stretch
Toe flexion	Great toe: MTP, 45°; IP, 90° Lateral four toes: MTP, 40°; PIP, 35°; DIP, 60°	Tissue stretch
Toe extension	Great toe: MTP, 70°; IP, 0° Lateral four toes: MTP, 40°; PIP, 0°; DIP, 30°	Tissue stretch

Sources: Rasmussen O: Stability of the ankle joint. Acta Orthop Scand 1985;(Suppl)211:56–78.
Seto JL, Brewster CE: Treatment approaches following foot and ankle injury. Clin Sports Med 1985;13:295.

Active dorsiflexion is initially performed with the knee flexed. Care must be taken to prevent pronation at the subtalar and oblique mid-tarsal joint during dorsiflexion. This can be achieved by slightly inverting the foot to lock the longitudinal arch.[19] Passive overpressure is applied. With the knee flexed to 90°, the length of the soleus muscle is examined. Passive overpressure into dorsiflexion when the knee is flexed, assesses the joint motion, as well as the soleus length. The soleus is implicated if pain is produced in this test, especially if resisted plantar flexion is painful or more painful with the knee flexed than with the knee extended.

To assess the length of the gastrocnemius, the patient is positioned in supine with the knee extended, and the ankle is positioned in subtalar neutral. The patient is then asked to dorsiflex the ankle. Passive overpressure into dorsiflexion is applied. The normal range is approximately 20°.[22] If the gastrocnemius is shortened, dorsiflexion of the ankle will be reduced as the knee is extended and increased as the knee is flexed. A muscular end-feel should be felt with the knee extended, and a capsular end-feel should be felt with the knee flexed.

Plantarflexion   The patient is positioned in supine, with the leg supported by a pillow, while the clinician stands at the foot at the table, facing the patient. The patient is asked to plantar flex the ankle. Plantar flexion of the ankle is approximately 30°–50°.[23] When tested in weight bearing with the unilateral heel raise, heel inversion should be seen to occur. Failure of the foot to invert may indicate instability of the foot or ankle, or posterior tibialis dysfunction, or adaptive shortening.[24]

Hindfoot Inversion (Supination) and Hindfoot Eversion (Pronation)
Subtalar joint motion is extremely important to normal foot function. A loss of eversion (pronation) causes weight bearing to occur along the lateral side of the ankle joint. The patient is positioned in prone. Both hindfoot inversion and hindfoot eversion are tested by lining up the longitudinal axis of the leg and vertical axis of the calcaneus. Two-thirds to one-third inversion to eversion should exist, but the calcaneus should move at least to vertical passively and functionally. Passive motion of hindfoot inversion (supination) is normally 20°.[23] The amount of hindfoot eversion (pronation) is normally 10°.[23]

Great Toe Motion   The patient is positioned in supine, with the leg supported by a pillow, while the clinician stands at the foot at the table, facing the patient. Active extension of the great toe is performed and assisted passively without dorsiflexing the first ray. Extension of the great toe occurs primarily at the MTP joint. Passive extension of the great toe at the MTP joint should demonstrate elevation of the medial longitudinal arch (windlass effect), and external rotation of the tibia.[25] MTP joint extension of between 55° and 90° is necessary at terminal stance,[26–28] depending on length of stride, shoe flexibility, and toe-in/toe-out foot placement angle.[29] Forty-five degrees of first MTP flexion, and 90° of interphalangeal (IP) joint flexion are considered normal.[19]

Strength Testing

Isometric tests are carried out in the extreme range of the joint, and if positive, in the neutral range. The straight plane motions of ankle dorsiflexion, plantar flexion, inversion, and eversion are tested initially. Pain with any of these tests requires a more thorough examination of the individual muscles. The individual isometric muscle tests can give the clinician information about patterns of weakness other than from spinal nerve root or peripheral nerve palsies and can also help to isolate the pain generators. Weakness on isometric testing needs to be analyzed for the type (increasing weakness with repeated contractions of the same resistance indicating a palsy versus consistent weakness with repeated contractions, which could suggest a deconditioned muscle or a significant muscle tear) and the pattern of weakness (spinal nerve root, nerve trunk, or peripheral nerve). A painful weakness is invariably a sign of serious pathology, and depending on the pattern, could indicate a fracture or a tumor. However, if a single motion is painfully weak, this could indicate muscle inhibition caused by pain.

Ankle

- *Gastrocnemius and plantaris muscles.* If no weakness is apparent, a test is performed in the functional position, standing with the knee extended and the opposite foot off the floor. Technically, one heel raise through full range of motion while standing with support on one leg scores a ³⁄₅ (fair) with manual muscle testing with five single-limb heel raises scoring a ⁴⁄₅ (good) and 10 single-limb heel raises scoring a ⁵⁄₅ (normal). From a functional viewpoint, a wider range of scoring can sometimes prove more useful (Table 12-8).
- *Soleus muscle.* The soleus muscle produces plantar flexion of the ankle joint regardless of the position of the knee. To determine the individual functioning of the soleus as a plantar flexor, the knee is flexed to minimize the effect of the gastrocnemius muscle. To test the soleus, the patient stands with some degree of knee flexion, and then rises up on toes. Ten to fifteen raises performed in this fashion are considered normal, five to nine raises are graded as fair, one to four raises are graded as poor, and zero repetitions is graded as nonfunctional (see Table 12-8).
- *Tibialis anterior muscle.* The tibialis anterior muscle produces the motion of dorsiflexion and inversion. The knee must remain flexed during the test to allow complete dorsiflexion. The patient's foot is positioned in dorsiflexion and inversion. The leg is stabilized, and resistance is applied to the medial dorsal aspect of the forefoot into plantar flexion and eversion.
- *Tibialis posterior muscle.* The tibialis posterior muscle produces the motion of inversion in a plantar-flexed position. The leg is stabilized in the anatomic position, with the ankle in slight plantar flexion. Resistance is applied to the medial border of the forefoot into eversion and dorsiflexion.
- *Fibularis (peroneus) longus, fibularis (peroneus) brevis, and fibularis (peroneus) tertius muscles.* The lateral compartment muscles and the fibularis (peroneus) tertius muscle produce the motion of eversion. The patient is positioned in supine with the foot over the edge of the table and the ankle in the anatomic position. Resistance is applied to the lateral border of the forefoot. Pain elicited on the lateral aspect of the midfoot with resisted eversion of the foot and plantarflexion of the first ray could indicate a complete rupture of the fibularis (peroneus) longus tendon.[13]
- *Digits.* Grades for the toes differ from the standard format because gravity is not considered a factor.

O:	No contraction.
Trace or 1:	Muscle contraction is palpated, but no movement occurs.
Poor or 2:	Subject can partially complete the range of motion.
Fair or 3:	Subject can complete the test range.
Good or 4:	Subject can complete the test range, but is able to take less resistance on the test side than on the opposite side.
Normal or 5:	Subject can complete the test range and take maximal resistance on the test side as compared with the normal side.

TABLE 12-8 Functional Testing of the Foot and Ankle

Starting position	Action	Functional test	
Standing on one leg	Lift toes and forefeet off ground (dorsiflexion)	10 to 15 repetitions:	Functional
		5 to 9 repetitions:	Functionally fair
		1 to 4 repetitions:	Functionally poor
		0 repetitions:	Nonfunctional
Standing on one leg	Lift heels off ground (plantar flexion)	10 to 15 repetitions:	Functional
		5 to 9 repetitions:	Functionally fair
		1 to 4 repetitions:	Functionally poor
		0 repetitions:	Nonfunctional
Standing on one leg	Lift lateral aspect of foot off ground (ankle eversion)	5 to 6 repetitions:	Functional
		3 to 4 repetitions:	Functionally fair
		1 to 2 repetitions:	Functionally poor
		0 repetitions:	Nonfunctional
Standing on one leg	Lift medial aspect of foot off ground (ankle inversion)	5 to 6 repetitions:	Functional
		3 to 4 repetitions:	Functionally fair
		1 to 2 repetitions:	Functionally poor
		0 repetitions:	Nonfunctional
Seated	Pull small towel up under toes or pick up and release small object (i.e., pencil, marble, cotton ball) (toe flexion)	10 to 15 repetitions:	Functional
		5 to 9 repetitions:	Functionally fair
		1 to 4 repetitions:	Functionally poor
		0 repetitions:	Nonfunctional
Seated	Lift toes off ground (toe extension)	10 to 15 repetitions:	Functional
		5 to 9 repetitions:	Functionally fair
		1 to 4 repetitions:	Functionally poor
		0 repetitions:	Nonfunctional

Source: Palmer ML, Epler M: Clinical Assessment Procedures in Physical Therapy, pp 68–73. Philadelphia, PA, JB Lippincott, 1990.

- *Flexor hallucis brevis and longus muscles.* The flexor hallucis brevis and flexor hallucis longus muscles produce MTP joint flexion and IP joint flexion. The foot is maintained in midposition. The first metatarsal is stabilized, and resistance is applied beneath the proximal and distal phalanx of the great toe into toe extension.
- *Flexor digitorum brevis and longus muscles.* The flexor digitorum longus and brevis muscles produce IP joint flexion. The motion is tested with the foot in the anatomic position. If the gastrocnemius muscle is shortened preventing the ankle from assuming the anatomic position, the knee is flexed. The toes may be tested simultaneously. The foot is held in the midposition and the metatarsals are stabilized. Resistance is applied beneath the distal and proximal phalanges.

- *Extensor hallucis longus and brevis muscles.* The extensor hallucis longus and the extensor hallucis brevis muscles produce the motion of extension of the IP and MTP joints. The foot is maintained in midposition. Resistance is applied to the dorsum of both phalanges of the first digit into toe flexion.
- *Extensor digitorum longus and brevis muscles.* The extensor digitorum longus and the extensor digitorum brevis muscles produce the motion of extension at the MTP and IP joints of the lateral four digits from a flexed position. Resistance is applied to the dorsal surface of the proximal and distal phalanges into toe flexion.

Intrinsic Muscles of the Foot The intrinsic muscles of the foot are tested with the patient in either the supine or sitting position. Most subjects are unable to voluntarily contract the intrinsic muscles of the foot individually.

- *Abductor hallucis muscle.* The metatarsals are stabilized and resistance is applied medially to the distal end of the first phalanx.
- *Adductor hallucis muscle.* The metatarsals are stabilized and resistance is applied to the lateral side of the proximal phalanx of the first digit.
- *Lumbrical muscles.* The lateral four metatarsals are stabilized and resistance is applied to the middle and distal phalanges of the lateral four digits.
- *Plantar interossei muscles.* The lateral three metatarsals are stabilized and resistance is applied to the middle and distal phalanges.
- *Dorsal interossei and abductor digiti minimi muscles.* The metatarsals are stabilized and resistance is applied:
  - Dorsal interossei: Applied to the middle and distal phalanges
  - Abductor digiti minimi: Applied to the lateral side of the proximal phalanx of the fifth digit

Functional Examination

(see Table 12-8)

Passive Articular Mobility

Passive articular mobility tests assess the accessory motions available between the joint surfaces. These include tests of the accessory glides of the joint, and tests involving joint compression and joint distraction. As with any other joint complex, the quality and quantity of joint motion must be compared with the results from the uninvolved side to determine the level of joint involvement, so that comparisons can be made. For these tests, the patient is positioned in supine or side lying.

Long-Axis Distraction The clinician stabilizes the proximal segment and applies traction to the distal segment. This test is performed at the talocrural joint (Figure 12-5), the subtalar joint (Figure 12-6), the MTP joints, and the IP joints.

Anterior-Posterior Glide To test the anterior movement, the clinician stabilizes the tibia and fibula and draws the talus and foot forward (Figure 12-7). Pushing the talus and foot together in a posterior direction on the tibia and fibula (Figure 12-8) tests the posterior movement.

The anterior-posterior glides can also be applied to the midtarsal, tarsometatarsal, MTP, and IP joints.

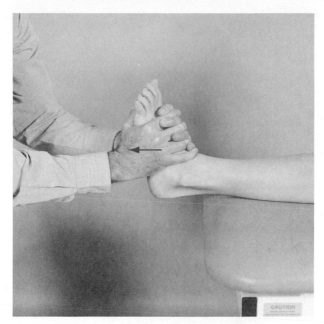

FIG. 12-5 Long axis distraction of the talocrural joint. (*Reproduced with permission from Dutton M: Orthopaedic Examination, Evaluation, and Intervention, p 871 (Fig. 19-30). New York, McGraw-Hill 2004.*)

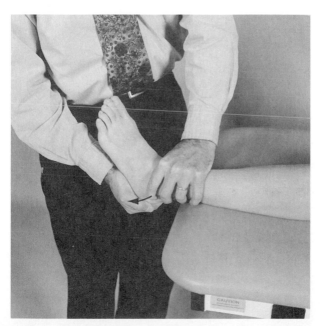

FIG. 12-6 Long axis distraction of the subtalar joint. (*Reproduced with permission from Dutton M: Orthopaedic Examination, Evaluation, and Intervention, p 871 (Fig. 19-31). New York, McGraw-Hill 2004.*)

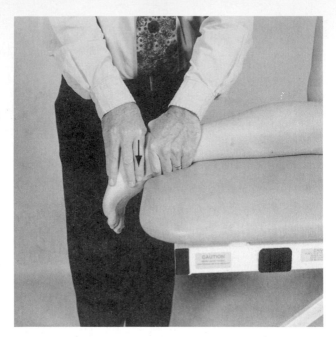

FIG. 12-7 Anterior glide of the talus. (*Reproduced with permission from Dutton M: Orthopaedic Examination, Evaluation, and Intervention, p 871 (Fig. 19-32). New York, McGraw-Hill 2004.*)

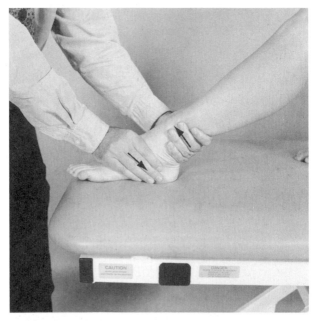

FIG. 12-8 Posterior glide of the talus. (*Reproduced with permission from Dutton M: Orthopaedic Examination, Evaluation, and Intervention, p 871 (Fig. 19-33). New York, McGraw-Hill 2004.*)

Tibial Excursion   Tibial excursion in an anterior and posterior direction occurs during dorsiflexion and plantar flexion respectively. This motion may be assessed in the non-weight-bearing position. The calcaneus and talus are fixed, and the tibia and fibula are glided in an anterior and posterior direction (Figure 12-9).[30]

Abduction-Adduction (Subtalar)   The patient is positioned in supine, with the knee slightly flexed and supported by a pillow. The clinician faces the patient. The clinician grasps the forefoot and places it into adduction and abduction. The amount and quality of the motions, as compared with the other foot, are compared. The range of adduction is generally twice that of abduction, approximately 30° and 15° respectively.[3]

Calcaneal Inversion–Eversion   The patient is positioned in supine, with the knee slightly flexed and supported by a pillow, while the clinician faces the patient. The clinician grasps the calcaneus in one hand, while the other hand is placed on the forefoot, to lock the talus. The calcaneus is passively inverted (varus) and everted (valgus) on the talus. The amount and quality of the motions, as compared with the other foot, are compared. Although some differences exist, generally, calcaneal eversion will measure 5°–10°, while calcaneal inversion will measure 20°–30°.[19,23,31]

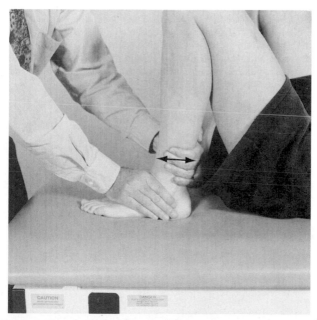

FIG. 12-9   Tibial excursion. (*Reproduced with permission from Dutton M: Orthopaedic Examination, Evaluation, and Intervention, p 872 (Fig. 19-34). New York, McGraw-Hill 2004.*)

Transverse Tarsal Joints (Talonavicular and Calcaneocuboid) The patient is positioned in supine with the knee flexed approximately 60° and the heel resting on the table. Using one hand, the clinician grasps and fixes the talus and calcaneus at the level of the talar neck. The other hand grasps the navicular using the navicular tubercle as a landmark (Figure 12-10) and then glides the cuboid dorsally or plantarly on the calcaneus.

Midtarsal Joint Motion The rotational movements of the midtarsal joint, which allow the forefoot to twist on the rearfoot, can be observed in the non-weight-bearing position. The clinician stabilizes the calcaneus with one hand, while inverting and everting the foot with the other hand.[30]

Cuboid Motion The patient is positioned in prone and the patient's knee is flexed. Using one hand, the clinician grasps calcaneus, locking it, while with the thumb and index of the other hand, the clinician grasps the cuboid and moves it dorsally and ventrally. The clinician notes the quality and quantity of motion.

Navicular Motion The patient is positioned in supine with the knee flexed approximately 60° and the heel resting on the table. Using one hand, the clinician grasps and fixes the navicular. With the other hand, the clinician grasps the cuneiforms and moves them dorsally and ventrally (Figure 12-11). The quality and quantity of motion is noted and compared with the other side.

Cuneiform Motion The patient is positioned in supine with the knee flexed approximately 60° and the heel resting on the table. The clinician grasps and locks the cuneiforms, and then moves the metatarsal joints on the navicular.

First MTP Joint (First Ray) Motion The patient is positioned in supine, with the clinician seated at the foot of the table facing away from the patient. The foot to be examined is positioned on a pillow in the clinician's lap. The clinician grasps and locks the first MTP joint, before grasping the great toe first metatarsal joint and moving it into extension and flexion (dorsally and ventrally respectively) (Figure 12-12).

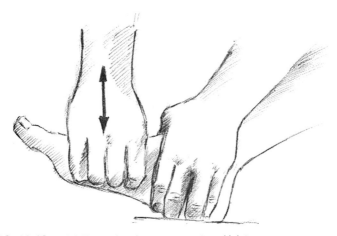

FIG. 12-10   Mobility testing the transverse tarsal joints.

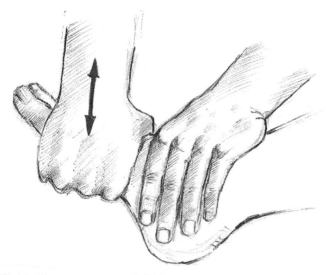

FIG. 12-11   Mobility testing the naviculocuneiform joints.

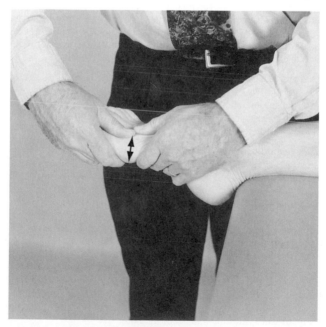

FIG. 12-12   Testing the first MTP joint motion. (*Reproduced with permission from Dutton M: Orthopaedic Examination, Evaluation, and Intervention, p 874 (Fig. 19-40). New York, McGraw-Hill 2004.*)

Limited range may result from a combination of biomechanical factors such as excessive pronation or joint glide restriction.[32] To examine the conjunct rotation of the metatarsals, the clinician locks the second metatarsal to evaluate the first, and locks the third to evaluate the second. The quantity and quality of motion is noted and compared to the other side.

Fifth Metatarsal Motion The patient is positioned in prone. Using one hand, the clinician grasps the cuboid and stabilizes it. With the other hand, the clinician grasps the fifth metatarsal and moves it dorsally and ventrally. To examine rotary motion of the metatarsal, the clinician locks the fourth metatarsal and examines motion of the fifth. To examine motion of the fourth metatarsal, the third metatarsal is locked. The quality and quantity of motion is noted and compared with the other side.

Phalangeal Motion The patient is positioned in supine, with the clinician seated at the foot of the table facing away from the patient. The foot to be examined is positioned on a pillow in the clinician's lap. The clinician grasps the metatarsal and locks it with one hand. With the other hand the first phalanx articulating with that metatarsal is grasped. After applying slight traction, the clinician examines the dorsal, ventral, abduction, adduction, and rotary motions. The quantity and quality of motion is noted and compared to the other side.

Special Tests

Special tests are merely confirmatory tests and should not be used alone to form a diagnosis. Selection for their use is at the discretion of the clinician and is based on a complete patient history. The results from these tests are used in conjunction with the other clinical findings and should not be used alone to form a diagnosis. To assure accuracy with these tests, both sides should be tested for comparison.

Ligamentous Stress Tests The examination of the ligamentous structures in the ankle and foot is essential, not only because of their vast array, but also because of the amount of stability that they provide. Positive results for the ligamentous stability tests include excessive movement as compared with the same test on the uninvolved extremity, pain, depending on the severity, or apprehension.

- *Mortise/syndesmosis.* Although other tests are mentioned, only the squeeze test (see next) has been found to have moderately "good" validity and "good" reliability respectively.[33] The Kleiger (external rotation) test (see later), although used primarily to determine the presence of a sprain of the medial (deltoid) ligaments, is also a reliable test for detecting the presence of syndesmotic sprains.[33]
- *Squeeze (distal tibiofibular compression) test.* In a study using fresh human cadavers, the squeeze test produced motion at the distal tibiofibular joint, causing the tibia and fibula to separate.[34] To perform the squeeze test, the clinician squeezes the tibia and fibula together at a point about 6–8 inches below the knee in the midshaft of the lower leg.[35] Pain felt in the anterolateral aspect of the distal third of the leg may indicate a compromised syndesmosis, if the presence of a tibia or fibula fracture or both, calf contusion, or compartment syndrome has been ruled out.[8,36]
- *Clunk (cotton) test.* The patient is positioned in supine with his or her foot over the end of the bed. One hand is used to stabilize the distal leg, while the clinician uses the other hand to grasp the heel and move the calcaneus

medially and laterally.[37] A clunk can be felt as the talus hits the tibia and fibula if there has been significant mortise widening.[2]

Alternatively, the patient can be positioned in supine with his or her knee flexed to the point where the ankle is in the position of full dorsiflexion. The clinician applies over pressure into further dorsiflexion by grasping the femoral condyles with one hand and leaning down into the table. The clinician uses the other hand to pull the tibia (crura) anteriorly. Because the ankle is in its close packed position, no movement should be felt.

- *Posterior drawer test.* The posterior drawer test can also be used to test for the presence of instability at the inferior tibiofibular joint. The patient is supine. The hip and knee are fully flexed to provide as much dorsiflexion of the ankle as possible. This drives the wide anterior part of the talus back into the mortise. An anterior stabilizing force is then applied to the cruris, and the foot and talus are translated posteriorly. If the inferior tibiofibular joint is stable, there will be no drawer available, but if there is instability, there will be a drawer.

- *Lateral collaterals.* The lateral collaterals resist inversion and consist of the anterior talofibular, calcaneofibular, and posterior talofibular. An additional function of the lateral ligaments of the ankle is to prevent excessive varus movement, especially during plantar flexion. In extreme plantar flexion, the mortise no longer stabilizes the broader anterior part of the talus, and varus movement of the ankle is then possible. The degree of displacement with these tests can be graded from 1+ to 3+ in excessive movement as compared to the uninvolved ankle.

- *The anterior drawer test.* The anterior drawer stress test is performed to estimate the stability of the ATFL.[38–41] The test is performed with the patient sitting at the end of the bed or lying supine with his or her knee flexed to relax the gastrocnemius-soleus muscles and the foot supported perpendicular to the leg.[41,42] The clinician uses one hand to stabilize the distal aspect of the leg, while the other hand grasps the patient's heel and positions the ankle in 10° to 15° of plantar flexion. The heel is very gently pulled forward, and, if the test is positive, the talus, and with it the foot, rotates anteriorly out of the ankle mortise, around the intact medial (deltoid) ligament, which serves as the center of rotation. Comparisons are made to the contralateral ankle to avoid any false positives. Opinions vary as to how much difference in displacement is normal, with standards ranging from greater than 2 millimeter[43] to greater than 4 millimeters.[1,38,44,45] This test has limited reliability, particularly if it is negative, or if it is performed without anesthesia in the presence of muscle guarding.[46]

The Dimple Sign

If pain and spasm are minimal, the presence of "a dimple" located just in front of the tip of the lateral malleolus, during the anterior drawer test is a positive indication for a rupture of the ATFL.[47] This results from a negative pressure created by the forward movement of the talus, which draws the skin inward at the side of ligament rupture.[48] This dimple sign is also seen with a combined rupture of the ATFL and CFLs.[47] However, sign is only present within the first 48 hours of injury, and cannot be elicited in ankles examined at 7 days or more after injury, because of organized hematoma and repair tissue blocking the communication between the joint and the subcutaneous tissues.[47]

Gungor Test[49]   The Gungor test can be used to evaluate the anterior displacement of the talus from the ankle mortise. This test is preferable to the anterior drawer test if the ankle is swollen and the patient is guarding.[12] The patient is positioned in prone with the ankle hanging past the end of the examination table and the toes facing downward. The heel is then pressed downward to force the talus anteriorly within the ankle mortise. A positive sign is noted when the skin becomes taut and the Achilles tendon becomes increasingly defined.[49]

Talar Tilt   The talar tilt test is considered the best test to assess the integrity of the CFL.[12] With an inverted ankle, strain on the CFL is highest in dorsiflexion; thus, when the ankle is dorsiflexed or in a neutral position, the CFL is the lateral ligament most often injured in inversion sprains.[50] Although isolated CFL tears are uncommon, CFL tears in combination with ATFL tears are the second most common injury pattern (20% of injuries).[50,51] Midsubstance rupture of the CFL remains the most common injury pattern, although a number of fibula or calcaneus avulsion-type injury patterns exist.[51] To perform this test, the clinician medially supports the tibia with one hand, and forcibly inverts the lateral aspect of the heel with the other hand. If comparison of the medial and lateral aspects of the ankle while the foot is everted and inverted demonstrates a difference of greater than 25% between the medial and lateral openings, a positive talar tilt test is noted.[1] Other findings may include a soft end-feel, or lateral dimpling.[52]

Anterior Talofibular Ligament Test   The patient is positioned in supine. The cruris is gripped with the stabilizing hand, using a lumbrical grip, while the other hand grasps over the mortise and onto the neck of talus, so that the index fingers are together at the point between fibular and talus. The clinician moves the patient's foot into plantarflexion and full inversion, and a force is applied in an attempt to adduct (distract) the calcaneus, thereby gapping the lateral side of the ankle. Pain on the lateral aspect of the ankle with this test or displacement depending on severity, or both may indicate a sprain of the ligament.

Calcaneofibular Ligament   The inversion stress maneuver is a test that attempts to assess CFL integrity.[39] The patient is positioned supine. The cruris is gripped with the stabilizing hand, while the moving hand cups the heel. The ankle is dorsiflexed via the calcaneus to a right angle (total dorsiflexion is impractical) and inverted. An adduction, and anterior-medial translation of the calcaneus is then applied tending to gap the lateral side of the joint. Pain on the lateral aspect of the ankle with this test or displacement depending on severity, or both may indicate a sprain of the ligament.

Posterior Talofibular   The patient is either prone or supine, and the cruris is gripped or the fibular stabilized. The patient's leg is stabilized in internal rotation, and the foot is placed in full dorsiflexion. The clinician externally rotates the heel or calcaneus, thereby moving the talar attachment of the ligament away from the malleolus. Pain on the lateral aspect of the ankle with this test or displacement depending on severity, or both may indicate a sprain of the ligament.

- *Medial (deltoid) ligament complex.* The medial (deltoid) ligaments function to resist eversion. Given their strength, these ligaments are only usually injured as the result of major trauma.

Kleiger (External Rotation) Test   The Kleiger (external rotation) test[35,53,54] is a general test to assess the integrity of the medial (deltoid) ligament complex, but can also implicate the syndesmosis if pain is produced over the anterior or posterior tibiofibular ligaments and the interosseous membrane.[33,36,55] If this test is positive, further testing is necessary to determine the source of the symptoms. Information about the mechanism of injury can afford the clinician some clues. Trauma involving external rotation tends to disrupt the deep medial (deltoid) ligaments before disruption of the superficial medial (deltoid) ligaments.[12] In contrast, trauma involving abduction disrupts the superficial medial (deltoid) ligaments, while the deep ligaments remain intact.[56]

The patient sits with his or her legs dangling over the end of the bed, with the knee flexed to 90°, and foot relaxed. The clinician stabilizes the lower leg with one hand and, using the other hand, grasps the foot and rotates it laterally (Figure 12-13). Pain on the medial and lateral aspect of the ankle or displacement of the talus from the medial malleolus or both, depending on severity, with this test may indicate a tear of the medial (deltoid) ligament.

Patla's Test for Tibialis Posterior Length[24]   The patient is positioned in prone, with the knee flexed to 90°. The clinician stabilizes the calcaneus in eversion and the ankle in dorsiflexion with one hand. With the other hand, the clinician contacts the plantar surface of the bases of the second, third, and fourth metatarsals with the thumb, while the index and middle fingers contact

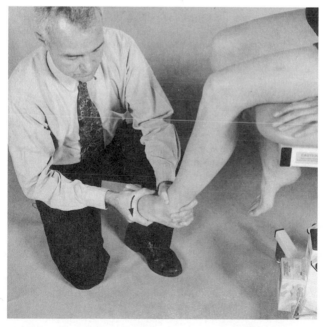

FIG. 12-13   Kleiger test. (*Reproduced with permission from Dutton M: Orthopaedic Examination, Evaluation, and Intervention, p 876 (Fig. 19-44). New York, McGraw-Hill 2004.*)

the plantar surface of the navicular. The clinician then pushes the navicular and metatarsal heads dorsally and compares the end-feel and patient response with the uninvolved side. A positive test is indicated with reproduction of the patient's symptoms.

Feiss Line[57]   The Feiss line test is used to assess the height of the medial arch, using the navicular position. With the patient nonweight bearing, the clinician marks the apex of the medial malleolus and the plantar aspect of the first MTP joint, and a line is drawn between the two points. The navicular is palpated on the medial aspect of the foot, and an assessment is made as to the position of the navicular relative to the imaginary line. The patient is then asked to stand with his or her feet about 3–6 inches apart. In weight bearing the navicular normally lies on, or very close to, the line. If the navicular falls one third of the distance to the floor, it represents a first-degree flatfoot; if it falls two-thirds of the distance, it represents a second-degree flatfoot, and if it rests on the floor, it represents a third-degree flatfoot.

Tendon Tests

- *Fibularis (peroneal) longus tendon subluxation.*[58] To test for fibularis (peroneal) longus tendon subluxation, the patient is positioned in prone with the knee of the involved leg flexed to approximately 90°. After inspection of the posterior lateral fibula for any obvious dislocation, the ankle is actively dorsiflexed and everted against resistance. This test dramatically recreates the fibularis longus tendon dislocation if positive.[12]
- *Thompson test for acute Achilles tendon rupture.* In this test, the patient is positioned in prone, or in kneeling with the feet over the edge of the bed. With the patient relaxed, the clinician gently squeezes the calf muscle (Figure 12-14) and observes for the production of plantarflexion. An absence of plantarflexion indicates a complete rupture of the Achilles tendon.[59] Although this test may be good for detecting acute Achilles tendon ruptures, it does not accurately detect chronic ruptures.[12,60]
- *Matles test for chronic Achilles tendon rupture.* The Matles test is the preferred test for detecting a chronic rupture of the Achilles tendon.[60] The patient is positioned in prone. The patient is asked to bend the knee to approximately 90°. As the patient flexes the knee, the clinician observes the position of the foot and ankle. Normally the foot is slightly plantarflexed as the knee is flexed to 90°. However, if there is an Achilles tendon rupture, the involved foot will either be in a neutral or a dorsiflexed position.[12,60]
- *"Too many toes" sign for posterior tibialis tendon dysfunction.* This is more an observation than a test. The patient is asked to stand in a normal relaxed position while the clinician views the patient from behind. If the heel is in valgus, the forefoot abducted, or the tibia externally rotated more than normal, the clinician will observe more toes on the involved side than on the normal side.[61]
- *Anterior tibialis tendon rupture test.* Although not a specific test in the true sense, a combination of clinical findings can strongly suggest the presence of an anterior tibialis tendon rupture. These include:[12,62–64]
  - A palpable defect between the extensor retinaculum and the insertion site of the tendon
  - A retracted bulbous proximal stump of the tendon on the anteromedial aspect of the ankle

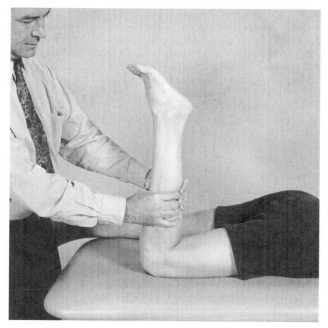

FIG. 12-14   Thompson test. (*Reproduced with permission from Dutton M: Orthopaedic Examination, Evaluation, and Intervention, p 876 (Fig. 19-45). New York, McGraw-Hill 2004.*)

- Inability to perform active dorsiflexion beyond ankle and subtalar joint neutral position
- Diminished ankle dorsiflexion by 10° to 15° from normal, especially with flexion of the hallux
- Some degree of foot-drop or a steppage-type gait, unless there is substitution of the extensor hallucis longus or other toe extensors
- Evidence of foot slap with gait
- Difficulty with heel walking

Articular Stability Tests

- *Navicular drop test.* The navicular drop test is a method by which to assess the degree to which the talus plantarflexes in space on a calcaneus that has been stabilized by the ground, during subtalar joint pronation.[65,66] The clinician palpates the position of the navicular tubercle as the patient's foot is nonweight bearing but resting on the floor surface with the subtalar joint maintained in neutral. The clinician then attempts to quantify inferior displacement of the navicular tubercle as the patient assumes 50% weight bearing on the tested foot.[29] A navicular drop, which is greater than 10 millimeter from the neutral position to the relaxed standing position, suggests excessive medial longitudinal arch collapse of abnormal pronation.[66,67]

- *Talar rock.* The talar rock[68] is an articular stability test for the subtalar joint. The test is performed with the patient positioned in side lying, his or her hip and knee flexed. The clinician sits on the table with his or her back to the patient, and places both hands around the ankle just distal to the malleoli. The clinician applies a slight distraction force to the ankle, before applying a rocking movement to the foot in an upward or downward direction. A "clunk" should be felt at the end of each of the movements.

- *Passive foot rotation.* This test assesses the integrity of the midtarsal and tarsometatarsal joints. A rotational movement is applied manually to the midtarsal and tarsometatarsal joints. At the midtarsal joint, the proximal row of the tarsal bones (navicular, calcaneus, and talus) is stabilized, and the distal row (cuneiforms and cuboid) is rotated in both directions. At the tarsometatarsal joints, the distal row of the tarsals is stabilized and the metatarsals are rotated in both directions.

Neurovascular Status

- *Homan's sign.* The patient is positioned in supine with his or her knee extended. The clinician stabilizes the thigh with one hand, and passively dorsiflexes the patient's ankle with the other. Pain in the calf with this maneuver may indicate a positive Homan's sign for deep vein thrombophlebitis, especially if there are associated signs including pallor and swelling in the leg and a loss of the dorsal pedis pulse.

- *Buerger's test.* The patient is positioned in supine with the knee extended. The clinician elevates the patient's leg to about 45° and maintains it there for at least 3 minutes. Blanching of the foot is positive for poor arterial circulation, especially if, when the patient sits with the legs over the end of the bed, it takes 1–2 minutes for the limb color to be restored.

- *Morton's test.*[69] The patient is positioned in supine. The clinician grasps the foot around the metatarsal heads and squeezes the heads together. The reproduction of pain with this maneuver indicates the presence of a neuroma, or a stress fracture.

- *Duchenne test.*[69] The patient is positioned in supine with his or her legs straight. The clinician pushes through the sole on the first metatarsal head, and pushes the foot into dorsiflexion. The patient is asked to plantarflex the foot. If the medial border dorsiflexes and offers no resistance while the lateral border plantarflexes, a lesion of the superficial fibular (peroneal) nerve, or a lesion of the L4, 5, and S1 nerve root is indicated.

- *Tinel's sign.* There are two locations around the ankle from where the Tinel's sign can be elicited. The anterior tibial branch of the deep fibular (peroneal) nerve can be tapped on the anterior aspect of the ankle. The posterior tibial nerve may be tapped behind the medial malleolus at the entrance to the tarsal tunnel. Tingling or paresthesia with these tests is considered a positive finding for peripheral nerve entrapment.

- *Dorsal pedis pulse.* The dorsal pedis pulse can be palpated just lateral to the tendon of the extensor hallucis longus over the dorsum of the foot.

Neurologic Tests

Symptoms are commonly referred to the leg, foot, and ankle from the lumbar spine, pelvis, hip, or knee. Important neurologic structures that pass through the ankle and terminate in the foot are the saphenous, superficial fibular (peroneal), deep fibular (peroneal), posterior and anterior tibial nerves, and the sural nerve. Symptoms can also be referred to the foot and ankle from the L4-S2 nerve roots (sciatic) but also from a host of other conditions. The applicable sensory, motor, and reflex testing should be performed if a disorder related to a spinal nerve root (L4-S2), or peripheral nerve is suspected. A neurogenic cause of foot pain must be considered in a patient, especially if the pain is refractory. The patient usually complains of pain that is poorly localized, which is aggravated by activity but may also occur at rest. Any difference in sensation between extremities should be noted and can be mapped out in more detail using a pinwheel. The segmental and peripheral nerve innervations are listed in Chapter 3. Common reflexes tested in this area are the Achilles reflex (S1-2), and the posterior tibial reflex (L4-5).

The pathologic reflexes (Babinski and Oppenheim) are tested if an upper motor neuron lesion is suspected.

Imaging Studies

Various imaging studies can be used to assist in the diagnosis on foot and ankle injuries.

Radiography Standard radiographs are usually the first imaging test to be performed (Table 12-9). These tests are performed if osseous pathology is suspected. Bone tenderness in the posterior half of the lower 6 centimeters of the fibula or tibia, and an inability to bear weight immediately after injury are indications to obtain radiographs to rule out fracture of the ankle.[70–72]

If there is bone tenderness over the navicular or fifth metatarsal or both, and an inability to bear weight immediately after injury then radiographs of the foot are indicated.[70,71]

Other roentgenographic techniques include arthrography, peroneal (fibularis) tenography, and magnetic resonance imaging (MRI). These tests are primarily used to highlight soft tissue injuries.

EXAMINATION CONCLUSIONS—THE EVALUATION

Following the examination, and once the clinical findings have been recorded, the clinician must determine a specific diagnosis or a working hypothesis, based on a summary of all the findings. This diagnosis can be structure related (medical diagnosis) (Table 12-10), or a diagnosis based on the preferred practice patterns as described in the *Guide to Physical Therapist Practice*.[73]

TABLE 12-9 Ottawa Ankle Rules for Foot and Ankle Radiographic Series in Patients with Acute Ankle Injury

An ankle radiographic series is required only if patient has pain in malleolar zone and any one of the following findings:	A foot radiographic series is required only if patient has pain in midfoot zone and any one of the following findings:
Bone tenderness at the posterior edge or tip of the lateral malleolus	Bone tenderness at the base of the fifth metatarsal
Bone tenderness at the posterior edge or tip of the medial malleolus	Bone tenderness at the navicular
Inability to bear weight both immediately and in emergency department	Inability to bear weight both immediately and in emergency department

Source: Stiell IG, et al.: Decision rules for the use of radiography in acute ankle injuries: Refinement and prospective validation. JAMA 1994;269:1127–1132.

TABLE 12-10 Differential Diagnosis of Common Causes of Leg, Foot, and Ankle Pain

Condition	Patient age	Mechanism of injury	Area of symptoms	Symptoms aggravated by	Observation	AROM	PROM	Resisted	Special tests	Tenderness with Palpation
Gastrocnemius strain	20–40	Sudden overload	Upper calf	Heel raise	Antalgic gait	Painful and limited DF	Pain with overpressure into DF Restricted range of DF with knee extended	Pain on PF		Mid to upper calf
Plantar fascitis	20–60	Gradual with no known cause	Sole of foot (under heel)	Weight bearing especially first thing in the morning	Unremarkable Flattened arches Pronated foot	Full and pain free	Pain with overpressure into great toe extension	Weak foot intrinsics	Pressure applied over plantar fascial insertion site on the calcaneus	Plantar aspect of heel
Achilles tendinitis	20–40	Overuse	Posterior ankle	Jumping, running	Minor swelling of posterior ankle	Painful and limited DF	Pain with overpressure into DF Restricted range of DF with knee extended	Pain on PF		Posterior ankle
Posterior tibialis tendinitis	20–40	Overuse with a flat pronated foot	Medial ankle, along the course of the tendon	Activities involving weight bearing plantar flexion	Possible peritendinous swelling over medial ankle	Pain on eversion Pain on PF	Pain with overpressure into eversion Pain with overpressure into PF	Pain on resisted inversion with the foot plantarflexed	Rule out tear with heel raise symmetry	Medial ankle
Morton's neuroma	40–60	Gradual with no known cause	Sole of foot	Weight bearing	Pronated foot Flattened arches	Full and pain free	Pain with overpressure into toe extension	Strong and painless		Web spaces of toes

									Palpation	
Retrocalcaneal bursitis	Varies	Direct irritation of bursa, usually from shoe			Possible swelling, erythema of hindfoot	Usually unremarkable	Usually unremarkable	Usually unremarkable		Just above the insertion site of the Achilles tendon on the calcaneus
Anterior tibialis tendinitis	15–45	Overuse	Anterior lower leg	Activities involving repetitive dorsiflexion	Unremarkable	Pain combined PF and inversion	Pain with over-pressure into PF	Pain on DF		Antero-lateral lower leg
Tarsal tunnel syndrome	25–50	Posttraumatic, neoplastic, inflammatory, rapid weight gain, fluid retention, abnormal foot/ankle mechanics, or a valgus foot deformity	Medial malleolus, distribution of posterior tibial nerve up the leg, or down into the medial arch, plantar surface of the foot and toes	Excessive dynamic pronation in walking or running	Pronated foot, pes planus, possible swelling	Full and pain free	Pain with extreme plantar flexion and eversion	Weak toe flexion (late)	Positive Tinel's over tarsal tunnel	No tenderness usually

(Continued)

403

TABLE 12-10 Differential Diagnosis of Common Causes of Leg, Foot, and Ankle Pain (*Continued*)

Condition	Patient age	Mechanism of injury	Area of symptoms	Symptoms aggravated by	Observation	AROM	PROM	Resisted	Special tests	Tenderness with Palpation
Midfoot sprain	15–40	High impact landing sports Foot twisted when in fixed position	Midfoot	Walking on toes	Usually unremarkable	Usually unremarkable	Usually unremarkable	Usually unremarkable	Weight-bearing lateral and anterior-posterior radiographs	Generalized tenderness of midfoot
Medial tibial stress syndrome	15–30	Overuse	Anterior lower leg Posterior-medial lower leg	Exercise involving involved lower extremity		Pain combined PF and inversion	Full and pain free	Pain on PF Pain on eversion		Posteromedial calf
Metatarsal stress fracture	15–45	Overuse	Forefoot	Weight-bearing activities	Possible edema over fracture site	Usually unremarkable	Usually unremarkable	Usually unremarkable	Palpation, ultrasound, tuning fork, bone scan, MRI, CT scan	Maximal point tenderness over the bone at the fracture site

Referred	Varies	Symptoms can be referred from the lumbar spine, hip, knee, or from systemic diseases such as diabetes mellitus (DM), spondyloarthropathy (Reiter's syndrome)	May be dermatomal if spinal nerve involved; stocking-like if DM, bilateral heels if Reiter's	Activities unrelated to foot and ankle; unrelated to activity	Varies, but may be unremarkable	Usually unremarkable	Usually unremarkable	Usually unremarkable, but weakness may be present if spinal nerve root involved	Sensation, DTR, lab tests	Tenderness of joint if spondyloarthropathy

DF = dorsiflexion; DTR = deep tendon reflex; PF = planter flexion.

REFERENCES

1. Childs S: Acute ankle injury. Lippincotts Prim Care Pract 1999;3:428–440.
2. Adamson C, Cymet T: Ankle sprains: evaluation, treatment, rehabilitation. Maryland Med J 1997;46:530–537.
3. Bordelon RL: Clinical assessment of the foot. In Donatelli RA (ed): Biomechanics of the Foot and Ankle, pp 85–98. Philadelphia, PA, WB Saunders, 1990.
4. Brostrom L: Sprained ankles: III. Clinical observations in recent ligament ruptures. Acta Chir Scand 1965;130:560–569.
5. Cox JS: The diagnosis and management of ankle ligament injuries in the athlete. Athl Training 1982;18:192–196.
6. Safran MR, et al.: Lateral ankle sprains: a comprehensive review, part 2: treatment and rehabilitation with an emphasis on the athlete. Med Sci Sports Exerc 1999; 31(7 Suppl):S438–S447.
7. Safran MR, et al.: Lateral ankle sprains: a comprehensive review, part 1: etiology, pathoanatomy, histopathogenesis, and diagnosis. Med Sci Sports Exerc 1999; 31(7 Suppl):S429–S437.
8. Marder RA: Current methods for the evaluation of ankle ligament injuries. J Bone Joint Surg 1994;76A:1103–1111.
9. Magee DJ: Lower Leg, Ankle, and Foot. In Magee DJ (ed): Orthopedic Physical Assessment, pp 765–845. Philadelphia, PA, WB Saunders, 2002.
10. Kelikian H, Kelikian AS: Disorders of the Ankle. Philadelphia, PA, WB Saunders, 1985.
11. Winkel D, Matthijs O, Phelps V: Examination of the Ankle and Foot. In Winkel D, Matthijs O, Phelps V (eds): Diagnosis and Treatment of the Lower Extremities, pp 375–401. Maryland, MD, Aspen, 1997.
12. Lee TK, Maleski R: Physical examination of the ankle for ankle pathology. Clin Podiatr Med Surg 2002;19:251–269.
13. Sammarco GJ, Mangone PG: Diagnosis and treatment of peroneal tendon injuries. Foot Ankle Surg 1986;6:197–205.
14. Guhl JF: Soft tissue (synovial) pathology. In Ankle Arthroscopy: Pathology and Surgical Technique, pp 93–135. Thorofare, NJ, Slack, 1993.
15. Reid DC: Sports Injury Assessment and Rehabilitation. New York, Churchill Livingstone, 1992.
16. Hertling D, Kessler RM: Management of Common Musculoskeletal Disorders: Physical Therapy Principles and Methods, 3rd ed., Philadelphia, PA, Williams & Wilkins, 1996.
17. Baxter DE: The heel in sport. Clin Sports Med 1994;13:683–693.
18. Appling SA, Kasser RJ: Foot and ankle. In Wadsworth C (ed): Current Concepts of Orthopedic Physical Therapy—Home Study Course, La Crosse, WI, Orthopaedic Section, APTA, 2001.
19. Mann RA: Biomechanical approach to the treatment of foot problems. Foot Ankle 1982;2:205–212.
20. Brand RL, Collins MDF: Operative management of ligamentous injuries to the ankle. Clin Sports Med 1982;1:117–130.
21. Leith JM, et al.: Valgus stress radiography in normal ankles. Foot Ankle Int 1997;18:654–657.
22. Leach RE, Dizorio E, Harvey RA: Pathologic hindfoot conditions in the athlete. Clin Orthop 1983;177:116–121.
23. Root M, Orien W, Weed J: Clinical Biomechanics: Normal and Abnormal Function of the Foot. Vol. II. Clinical Biomechanics, Los Angeles, 1977.
24. Patla CE, Abbott JH: Tibialis posterior myofascial tightness as a source of heel pain: diagnosis and treatment. J Orthop Sports Phys Ther 2000;30:624–632.
25. Rose GK, Welton GA, Marshall T: The diagnosis of flat foot in the child. J Bone Joint Surg 1985;67B:71–78.
26. Bojsen-Möller F, Lamoreux L: Significance of dorsiflexion of the toes in walking. Acta Orthop Scand 1979;50:471–479.

27. Buell T, Green DR, Risser J: Measurement of the first metatarsophalangeal joint range of motion. J Am Podiat Med Assn 1988;78:439–448.

28. Joseph J: Range of movement of the great toe in men. J Bone Joint Surg 1954; 36B:450–457.

29. Gross MT: Lower quarter screening for skeletal malalignment—suggestions for orthotics and shoewear. J Orthop Sports Phys Ther 1995;21:389–405.

30. Donatelli R: Normal anatomy and pathophysiology of the foot and ankle. In Wadsworth C (ed): Contemporary Topics on the Foot and Ankle. La Crosse, WI, Orthopedic Section, APTA, 2000.

31. Inman VT: The Joints of the Ankle, pp 31–74. Baltimore, MD, Williams & Wilkins, 1991.

32. Katcherian DA: Pathology of the first ray. In Mizel MS, Miller RA, Scioli MW (eds): Orthopaedic Knowledge Update, Foot and Ankle, pp 157–159. Rosemont, IL, American Academy of Orthopaedic Surgeons, 1998.

33. Alonso A, Khoury L, Adams R: Clinical tests for ankle syndesmosis injury: reliability and prediction of return to function. J Orthop Sports Phys Ther 1998;27: 276–284.

34. Teitz CC, Harrington RM: A biomechanical analysis of the squeeze test for sprains of the syndesmotic ligaments of the ankle. Foot Ankle Int 1998;19:489–492.

35. Brosky T, et al.: The ankle ligaments: consideration of syndesmotic injury and implications for rehabilitation. J Orthop Sports Phys Ther 1995;21:197–205.

36. Hopkinson WJ, et al.: Syndesmosis sprains of the ankle. Foot Ankle Int 1990;10:325.

37. Peng JR: Solving the dilemna of the high ankle sprain in the athlete. Sports Med Arthrosc Rev 2000;8:316–325.

38. Anderson KJ, Lecocq JF: Operative treatment of injury to the fibular collateral ligaments of the ankle. J Bone Joint Surg 1954;36A:825–832.

39. Hollis JM, Blaiser RD, Flahiff CM: Simulated lateral ankle ligamentous injury: change in ankle stability. Am J Sports Med 1993;23:672–677.

40. Johnson EE, Markolf K: The contribution of the anterior talofibular ligament to ankle laxity. J Bone Joint Surg 1983;65A:81–88.

41. Landeros O, Frost HM, Higgins CC: Anteriorly unstable ankle due to trauma: a report of 29 cases. J Bone Joint Surg 1966;48A:1028.

42. Landeros O, Frost HM, Higgins CC: Post traumatic anterior ankle instability. Clin Orthop 1968;56:169–178.

43. Wedmore IS, Charette J: Emergency department evaluation and treatment of ankle and foot injuries. Emerg Med Clin North Am 2000 18:86–114.

44. Gould N, Selingson D, Gassman J: Early and late repair of lateral ligaments of the ankle. Foot Ankle 1980;1:84–89.

45. Staples OS: Rupture of the fibular collateral ligaments of the ankle. J Bone Joint Surg 1975;57A:101–107.

46. Frost HM, Hanson CA: Technique for testing the drawer sign in the ankle. Clin Orthop 1977;123:49–51.

47. Aradi AJ, Wong J, Walsh M: The dimple sign of a ruptured lateral ligament of the ankle: Brief report. J Bone Joint Surg [Br] 1988;70-B:327–328.

48. van Dijk, CN, et al.: Physical examination is sufficient for the diagnosis of sprained ankles. J Bone Joint Surg [Br] 1996;78-B:958–962.

49. Birrer RB, et al.: Managing ankle injuries in the emergency department. J Emerg Med 1999;17:651–660.

50. Martin LP, et al.: Elongation behavior of calcaneofibular and cervical ligaments during inversion loads applied in an open kinetic chain. Foot Ankle Intl 1998;19: 232–239.

51. Sugimoto K, et al.: Subtalar arthrography in recurrent instability of the ankle. Clin Orthop 2002;394:169–176.

52. Beynnon BD, et al.: Ankle ligament injury risk factors: a prospective study of college athletes. J Ortho Res 2001;19:213–220.

53. Kleiger B: Mechanisms of ankle injury. Orthop Clin North Am 1974;5: 127–146.

54. Hockenbury RT, Sammarco GJ: Evaluation and treatment of ankle sprains—clinical recommendations for a positive outcome. Phys Sports Med 2001;24:57–64.
55. Katznel A, Lin M: Ruptures of the ligaments about the tibiofibular syndesmosis. Injury 1984;25:170–172.
56. Rasmussen O, Kroman-Andersen C: Experimental ankle injuries: analysis of the traumatology of the ankle ligaments. Acta Orthop Scand 1983;54:356–362.
57. Palmer ML, Epler M: Clinical Assessment Procedures in Physical Therapy. Philadelphia, PA, JB Lippincott, 1990.
58. Safran MR, O'Malley D Jr, Fu FH: Peroneal tendon subluxation in athletes: new exam techniques, case reports, and review. Med Sci Sports Exerc 1999;31:S487–S492.
59. Thompson TC, Doherty JH: Spontaneous rupture of tendon of Achilles: a new clinical diagnostic test. J Trauma 1962;2:126.
60. Maffulli N: The clinical diagnosis of subcutaneous tear of the Achilles tendon. A prospective study in 174 patients. Am J Sports Med 1998;26:266–270.
61. Johnson KA: Posterior tibial tendon. In Baxter DE (ed): The Foot and Ankle in Sport. St Louis, MO, Mosby, 1995.
62. Kausch T, Rutt J: Subcutaneous rupture of the tibialis anterior tendon: review of the literature and a case report. Arch Orthop Trauma Surg 1998;117:290–293.
63. Miller RR, Mahan KT: Closed rupture of the anterior tibial tendon: a case report. J Am Pod Med Assn 1998;88:394–399.
64. Omari AM, Lee AS, Parsons SW: The clinical presentation of chronic tibialis anterior tendon insufficiency. Foot Ankle Surg 1999;5:251–256.
65. Picciano AM, Rowlands MS, Worrell T: Reliability of open and closed kinetic chain subtalar joint neutral positions and navicular drop test. J Orthop Sports Phys Ther 1993;18:553–558.
66. Mueller MJ, Host JV, Norton BJ: Navicular drop as a composite measure of excessive pronation. J Am Podiat Med Assn 1993;83:198–202.
67. Brody DM: Techniques in the evaluation and treatment of the injured runner. Orthop Clin North Am 1982;13:541–558.
68. Mennell JM: Foot pain. Boston, MA, Little, Brown, 1969.
69. Evans RC: Illustrated Essentials in Orthopedic Physical Assessment. St Louis, MO, Mosby-Year Book, 1994.
70. Stiell IG, et al.: Decision rules for the use of radiography in acute ankle injuries: Refinement and prospective validation. JAMA 1994;269:1127–1132.
71. Stiell IG, et al.: Implementation of the Ottawa Ankle Rules. JAMA 1994;271: 827–832.
72. Leddy JJ, et al.: Prospective evaluation of the Ottawa Ankle Rules in a University Sports Medicine Center. With a modification to increase specificity for identifying malleolar fractures. Am J Sports Med 1998;26:158–165.
73. Guide to physical therapist practice. Phys Ther 2001;81:S13–S95.

13 | The Craniovertebral Junction

OVERVIEW

The craniovertebral (CV) junction is a collective term that refers to the region of the cervical spine where the skull and vertebral column articulate. It comprises the bony structures of the foramen magnum, occiput, atlas, axis, and their supporting ligaments (see *Orthopaedic Examination, Evaluation, and Intervention*, pp 990–998). This complex is perhaps the most complicated series of articulations in the human body, as it has to serve as a transition zone between the normal vertebral joint structures and the completely different skull.

EXAMINATION

The primary objective of the examination of this region is to rule out any serious injury, especially if the patient reports any recent trauma to the head or neck (see *Orthopaedic Examination, Evaluation, and Intervention*, pp 998–1012). The differential diagnosis for head and facial pain is outlined in Table 13-1 (see *Orthopaedic Examination, Evaluation, and Intervention*, pp 222–229). The initial examination should focus on general appearance (including skin lesions such as rashes), vital signs (pulse, blood pressure, and temperature), mental status and speech, gait, balance and coordination, and, if deemed appropriate, cranial nerve and long tract examination, visual fields, acuity and ophthalmoscopic fundus examination, and skull palpation.[1] Once serious injury has been ruled out, a detailed assessment of the CV joints can be performed. In addition, because of their close relationship, the cervical spine and the temporomandibular joint should be assessed as part of a comprehensive examination of this area, as symptom referral from these regions is common.

The specific examination of the CV joints is best performed in a sequential manner (Figure 13-1). In general, the occipito-atlantal (O-A) joint is examined and treated before the atlanto-axial (A-A) joint to avoid confusion between findings from the combined test of both joints. The examination and any intervention are terminated if any serious signs and symptoms are produced. In these instances, an appropriate referral is made.

History

Owing to the proximity of the cranial structures, the clinician should develop the habit of quickly screening patients with neck and head pain for their ability to orient to time, place, and name; concentrate; reason and process information; make judgments; communicate effectively; and recall information. A number of signs and symptoms warrant a full neurologic and general physical examination (Table 13-2).[1] The clinician must always be alert to the potential coincidental occurrence of secondary headache syndromes (refer to Chapter 14). These include headache associated with trauma, vascular disease, nonvascular intracranial disorders, substance use or withdrawal, noncephalic infections, metabolic disorders, disorders of facial or cranial structures, and cranial neuralgia (see *Orthopaedic Examination, Evaluation, and Intervention*, p 225).[2]

TABLE 13-1 Possible Causes of Head and Facial Pain

- Trauma
- Headache
- Occipital neuralgia
- Osteoarthritis
- Rheumatoid arthritis and related rheumatoid arthritis variants (dermatomyositis, temporal arteritis)
- Lyme disease
- Fibromyalgia
- Arteriovenous malformation
- Intracranial infection (meningitis)
- Cerebrovascular disease
- Tumor
- Encephalitis
- Systemic infections
- Multiple sclerosis
- Miscellaneous

Dizziness (vertigo) and nystagmus are nonspecific neurologic signs that require a careful diagnostic workup (see Table 13-2).

A report of vertigo, although potentially problematic, is not in of itself a contraindication to the continuation of the examination. Differential diagnosis for complaints of dizziness includes primary central nervous system diseases, vestibular and ocular involvement, and, more rarely, metabolic disorders.[3] Careful questioning can help in the differentiation of central and peripheral causes of vertigo.

- Central vertigo is usually a result of a disturbance of the vestibular system, which can produce sensations of head and body rotations, to and fro movements, or up and down movements.
- Peripheral vertigo is manifested with general complaints such as unsteadiness, lightheadedness.

Cervical vertigo may be produced by localized muscle changes and receptor irritation.[4] Dizziness provoked by head movements or head positions could indicate an inner ear dysfunction. Dizziness provoked by specific cervical motions, particularly extension or rotation may also indicate a vertebral artery compromise.

Systems Review

The CV region houses many vital structures. These include the spinal cord, the vertebral artery, and the brain stem. It is extremely important for the clinician to approach this area with caution and to rule out the presence of serious pathology. CV and cranial dysfunction can be responsible for a number of signs and symptoms that may either be benign or indicate the presence of serious pathology (Table 13-3).

The cranial nerves should be assessed, particularly if there are complaints about vision, or the patient appears to have problems with speech or swallowing or both. Patients with referred pain in the region of the trigeminal nerve commonly have an underlying disorder of the upper cervical spine, such as A-A instability caused by rheumatoid arthritis.[5,6]

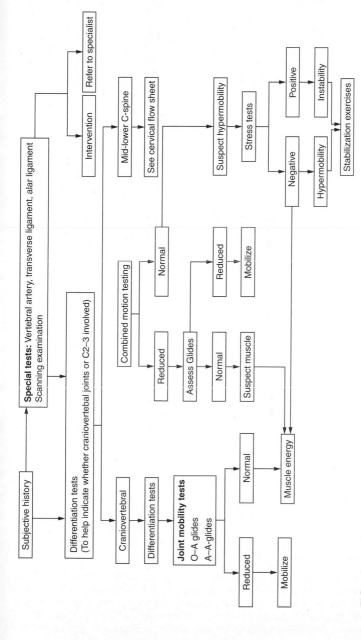

FIG. 13-1 Algorithm for the examination of the CV region.

411

TABLE 13-2 Signs and Symptoms Requiring Neurologic Assessment

- Headaches that are sudden, severe, and diffuse
- Headaches that awaken one from sleep
- Headaches associated with projectile vomiting, but no nausea
- Unilateral pulsating pain in synchrony with the heartbeat
- Headaches that worsen with activity or exertion
- Headaches that begin or worsen with recumbency
- Focal tenderness over the temporal artery in someone over the age of 60
- Sudden, intense, sharp pain of short duration that is either spontaneous or triggered by a mild stimulus
- Severe pain around the sinuses or teeth
- Headaches associated with other symptoms
- Cognitive impairment
- Visual disturbances (i.e., blindness, diplopia, distortions, spots, or loss of vision on one side)
- Numbness or altered sensation
- Loss of strength or coordination
- Loss or alteration of smell, taste, or hearing
- Fever or associated systemic illness
- Difficulty swallowing
- Loss or impairment of voice, chronic cough

Source: Isaacs E, Bookout M: Screening for pathological origins of head and facial pain. In Boissonnault WG (ed): Examination in Physical Therapy Practice: Screening for Medical Disease, pp 175–189. Philadelphia, PA, WB Saunders, 1995.

Tests and Measures

The examination of the CV region progresses from the application of gentle stresses to the use of more assertive tests.

Observation

The patient is observed in the sagittal, coronal, and transverse planes (see *Orthopaedic Examination, Evaluation, and Intervention*, p 1002).

Active Range of Motion

Rotation   The patient is asked to perform active neck rotation. Neck and head rotation could be considered as the functional motion of the CV joints, particularly the A-A joints. If the patient's symptoms and loss of motion are not reproduced with active rotation, it is doubtful that damage to tissues making up the CV joints is significant, or even present. An inability to rotate the head any amount in either direction is potentially a very serious sign. Every measure must be taken to determine the cause of this inability to move. In addition to the presence of serious injury, other conditions that can be provoked by cervical rotation include vertebral artery compromise—cervical rotation is the most likely (single) motion to reproduce signs or symptoms of vertebral artery compromise.[7–10]

Short Neck Flexion   Active neck flexion tests cranial nerve XI and the C1 and C2 myotomes as well as muscle strength, and the patient's willingness to move. The clinician instructs the patient to place his or her chin on the "Adam's apple" (Figure 13-2). This maneuver simulates flexion at the CV joints. If this maneuver produces tingling in the feet, or electric shock sensations down the

TABLE 13-3 Examination Findings and the Possible Conditions Causing Them[1]

Findings	Possible condition
Dizziness	Upper cervical impairment, vertebrobasilar ischemia, CV ligament tear. May also be relatively benign
Quadrilateral paresthesia	Cord compression, vertebrobasilar ischemia
Bilateral upper limb paresthesia	Cord compression, vertebrobasilar ischemia
Hyperreflexia	Cord compression, vertebrobasilar ischemia
Babinski or clonus sign	Cord compression, vertebrobasilar ischemia
Consistent swallow on transverse ligament stress tests	Instability, retropharyngeal hematoma, rheumatoid arthritis
Nontraumatic capsular pattern	Rheumatoid arthritis, ankylosing spondylitis, neoplasm
Arm pain lasting >6–9 months	Neoplasm
Persistent root pain <30 years	Neoplasm
Radicular pain with coughing	Neoplasm
Pain worsening after 1 month	Neoplasm
>1 level involved	Neoplasm
Paralysis	Neoplasm or neurologic disease
Trunk and limb paresthesia	Neoplasm
Bilateral root signs and symptoms	Neoplasm
Nontraumatic strong spasm	Neoplasm
Nontraumatic strong pain in the elderly patient	Neoplasm
Signs worse than symptoms	Neoplasm
Radial deviator weakness	Neoplasm
Thumb flexor weakness	Neoplasm
Hand intrinsic weakness or atrophy or both	Neoplasm, thoracic outlet syndrome, carpal tunnel syndrome
Horner's syndrome	Superior sulcus tumor, breast cancer, cervical ganglion damage, brainstem damage
Empty end-feel	Neoplasm
Severe posttraumatic capsular pattern	Fracture
Severe posttraumatic spasm	Fracture
Loss of range of motion (ROM) posttrauma	Fracture
Posttraumatic painful weakness	Fracture

Source: Meadows J: Orthopedic Differential Diagnosis in Physical Therapy. New York, McGraw-Hill, 1999.

neck (Lhermitte's sign) it is highly indicative of serious pathology. Although Lhermitte's sign is not a specific symptom, it is commonly encountered in meningitis and cervical spinal cord demyelination caused by multiple sclerosis (see *Orthopaedic Examination, Evaluation, and Intervention,* pp 1266–1267).[11] The sign has been found in many other conditions that cause a traumatic or compressive cervical myelopathy, such as cervical spondylosis, cervical instability, and epidural or subdural tumors.[9,12] If the patient reports a pulling sensation during short neck flexion the cervicothoracic junction may be at fault.

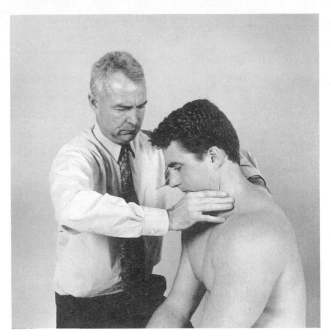

FIG. 13-2 Short neck flexion with over pressure. (*Reproduced with permission from Dutton M: Orthopaedic Examination, Evaluation, and Intervention, p 1003 (Fig. 22–8). New York, McGraw-Hill, 2004.*)

Placing the neck in short neck flexion places the short neck *extensors* (C1), which are innervated by the spinal accessory nerve, on stretch. The clinician applies overpressure and tests the short neck extensors by asking the patient to resist. Positive findings with this test are severe pain, nausea or muscle spasm or both, cord signs, the latter of which may indicate a dens fracture, or a tumor.[9] Thus, if a patient is able to flex his or her neck, a cervical fracture or a transverse ligament compromise can be provisionally ruled out.

Short Neck Extension To ensure that short neck extension occurs around the correct axis, the clinician instructs the patient to lift his or her chin toward the ceiling (Figure 13-3). A total inability to perform this motion (in the presence of other motions) often signals the presence of major tearing of anterior cervical structures. If this test produces tingling in the feet, it is highly suggestive of compression to the spinal cord. This compression may be because of "buckling" of the ligamentum flavum caused by loss of its elasticity. A loss of balance or a drop attack with this maneuver would strongly suggest a compromise of the vertebrobasilar system. A drop attack is defined as a loss of balance without a loss of consciousness. Overpressure is applied as the clinician attempts to lift the patient's chin in the direction of the ceiling. The short neck *flexors* (C1), which are innervated by the spinal accessory nerve, can be tested in this position by lifting the patient's chin toward the ceiling while the patient resists.

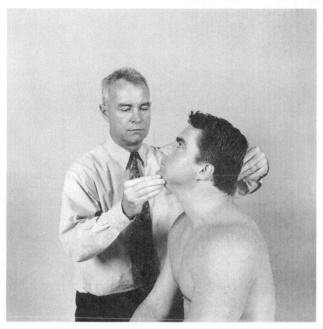

FIG. 13-3 Short neck extension with overpressure and resistance. (*Reproduced with permission from Dutton M: Orthopaedic Examination, Evaluation, and Intervention, p 1003 (Fig. 22–9). New York, McGraw-Hill, 2004.*)

Palpation

Examination of the skin overlying the spine has been found to be very helpful toward making a diagnosis as certain skin changes in a particular location may point in the direction of a dysfunctional spinal area.[13] The skin is assessed for its thickness, moisture and ease of displacement in all directions. Abnormal autonomic skin reactions, such as erythematous changes, increased sweat production, and pain that can be induced with minimal palpatory pressure, may indicate a segmental dysfunction.[14] However, Horner's syndrome must also be ruled out (see *Orthopaedic Examination, Evaluation, and Intervention*, p 64).

Palpation may be started at that area indicated by the patient as painful. These painful sites must be correctly localized. The following bony landmarks in this region should be palpated.

Occiput The clinician locates the external occipital protuberance, which is the most prominent bony structure at the occiput in the midline. By following the external occipital protuberance laterally, the clinician can locate the superior nuchal line. The semispinalis capitis muscle is located about 1½ finger widths below the superior nuchal line.[14]

Mastoid The mastoid processes are located behind the ear. Once located, the clinician moves the fingers inferiorly toward the tip of the mastoid process. Starting from the medial tip of the mastoid process, the palpating finger is moved superiorly to the upper pole of the mastoid sulcus, an important area in the examination of the irritation zones of the occiput and C1.[14]

Atlas By placing the palpating fingers between the mastoid process and the descending ramus of the mandible, the transverse process of the atlas can be located. The inferior oblique and the superior oblique both have attachments to this site.

Axis The spinous process of C2 is the first prominent bony landmark that is accessible to palpation below the external occipital protuberance of the occiput. The spinous process of C2 serves as the origin of the inferior oblique muscle and the rectus capitis posterior major muscle.

Differing Philosophies

The next stage in the examination process depends on the clinician's background. For those clinicians heavily influenced by the muscle energy techniques of the osteopaths,[15] position testing is used to determine which segment to focus on. Other clinicians omit the position tests and proceed to the combined motion and passive physiologic tests.

Positional Tests The patient is sitting, the clinician standing behind them. With the index and middle finger of both hands, the clinician palpates the distance between the transverse processes of the atlas and the mastoid processes of the temporal bones.

Flexion

- *Occipito-atlantal joint.* With the index and long finger of one hand, the clinician palpates the mastoid process and the transverse process of C1. The patient is asked to flex the O-A joint complex. The clinician assesses the position of the occiput relative to the atlas. The other side is then tested and a comparison is made. The side to which the occiput is side-flexed in flexion is the side of the shortest distance.
- *Atlanto-axial joint.* Positional testing of this joint is performed by bilaterally palpating the posterior arch of the atlas in the suboccipital gutter and the lamina of the axis with the index and middle finger. The joint is flexed around its axis. The clinician assesses the position of the C1 vertebra relative to C2 by noting the position of the posterior arch relative to the corresponding lamina of C2. The other side is then tested and a comparison is made. A posterior left posterior arch of C1 relative to the left lamina of C2 is indicative of a left rotated position of the C1-2 joint complex in flexion.

Extension

- *Occipito-atlantal joint.* The O-A joint complex is flexed around the appropriate axis. The clinician assesses the position of the occiput relative to the atlas by comparing the left with the right side. The side to which the occiput is side-flexed in extension is the side of the shortest distance.
- *Atlanto-axial joint.* Positional testing of this joint is performed by bilaterally palpating the posterior arch of the atlas in the suboccipital gutter and the lamina of the axis with the index and middle finger of both hands. The joint is extended around the appropriate axis. The clinician assesses the position of the C1 vertebra relative to C2 by noting the position of the posterior arch relative to the corresponding lamina of C2. A posterior left posterior arch of C1 relative to the left lamina of C2 is indicative of a left rotated position of the C1-2 joint complex in extension.

Passive Physiologic Mobility Testing of the Occiput, Atlas, and Axis Occipito-Atlantal Joint

When mobility testing this joint, the first point to remember is that the joint is capable of flexion, extension, but that side bending and rotation can also occur, albeit slight. The second point to keep in mind is that the arthrokinematics of this joint are the reverse of those occurring in the other zygapophysial joints, and that they occur in a different plane (horizontal).

With the patient in supine, the head is extended around the axis for the O-A joint (Figure 13-4). The head is then side-flexed left and right. As the side bending is performed, a gradual translation force is applied in the opposite direction to the side bending. The range of movement of the side bending is assessed from side to side, as is the end-feel of the translation. This procedure is then repeated for flexion.

During extension of the O-A joint, the occipital condyles glide anteriorly to the limit of their symmetrical extension range. During left side bending and right translation in extension, the coupled right rotation is produced. This rotation causes the right occipital condyle to return toward a neutral position, while the left condyle advances toward the extension barrier. If left side bending in extension is limited, then the limiting factor is on the left joint of the segment (ipsilateral to the side bending), which is preventing the advance of the condyle into its normal position. Thus, extension and right translation tests

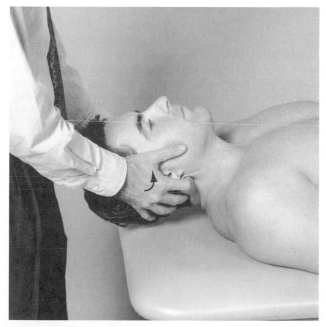

FIG. 13-4   Passive mobility testing of O-A extension. (*Reproduced with permission from Dutton M: Orthopaedic Examination, Evaluation, and Intervention, p 1006 (Fig. 22–14). New York, McGraw-Hill, 2004.*)

the anterior glide of the left O-A joint, while extension and left translation stresses the anterior glide of the right O-A joint (Table 13-4).

During flexion of the O-A joint, the occipital condyles glide posteriorly. The right rotation associated with left side bending causes the left condyle to move away from the flexion barrier toward the neutral position, while the right condyle is moved posteriorly further into the flexion barrier. Thus, flexion and translation to the right tests the posterior glide of the right O-A joint, while flexion and translation to the left tests the posterior glide of the left O-A joint (see Table 13-4).

It is apparent that the arthrokinematics and osteokinematics are tested simultaneously with these maneuvers, thus the cause of the restriction must be determined using the end-feel.[16]

Atlanto-Axial Joint The A-A joint can be tested in sitting or supine. In the seated test, the clinician stabilizes C2 with one hand and then rotates the patient's head with the other hand until an end-feel is perceived (Figure 13-5). With the patient positioned in supine, the clinician uses side bending of the head and neck around the CV axis, combined with rotation of the head and neck in the direction opposite to the side bending. If the head and neck are positioned in flexion during this maneuver, it could be argued that this better tests the anterior glide of the A-A joint ipsilateral to the side bend. Positioning the head in extension during this maneuver is not recommended because of the potential threat to the vertebral artery. The clinician assesses the amount of range available and the end-feel, and then compares the findings with the other side.

Combined Motion Testing Flexion and extension at the O-A joints involves a posterior and anterior gliding of the occipital condyles, respectively. The same gliding (although reciprocal in opposing facets) is utilized in rotation. At the A-A joint, flexion and extension primarily involve a "rolling" action of the condyles, with an insignificant amount of gliding. Therefore, CV flexion and extension will have a minimal effect on A-A rotation.[17] Thus, if a symptom or range of motion is drastically altered by CV flexion or extension, an assumption could be made that the dysfunction is at the O-A joint.[17]

The findings from the combined motion tests can be used to determine which joint glide is to be assessed. For example, if it was determined in the

TABLE 13-4 Movement Restrictions of the CV Joints and Their Probable Causes

Movement restricted	Possible reason
Flexion or right-side bending	Left flexion hypomobility Left extensor muscle tightness Left posterior capsular adhesions Left subluxation (into extension)
Extension or right-side bending	Right extension hypomobility Right flexor muscle tightness Right anterior capsular adhesions Right subluxation (into flexion)
Flexion or right-side bending motion greater than extension or left-side bending	Left capsular pattern • Arthritis • Arthrosis
Flexion or right-side bending equal to extension or left-side bending	Left arthrofibrosis (very hard) capsular end-feel
Right-side flex in flexion and extension	Probably an anomaly

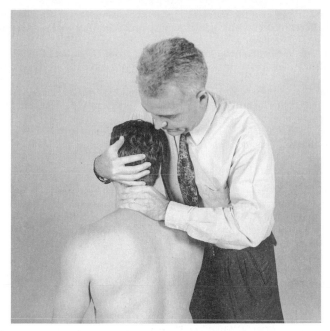

FIG. 13-5 Passive mobility testing of A-A rotation. (*Reproduced with permission from Dutton M: Orthopaedic Examination, Evaluation, and Intervention, p 1008 (Fig. 22–16). New York, McGraw-Hill, 2004.*)

combined motion testing that the *right* O-A joint is restricted or painful with flexion (a loss of its posterior glide), the O-A joint is positioned in its extreme of flexion and right rotation (the two motions associated with a posterior glide of the right O-A joint).

Linear Segmental Stress Testing

The CV region demonstrates a high degree of mobility, but little stability, with the ligaments affording little protection during a high-velocity injury. Instability of this region can result from a number of causes:

- *Trauma* (especially a hyperflexion injury to the neck)
- *Disease, including rheumatoid arthritis, psoriatic arthritis, ankylosing spondylitis.* Nontraumatic hypermobility or frank instability of the O-A joint has been reported in association with rheumatoid arthritis.[18]
- *History of corticosteroid use.* Prolonged exposure to this class of drug can produce a softening of the dens and transverse ligament by deteriorating the Sharpey fibers, which attach the ligament to the bone. Steroid use also promotes osteoporosis predisposing bones to fracture.
- *Recurrent upper respiratory tract infections (UTRI) or chronic sore throats in children.* Maladie de Grisel syndrome[19] is a spontaneous A-A dislocation, affecting children between 6 and 12 years. The outstanding symptom is a spontaneously arising torticollis. The most likely etiology seems to be

an inflammation of the retropharyngeal space, caused by upper respiratory tract infections or by adenotonsillectomy, producing pharyngeal hyperemia, and bone absorption.

- *Congenital*. Nontraumatic hypermobility or frank instability of the occipitoatlantal joint has been reported in association with congenital bony malformations.[20]
- *Down's syndrome*. Nontraumatic hypermobility or frank instability of the occipitoatlantal joint has been reported in children and adolescents with Down's syndrome.[21,22]
- Patient under the age of 9 who can often have an immature or absent dens
- *Osteoporosis*. Osteoporosis can lead to an increased susceptibility to fracture.

Indications for Stability Testing The following findings are considered to be indications to stability test the CV region:[9]

- History of neck trauma or any of the causes of instability listed previously
- Patient reports that his or her neck feels unstable
- The presence of the following signs/symptoms:
  - A lump in the throat
  - Lip paresthesia
  - Nausea/vomiting
  - Severe headache and muscle spasm
  - Dizziness

The patient is laid supine to remove any muscular influences. If the patient is unable to lie down, you may need to reconsider the appropriateness of performing these tests.

Longitudinal Stability General traction is applied to the entire cervical region. If this maneuver does not reproduce the signs or symptoms, C2 is stabilized so that the traction force may be directed at the CV region (Figure 13-6).

Anterior Shear—Transverse Ligament[9] The patient is positioned in supine with his or her head cradled in the clinician's hands. The clinician locates the anterior arches of C2 by moving around the vertebra from the back to the front using the thumbs. Once located, the clinician pushes down on the anterior arches of C2 with the thumbs toward the table, while the patient's occiput and C1, cupped in the clinician's hands, is lifted, keeping the head parallel to the ceiling, but in slight flexion (Figure 13-7). The patient is instructed to keep his or her eyes open and to count backward aloud. The position is held for approximately 15 seconds or until an end-feel is perceived.

Coronal Stability—Alar Ligament Rotation and side bending tighten the contralateral alar (rotation or side bending to the right tightens the left alar), whereas flexion typically tightens both alar ligaments.

The transverse process of C2 is palpated with one hand, while the patient's head is side bent or rotated (Figure 13-8). This is a test of immediacy. If the C2 spinous process does not move as soon as the head begins to rotate, laxity of the alar ligament should be suspected.

Transverse Shear[9] Transverse shearing of the CV joints is performed with the patient supine. The clinician stabilizes the mastoid, and C1 is moved in a transverse direction, using the soft part of the metacarpophalangeal joint of the

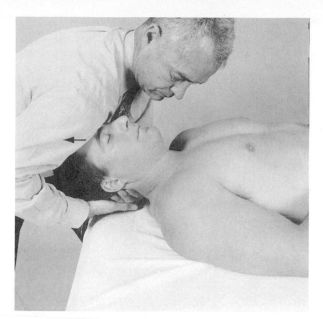

FIG. 13-6 Longitudinal stability testing. (*Reproduced with permission from Dutton M: Orthopaedic Examination, Evaluation, and Intervention, p 1009 (Fig. 22–17). New York, McGraw-Hill, 2004.*)

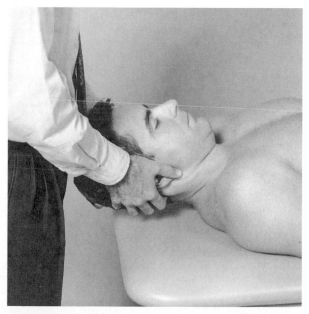

FIG. 13-7 Transverse ligament test. (*Reproduced with permission from Dutton M: Orthopaedic Examination, Evaluation, and Intervention, p 1010 (Fig. 22–18). New York, McGraw-Hill, 2004.*)

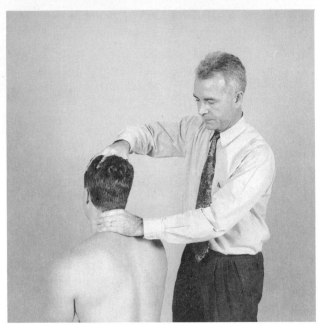

FIG. 13-8   Alar ligament test. *(Reproduced with permission from Dutton M: Orthopaedic Examination, Evaluation, and Intervention, p 1010 (Fig. 22–19). New York, McGraw-Hill, 2004.)*

index finger. The test is repeated with stabilization of C1 and then translation of the mastoid.

C1 and C2 can be tested similarly. The soft aspect of each second metacarpal head is placed on the opposite transverse processes and laminae of C1 and C2, with the palms facing each other. The clinician stabilizes C1 and then attempts to move C2 transversely using the soft part of metacarpophalangeals. No movement should be felt.

Neurologic Examination

The presence of neurologic symptoms in the head, neck, or upper limb warrants a full neurologic examination to assess the conduction of the central and peripheral nervous systems. The patient with a neck trauma can report seemingly bizarre symptoms, but these need to be heeded until the clinician can rule out serious pathology. In addition to deep tendon reflexes and sensory tests, the clinician should perform the spinal cord reflexes of Babinski and Hoffman. The presence of any upper motor neuron (UMN) sign or symptom requires an immediate medical referral. Cervical myelopathy, involving an injury to the spinal cord itself is associated with multisegmental paresthesias, UMN signs, and symptoms such as spasticity, hyperreflexia, visual and balance disturbances, ataxia, and sudden changes in bowel and bladder function.

Special Tests

Barre's Test   Barre's test can be used to test for vertebral artery insufficiency, especially if the patient is unable to lie supine.

The patient is seated with the arms outstretched, forearms supinated (Figure 13-9). The patient is asked to close his or her eyes and move the head and neck into maximum extension and rotation. A positive test is one in which one of the outstretched arms sinks toward the floor and pronates, indicating the side of the compromise.

Dix-Hallpike Test   This test can be used to help determine if the cause of the patient's dizziness is because of a vestibular impairment resulting from an accumulation of utricle debris (otoconia). This test is only usually performed if the vertebral artery test and instability tests do not provoke symptoms.

The test involves having the patient suddenly lie down from a sitting position with the head rotated in the direction that the clinician feels is the provocative position.[23] The end point of the test is when the patient's head overhangs the end of the table so that the cervical spine is extended (see *Orthopaedic Examination, Evaluation, and Intervention*, p 1011). A positive test is the reproduction of the patient's symptoms.

Modified Sharp-Purser Test   The patient is positioned in sitting. The patient is asked to segmentally flex the head and relate any signs or symptoms

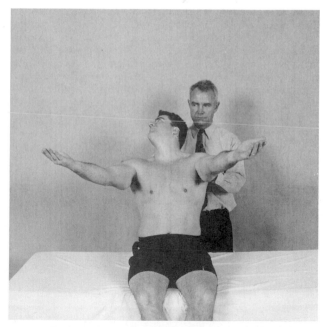

FIG. 13-9   Barre's vertebral artery test. (*Reproduced with permission from Dutton M: Orthopaedic Examination, Evaluation, and Intervention, p 1011 (Fig. 22–22). New York, McGraw-Hill, 2004.*)

that this might evoke to the clinician. In addition, a positive test is indicated if the patient hears or feels a "clunk." Local symptoms such as soreness etc. are ignored for the purposes of evaluating the test. If no serious signs or symptoms are provoked, the clinician stabilizes C2 with one hand, and applies a posteriorly oriented force to the head.

In the presence of a positive test, a provisional assumption is made that the symptoms are caused by excessive translation of the atlas compromising one or more of the sensitive structures listed above and the physical examination is terminated. No intervention should be attempted other than the issuing of a cervical collar to prevent CV flexion and an immediate referral to his or her physician.

Imaging Studies

Radiographs   The standard, initial cervical spine radiographic series in trauma patients includes a cross-table lateral view, an anteroposterior view, and an open-mouth view, the latter of which is used to help rule out a fracture of the dens.[24] The usefulness of the anteroposterior view has been questioned because it provides little additional information.[25] Although this three-view screening series can detect 65–95% of axis injuries,[26,27] the C2 vertebra often is obscured by overlying bony maxillary, mandibular, and dental structures; therefore, C2 fractures may be missed.[24] The clinician needs to be aware of the limitations of plain radiographs, as problems exist with both specificity and sensitivity. However, radiographs can provide a gross assessment of the severity of the degenerative changes of the spine.

Computed Tomography   Thin-section computed tomography (CT) is the best study for evaluating C2 bony fractures.[28] Sagittal reconstruction of CT images is important because axial images may not detect a transverse odontoid fracture.[24] Although CT is excellent in evaluating bony injuries, it can miss soft tissue and significant ligamentous injuries.[24] Recently, therefore, dynamic flexion/extension lateral fluoroscopic evaluation has been advocated in polytrauma patients to identify occult ligamentous instabilities and confirm that the cervical spine is uninjured.[29] As with any diagnostic study, the findings must be correlated with the history and physical examination.

EXAMINATION CONCLUSIONS—THE EVALUATION

Following the examination, and once the clinical findings have been recorded, the clinician must determine a specific diagnosis or a working hypothesis, based on a summary of all the findings. This diagnosis can be structure related (medical diagnosis), or a diagnosis based on the preferred practice patterns as described in the *Guide to Physical Therapist Practice*.[30]

REFERENCES

1. McCrory P: Headaches and exercise. Sports Med 2000;30:221–229.
2. Welch KM: A 47-year-old woman with tension-type headaches. JAMA 2001;286:960–966.
3. Mohn A, et al.: Celiac disease—associated vertigo and nystagmus. J Pediatr Gastroenterol Nutr 2002;34:317–378.
4. Dvorak J, Dvorak V: Differential diagnosis of vertigo. In Gilliar WG, Greenman PE (eds): Manual Medicine: Diagnostics, pp 67–70. New York, Thieme Medical, 1990.
5. Travell JG Simons DG: Myofascial Pain and Dysfunction—The Trigger Point Manual. Baltimore, MD, Williams & Wilkins, 1983.

6. Viikara-Juntura E: Examination of the Neck. Validity of Some Clinical, Radiological and Epidemiologic Methods. Helsinki, University of Helsinki, Institute of Occupational Health, 1988.
7. Hardin J Jr: Pain and the cervical spine. Bull Rheum Dis 2001;50:1–4.
8. Bland JH: New anatomy and physiology with clinical and historical implications. In Bland JH (ed): Disorders of the Cervical Spine, pp 71–79. Philadelphia, PA, WB Saunders, 1994.
9. Pettman E: Stress tests of the CV joints. In Boyling JD, Palastanga N (eds): Grieve's Modern Manual Therapy: The Vertebral Column, pp 529–538. Edinburgh, Churchill Livingstone, 1994.
10. Bogduk N: An anatomical basis for the neck-tongue syndrome. J Neurol Neurosurg Psychiatry 1981;44:202–208.
11. Kanchandani R Howe JG: Lhermitte's sign in multiple sclerosis: a clinical survey and review of the literature. J Neurol Neurosurg Psychiatry 1982;45:308–312.
12. Murphy DK Gutrecht JA: Lhermitte's sign in cavernous angioma of the cervical spinal cord. J Neurol Neurosurg Psychiatry 1998;65:954–955.
13. Greenman PE: Principles of Manual Medicine, 2nd ed. Baltimore, MD, Williams & Wilkins, 1996.
14. Dvorak J, Dvorak V: General principles of palpation. In Gilliar WG, Greenman PE (eds): Manual Medicine: Diagnostics, pp 71–75. New York, Thieme Medical, 1990.
15. Mitchell FL, Moran PS, Pruzzo NA: An Evaluation and Treatment Manual of Osteopathic Muscle Energy Procedures. Manchester, MO, Mitchell, Moran and Pruzzo, 1979.
16. Meadows JTS: Manual Therapy: Biomechanical Assessment and Treatment, Advanced Technique. Lecture and video supplemental manual. Calgary, Swodeam Consulting, 1995.
17. Pettman E: Level III course notes. Berrien Springs, Michigan: North American Institute of Manual Therapy, 2003.
18. Martel W: The occipito-atlanto-axial joints in rheumatoid arthritis. Am J Roentgenol 1961;86:223–240.
19. Parke WW, Rothman RH, Brown MD: The pharyngovertebral veins: an anatomical rationale for Grisel's syndrome. J Bone Joint Surg 1984;66A:568.
20. Georgopoulos G, Pizzutillo PD, Lee MS: Occipito-atlantal instability in children. J Bone Joint Surg 1987;69A:429–436.
21. El-Khoury GY, et al.: Posterior atlantooccipital subluxation in Down syndrome. Radiology 1986;159:507–509.
22. Brooke DC, Burkus JK, Benson DR: Asymptomatic occipito-atlantal instability in Down's syndrome. J Bone Joint Surg 1987;69A:293–295.
23. Meadows J: Orthopedic Differential Diagnosis in Physical Therapy. New York, McGraw-Hill, 1999.
24. Sasso RC: C2 dens fractures: Treatment options. J Spinal Disord 2001;14:455–463.
25. Freemyer B, et al.: Comparison of five-view and three-view cervical spine series in the evaluation of patients with cervical trauma. Ann Emerg Med 1989;18:818–821.
26. Schaffer MA, Doris PE: Limitation of the cross table lateral view in detecting cervical spine injuries: a retrospective analysis. Ann Emerg Med 1981;10:508–513.
27. Marchesi DG: Management of odontoid fractures. Orthopaedics 1997;20:911–916.
28. Blacksin MF, Lee HJ: Frequency and significance of fractures of the upper cervical spine detected by CT in patients with severe neck trauma. Am J Roentgenol 1995;165:1201–1204.
29. Harris MB, Waguespack AM, Kronlage S: "Clearing" cervical spine injuries in polytrauma patients: is it really safe to remove the collar? Orthopedics 1997; 20:903–907.
30. Guide to physical therapist practice. Phys Ther 2001;81:S13–S95.

14 | The Cervical Spine

OVERVIEW

The cervical spine is one of the key links in the upper kinetic chain as it is responsible for the control of head, and thus eye motion. The cervical spine is made up of seven vertebrae. C1 articulates with the occiput of the skull above and with C2 below (see *Orthopaedic Examination, Evaluation, and Intervention*, pp 1033–1045). The atlanto-occipital joint primarily allows flexion and extension, while the atlanto-axial articulation primarily provides rotation (refer to Chapter 13). Vertebrae C3 through C7 allow for varying degrees of flexion, extension, side bending, and rotation as an interdependent group. Movements of flexion center on C5 and C6 and extension movements center on C6 and C7.[1] Intervertebral disks are found from C2-3 and below and are subjected to significant deformation during flexion and extension (see *Orthopaedic Examination, Evaluation, and Intervention*, Chapter 20). Eight pairs of cervical spinal nerves exit bilaterally through the intervertebral foramina. Each spinal nerve is named for the vertebra above which it exits; for example, the C6 nerve exits above the C6 vertebra.

With stability being sacrificed for mobility, the cervical spine is rendered more vulnerable to both direct and indirect trauma. The cervical spine can be the source of many pain syndromes, including neck, upper thoracic and periscapular syndromes, cervical radiculopathy, and shoulder and elbow syndromes.[2] These syndromes may result from a vast array of causes, ranging from acute minor sprains to chronic degenerative changes.[3] These degenerative changes can occur at the cervical articulations or at the intervertebral disk. Disk degeneration may be painful in its own right, while herniation can lead to compression of the nerve root (radiculopathy) or spinal cord (myelopathy). Although most neck pain is transient and has an uncertain cause, more serious causes include deceleration injuries and inflammatory diseases.[4]

EXAMINATION

The cervical spine is an area with a high potential for serious injury, which makes this an area of the body that needs to be examined with caution, especially when there is a history of acute and recent trauma of the neck because of the potential for the examination itself to be harmful.[5] Although most conditions involving neck and upper limb symptoms can be diagnosed after a careful history and physical examination, in cases of significant trauma, imaging studies may be required to exclude a fracture or instability. Clearing tests for the cervical spine include:

- Vertebral artery tests (see *Orthopaedic Examination, Evaluation, and Intervention*, Chapter 21)
- Sharp-Purser test (Chapter 13)
- Articular stability tests (Chapter 13)
- Transverse ligament test (Chapter 13)
- Alar ligament test (Chapter 13)
- Temporomandibular joint

The examination must be graduated and progressive so that the testing can be discontinued at the first signs of serious pathology (see *Orthopaedic Examination, Evaluation, and Intervention*, pp 1045–1068).[5] An examination algorithm for the mid-lower cervical spine is outlined in Figure 14-1.

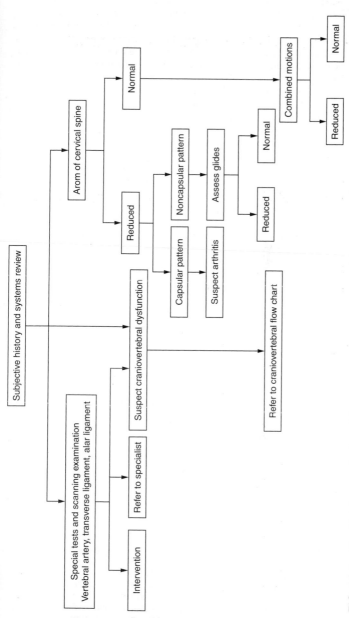

FIG. 14-1 Algorithm for examination of the cervical spine.

History

The patient's chief complaint should be ascertained. The history often gives the clinician clues as to the source of the patient's symptoms, the nature and location of the involved structure (Table 14-1), the severity of the condition, and the activities or positions that appear to aggravate or improve the patient's condition (Table 14-2). Determining the location of the pain can provide some clues as to the cause (Figure 14-2). In addition, asking the patient to describe his or her symptoms over a 24-hour period can provide the clinician with valuable information about positions and activities that aggravate or relieve the symptoms and the duration of the symptoms. Pain that increases with activity or within a few hours after activity, but settles down with rest or a change in position, is commonly referred to as mechanical pain. Conditions that have a mechanical origin are usually improved with rest, although they may worsen initially on retiring.[6] The patient's sleeping position and habits should be investigated. Pain caused by sustained positions may awaken the patient at night, but is usually relieved with a change of position. Patients who report difficulty sleeping because of pain may have an inflammatory condition. Cervical symptoms are often increased when a foam or very firm pillow is used.[7] Sleeping in the prone position requires adequate rotation. Some degree of cervical extension is also required depending on the number and type of pillow used. Pain that persists or worsens despite rest and intervention, pain that persists around the clock, or pain that worsens at night raises suspicion for a metabolic or neoplastic condition, or for psychosocial factors that prolong recovery.[8]

The chronicity of the symptoms can afford the clinician with some clues. Muscle strains usually resolve within a few days to a couple of weeks, ligament sprains may take up to a couple of months, and disk injuries or herniations with

TABLE 14-1 Pain Location and Possible Cause

Pain location	Possible cause
Localized pain	Muscle strain
	Ligament sprain
	Facet degeneration
	Disk degeneration
	Spinal nerve root irritation (C3)
	Shoulder impingement
Upper trapezius region	Spinal nerve root irritation (C4)
Shoulder and lateral upper arm	Spinal nerve root irritation (C5)
Radial forearm and thumb, and occasionally the index finger	Spinal nerve root irritation (C5, 6)
Posterior arm, dorsal (occasionally ventral) forearm, and the index and middle fingers	Spinal nerve root irritation (C7)
Medial arm, ulnar forearm, and the ring and little fingers	Spinal nerve root irritation (C8)
	Thoracic outlet syndrome
	Ulnar nerve neuropathy
Scapular region	Lower cervical nerve roots, disks, spinal longitudinal ligaments, and facet joints
	Thoracic outlet syndrome
Upper extremity in nondermatomal distribution	Cervical myelopathy
Head	Upper cervical spine

TABLE 14-2 Differential Diagnosis of Cervical Spondylosis, Cervical Myelopathy, Spinal Stenosis, Thoracic Outlet Syndrome, and Posterolateral Disk Herniation

	Cervical spondylosis (osteoarthritis)	Cervical myelopathy	Spinal stenosis	Thoracic outlet syndrome	Posterolateral cervical disk herniation
Pain	Unilateral	Not usually painful unless there is an associated radiculopathy	Unilateral or bilateral	May or may not be pain	Unilateral (commonly) or bilateral
Distribution of pain	Into affected dermatomes	Upper extremity (nondermatomal)	Usually several dermatomes affected	Upper extremity (nondermatomal)	Into affected dermatomes
Pain worsened by	Cervical extension	Cervical extension	Cervical extension	Shoulder retraction and depression	Cervical flexion
Pain relieved by	Positioning Cervical flexion	Positioning	Rest Cervical flexion	Diverse	Positioning
Age group affected	>45 years >60 years	40–60 years 50–70 years	11–70 years Most common: 30–60 years		17–60 years
Instability	Possible	Possible	No	No	No
Levels commonly affected	C5-6, C6-7	C4-5, 5-6	Varies	C8-T1	C5-6
Onset	Slow	Slow	Slow	Slow	Sudden
Deep tendon reflexes	Hyporeflexive	Hyporeflexive in UE Hyperreflexive in LE	Hyporeflexive	Unremarkable or hyporeflexive	Hyporeflexive
Diagnostic imaging	Diagnostic	MRI or CT myelography or both	MRI	Radiograph	Diagnostic when clinical signs support

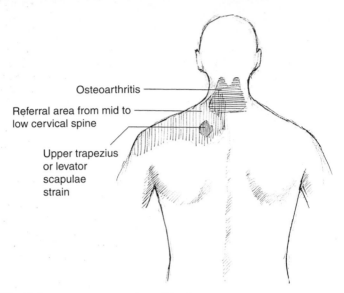

Osteoarthritis

Referral area from mid to low cervical spine

Upper trapezius or levator scapulae strain

FIG. 14-2 Pain location and possible diagnoses.

radiculopathy can take 3 to 6 months for full recovery.[8] It is important for the clinician to determine whether the patient has had successive onsets of similar symptoms in the past, as recurrent injury tends to have a detrimental affect on the potential for recovery. If it is a recurrent injury, the clinician should note how often and how easily, the injury has recurred, and the success or failure of previous interventions.

For the purposes of the examination, it is important to establish a baseline of symptoms so that the clinician is able to determine whether a particular movement aggravates or lessens the patient's symptoms. The patient should be asked to describe the symptoms (pain, paresthesia, numbness, weakness, stiffness), their location (head, neck, shoulder, arm, hand), and their nature (constant, intermittent, or variable). All symptoms presented should be recorded on a body diagram, even those that may initially appear unrelated. If pain is the major symptom, the clinician should attempt to quantify the pain using a pain rating scale. It is also appropriate at this time to establish the patient's goals.

Localized pain generally points to muscle strains, ligament sprains, and facet or disk (degenerative) processes, although these structures commonly radiate pain to the thoracic spine, the periscapular, the upper chest, or upper trapezius (see Table 14-1). Symptoms that radiate into the upper limbs frequently stem from cervical radiculitis, although myofascial radiation patterns occur occasionally.[8] Radicular or referred pain may be accompanied by sensorimotor symptoms.[9] The neurologic examination attempts to differentiate between nerve root and spinal cord compression (see Table 14-2). Other differential diagnostic considerations for upper limb symptoms include thoracic outlet syndrome (see *Special Tests*) and peripheral nerve entrapments.[10]

The cervical zygapophyseal (facet) joints can be responsible for a significant portion of chronic neck pain. Established referral zones for the cervical zygapophyseal joint[11,12] overlap both myofascial and dermatomal pain patterns. Cervical zygapophyseal joint pain is typically unilateral, and described by the patient as a dull ache. Occasionally, the pain can be referred into the craniovertebral or interscapular regions. Pain that is constant in nature and unrelated to rest or activity may be inflammatory in origin, in which case physical therapy, and specifically manual therapy, may be inappropriate.[13] Pain may also be referred to the tip of the acromion or scapular region via the cutaneous branches of the upper thoracic dorsal rami.[14] The rib articulations of cervicothoracic region may produce local pain, or refer pain to the suprascapular fossa or shoulder.[15]

The clinician must determine whether there are musculoskeletal symptoms elsewhere. It is well established that head, neck, and upper thoracic symptoms can be associated with other than local conditions. Neck pain accompanied by widespread musculoskeletal pain raises the strong possibility of fibromyalgia, while neck pain with synovitis of peripheral joints suggests an inflammatory arthropathy such as rheumatoid arthritis.[4] Generalized aching and the presence of trigger points characterize myofascial pain syndromes. In the cervical spine, myofascial pain can occur as a secondary tissue response to an intervertebral disk or zygapophyseal joint injury.[16]

Mechanism

The clinician must determine whether trauma occurred and the exact mechanism. In acute sprains and strains, patients typically relate an activity that precipitated the onset of their symptoms. This may have involved lifting or pulling a heavy object, an awkward sleeping position, a hyperextension injury, or a prolonged static posture. In whiplash-associated disorders, patients generally describe an accident in which they were unexpectedly struck from the rear, front, or side. Rotational injuries can also occur. If there were neurologic symptoms following the trauma (paresthesias, dizziness, ringing in the ears (tinnitus), visual disturbances, or loss of consciousness), more severe damage should be suspected.[17] If the patient reports electric shock-like symptoms when looking downward (neck flexion), the clinician should consider the possibility of inflammation or irritation of the meninges (Lhermitte's sign).[18–20]

The onset of symptoms may provide clues as to the type of tissue involved. Muscle or ligamentous pain may either occur immediately following trauma, or can be delayed for several hours or days.

Clinical Pearl

An insidious onset of symptoms could suggest postural, degenerative, or myofascial origins; a disease process, such as ankylosing spondylitis, cervical spondylosis, thoracic outlet syndrome, or facet syndrome. An insidious onset may also indicate the presence of a serious pathology such as a tumor.

Systems Review

General health questions provide information about the status of the cardiopulmonary system, the presence or absence of systemic disease, and information about medications the patient may be taking, which might impact the examination or intervention. Where applicable, the patient should be examined for central and peripheral neurologic deficit, neurovascular compromise, and serious skeletal injury such as fractures or craniovertebral ligamentous instability. Warning signs in the cervical region include:

- An unexplained weight loss, which could suggest cancer.
- Evidence of compromise to two or three spinal nerve roots.
- A gradual increasing of pain. Normally pain subsides over time.
- An expansion of symptoms in terms of the regions involved. The area of symptoms should decrease with time as healing occurs.
- Spasm with passive range of motion (PROM) of the neck.
- Visual disturbances. Such disturbances could indicate a cranial nerve involvement, or a cranial bleed.
- Painful and weak resistive testing.
- Hoarseness. Hoarseness may be the result of cranial nerve involvement or pharyngeal damage. In cases of a motor vehicle accident, hoarseness may occur as a reaction to the inhalation of the chemicals released by the deployment of the airbag.
- Horner's syndrome.
- T1 palsy (weakness and atrophy of the intrinsic muscles of the hand).
- Side bending away from the painful side causes pain (if this is the only motion that causes pain).

It must also be remembered that every cervical patient, especially the ones with a history of a hyperextension mechanism, are at potential risk for serious head and neck injuries, including compromise of the vertebral artery. The following signs and symptoms demand a cautious approach or an appropriate referral:

- Recent trauma of 6 weeks or less
- An acute capsular pattern of the neck. According to Cyriax,[21] the capsular pattern of the cervical spine is full flexion in the presence of limited extension, and symmetrical limitation of rotation and side bending. The presence of a capsular pattern may indicate arthritis.
- Severe movement loss of head and neck motion, whether capsular or noncapsular
- Strong spasm
- Paresthesia
- Segmental paresis
- Segmental or multisegmental hypo-, hyper- or areflexia (see next section)
- Other neurologic signs or symptoms or both
- Constant or continuous pain
- Moderate to severe radiating pain
- Moderate to severe headaches
- Tinnitus (ringing in the ear)
- History of loss of consciousness
- Memory loss or forgetfulness
- Difficulties with problem solving
- Reduced motivation
- Irritability
- Anxiety and/or depression
- Insomnia

> *Clinical Pearl*
>
> Symptoms that respond to mechanical stimuli in a predictable manner are usually considered to have a mechanical source. Symptoms that show no predictable response to mechanical stimuli are unlikely to be mechanical in origin, and their presence should alert the clinician to the possibility of a more sinister disorder or one of central initiation, autonomic, or affective nature.[13]

Neurologic Symptoms

The systems review must include questions that will elicit any symptoms that might suggest a central nervous system condition, or a vascular compromise to the brain. Cervical myelopathy, involving an injury to the spinal cord itself is associated with multisegmental paresthesias, upper motor neuron (UMN) signs and symptoms such as spasticity, hyperreflexia, visual and balance disturbances, ataxia, and sudden changes in bowel and bladder function (Tables 14-3, 14-4). The presence of any UMN sign or symptom requires an immediate medical referral.

Vascular Compromise

The existence of dizziness or seizures always warrants further investigation. It is not always an easy task for the clinician to determine if the presenting dizziness is caused by a disturbed afferent input from the cervical spine, which can be extremely rewarding to treat, or if the cause is more serious.[5] For example, dizziness provoked by head movements may indicate an inner ear or vertebral artery problem. A history of falling without loss of consciousness (drop attack) is strongly suggestive of vertebral artery compromise.[22] Testing of the vertebral artery should be considered if the observation and history reveal any of the signs and symptoms that have been linked, directly or indirectly to vertebral artery insufficiency, which include:

- Wallenberg's, Horner's, and similar syndromes
- Bilateral or quadrilateral paresthesia
- Hemiparesthesia
- Ataxia
- Nystagmus
- Drop attacks

TABLE 14-3 Clinical Presentation of Cervical Spondylotic Myelopathy

Common symptoms	Common signs
Clumsy or weak hands	Atrophy of the hand musculature
Leg weakness or stiffness	Hyperreflexia
Neck stiffness	Lhermitte's sign (electric shock-like sensation down the center of the back following flexion of the neck)
Pain in shoulders or arms	Sensory loss
Unsteady gait	

Source: Young WF: Cervical spondylotic myelopathy: A common cause of spinal cord dysfunction in older persons. Am Fam Phys 2000;62:1064–1070,1073.

TABLE 14-4 Conditions that Mimic Cervical Spondylotic
Myelopathy on Presentation

- Amyotrophic lateral sclerosis
- Extrinsic neoplasia (metastatic tumors)
- Hereditary spastic paraplegia
- Intrinsic neoplasia (tumors of spinal cord parenchyma)
- Multiple sclerosis
- Normal pressure hydrocephalus
- Spinal cord infarction
- Syringomyelia
- Vitamin B_{12} deficiency

Source: Young WF: Cervical spondylotic myelopathy: A common
cause of spinal cord dysfunction in older persons. Am Fam
Phys 2000;62:1064–1070,1073.

- Periodic loss of consciousness
- Lip anesthesia
- Hemifacial para/anesthesia
- Dysphasia
- Dysarthria

Headache or Facial Pain

A history of headaches may or may not be benign, depending on the frequency and severity. Differential diagnosis is important, especially in light of
the fact that there is considerable overlap between tension headaches, cervicogenic headaches, cervical, trigeminal and glossopharyngeal neuralgia,
Lyme disease, migraines without aura, and temporomandibular joint (TMJ)
dysfunction (see *Orthopaedic Examination, Evaluation, and Intervention*,
pp 223–225).[23] A determination must be made as to the location frequency and
intensity of the headaches, and whether a certain position alters the headache.
If the patient reports relief of pain and referred symptoms with the placement
of the hand or arm of the affected side on top of the head, this is Bakody's
sign and is usually indicative of a disk lesion of the C4 or C5 level.[24]

Cervicogenic headaches, which can be mild, moderate, or severe; tend to be
unilateral; and located in the suboccipital region with referral to the frontal,
retro-orbital, and temporal areas.[25,26] The more serious causes of headache without a history of trauma include spontaneous subarachnoid hemorrhage, meningitis, pituitary tumor, brain tumor, encephalitis (see *Orthopaedic Examination,
Evaluation, and Intervention*, p 1048).

Facial pain can be the consequence of temporomandibular dysfunction,
temporal arteritis, acute sinusitis, orbital disease, glaucoma, trigeminal neuralgia, referred pain, and herpes zoster (see *Orthopaedic Examination, Evaluation, and Intervention*, pp 222–229).

Balance Disturbance

Early indications of a balance disturbance can occur during the history or systems review with correct questioning. A simple question such as "Do you
have difficulty with walking or with balance?" can provide the clinician with
valuable information. Positive responses may indicate a cervical myelopathy
or a systemic neurologic impairment.[27] Myelopathy may occur with compression of the spinal cord, and is more likely to occur at the C5-6 level,
because in this region the spinal cord is at its widest and the spinal canal is at

its narrowest.[28] Usually narrowing of the spinal canal occurs during the end stages of degenerative disease, although structural anomalies such as a narrowed trefoil canal, or shortened pedicles, can result in congenital stenosis.[29] Depending on the cause, the onset of myelopathy can be sudden or gradual. The patient typically complains of symptoms in multiple extremities, and clumsiness when performing fine motor skills.

Tests and Measures

Observation

A major contributor to cervicogenic pain is a lack of postural control because of poor neuromuscular function.[23,30–32] Static observation of general posture, as well as the relationship of the neck on the trunk and the head on the neck is observed, while the patient is standing and sitting, both in the waiting area and in the examination room (see *Orthopaedic Examination, Evaluation, and Intervention*, pp 1048–1049).

The patient should have a smooth cervical lordosis with gentle transition into thoracic kyphosis. A "forward" head (ear forward of the acromion) or accentuated cervicothoracic hump creates a constant flexion moment of the head over the spine.[8] Similarly, flexed posturing at the hips from tight hip flexors results in a compensatory increase in the lumbar and cervical lordoses. Sustained postures, or fatigue overloading of the deep spinal and postural muscles, can result in increased joint compressive forces, and inefficient movement strategies.[33–36]

Thoracic outlet syndrome or other chronic strain patterns can be associated with obesity, or those patients with rounded shoulders, a hunched posture, or overdeveloped anterior chest wall muscles.

Active Range of Motion

The clinical examination of the mobility of the cervical spine should consist of a comparison between active and passive ranges, both in straight planes and with combined motions of the cervical spine. Knowledge of cervical anatomy and kinematics should assist the clinician in determining the structure responsible based on the pattern of movement restriction noted in the physical examination (see *Orthopaedic Examination, Evaluation, and Intervention*, pp 1049–1053). For example, active motion induced by the contraction of the muscles determines the so-called physiologic ROM,[37] whereas passively performed movement causes stretching of noncontractile elements, such as ligaments, and determines the anatomic ROM. Shoulder problems are often confused with a C5 or C6 radiculopathy or with a cervical spondylosis. If muscle strength and reflexes are normal, which makes a radiculopathy less likely, the key differentiating feature is pain with neck movement versus shoulder movement.

The ROM available at the cervical spine is the result of such factors as the shape and orientation of the zygapophyseal joint surfaces, the inherent flexibility of the restraining ligaments and joint capsules, and the height and pliability of the intervertebral disk (IVD).[29] In addition the ROM is influenced by the range available in the craniovertebral joints and upper thoracic joints.

In general, the patient should be able to touch chin to chest with mouth closed (flexion of about 60°), look almost straight up to the ceiling (extension of about 70°), rotate chin to approach the shoulder (rotation of about 80°), and bend the ear toward the shoulder (side bending of about 45°) (Figure 14-3).[8]

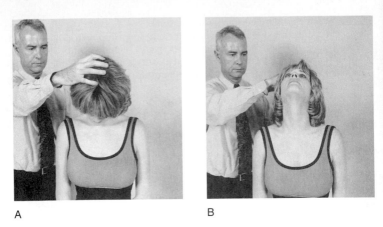

A   B

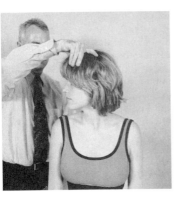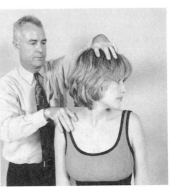

C   D

FIG. 14-3 Cervical active range of motion with passive overpressure and resistance. (*Reproduced with permission from Dutton M: Orthopaedic Examination, Evaluation and Intervention, p 1051 (Fig. 23-10). New York, McGraw-Hill 2004.*)

The inclinometer technique recommended by the American Medical Association may be used for an objective measurement of cervical motion (see *Orthopaedic Examination, Evaluation, and Intervention*, pp 1052–1053).[38] As with other joints in the body, the available ROM typically decreases with age, the only exception being the rotation available at C1-2, which may increase.[37] Considerable emphasis should be placed on the amount and quality of flexion available, and the symptoms it provokes, as flexion is the only motion tolerated well by the cervical spine. McKenzie[6] advocates the addition of neck protrusion and neck retraction to the ROM examination, or to specific motions, to determine if these additions affect the symptoms (see *Combined Motion Testing*).

Each of the motions is tested with a gentle overpressure (see Figure 14-3), applied at the end of range if the active range appears to full and pain free, although, with the exception of rotation, the weight of the head usually provides sufficient overpressure. It is necessary to apply overpressure even in the presence of pain to get an end-feel. If the application of overpressure produces pain, the presence of an acute muscle spasm is possible. Caution must be taken when using overpressure in the direction of rotation, especially if the rotation is combined with ipsilateral side bending and extension, as this can compromise the vertebral artery.[39] The clinician should evaluate the following:

- The quality and quantity of the motion. Quantity and quality of movement refers to the ability to achieve end range with curve reversal and without deviation from the intended movement plane.[40]
- The end-feel
- The symptoms provoked
- The willingness of the patient to move
- The presence of specific patterns of restriction

Combined Motion Testing

As normal function involves complex and combined motions of the cervical spine, combined motion testing can also be used.

Using a biomechanical model, a restriction of cervical extension, side bending, and rotation to the same side as the pain is termed a *closing* restriction. A restriction of the opposite motions (cervical flexion, side bending, and rotation to the opposite side of the pain) is termed an *opening* restriction. Opening restrictions are slightly more difficult to identify in the cervical spine because, frequently, there is no actual restriction of cervical flexion, but rather a restriction of rotation and side bending, along with reproduction of pain on the contralateral side.[41]

The results from these motions are combined with the findings from the history and the single plane motions to categorize the symptomatic responses into one of three syndromes: postural, dysfunction, or derangement. This information can guide the clinician as to which motions to use in the intervention.

Key Muscle Testing

A focused examination of the myotome or "key muscles" is essential in any active patient complaining of neck pain, because a patient can have a pure motor radiculopathy with few or no extremity symptoms. In an athlete, maximal force must be applied when testing the major muscle groups to detect early weakness. There are numerous smaller muscles throughout this area, so resistance needs to be applied gradually. By repetitively loading the patient's resisting muscle with rapid, consecutive impulses, more subtle weakness can be detected. Even if the pressure overpowers the patient, the key is detecting asymmetries in strength or differences from one key muscle to the next.

During the resisted tests, the clinician looks for relative strength and fatigability. The muscles tested below are also used during the Cyriax upper quarter scanning examination. Alternates are given for each "myotome" or key muscle.

Resisted Cervical Rotation   Resisted cervical rotation tests the C2 "myotome."

Resisted Cervical Side Bending   Resisted side bending tests the C3 "myotome."

Scapular Elevators (C2-4)   The clinician asks the patient to elevate his or her shoulders about one half of full elevation. The clinician applies a downward force on both shoulders while the patient resists (Figure 14-4).

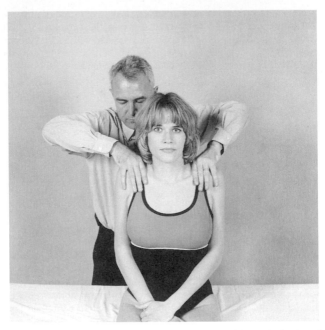

FIG. 14-4   Resisted shoulder elevation. (*Reproduced with permission from Dutton M: Orthopaedic Examination, Evaluation and Intervention, p 1054 (Fig. 23-12). New York, McGraw-Hill 2004.*)

Diaphragm (C4)   The clinician measures the amount of rib expansion that occurs with a deep breath using a tape measure. A comparison is made to a similar measurement at rest. Four measurement positions are used:

- Fourth lateral intercostal space
- Axilla
- Nipple line
- Tenth rib

Shoulder Abduction (C5)   The clinician asks the patient to abduct the arms to about 80°–90° with the forearms in neutral. The clinician applies a downward force on the humerus, while the patient resists (Figure 14-5).

Shoulder External Rotation (C5)   The clinician asks the patient to put the arms by the sides, with the elbows flexed to 90° and forearms in neutral. The clinician applies an inward force to the forearms (Figure 14-6).

Elbow Flexion (C6)   The clinician asks the patient to put the arms by the sides, with the elbows flexed to 90° and the forearms in neutral. The clinician applies a downward force to the forearms (Figure 14-7).

Wrist Extension (C6)   The clinician asks the patient to place the arms by the sides, with the elbows flexed to 90° and the forearms, wrists, and fingers in neutral. The clinician applies a downward force to the back of the patient's hands (Figure 14-8).

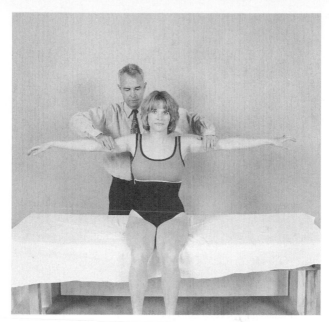

FIG. 14-5 Resisted shoulder abduction. (*Reproduced with permission from Dutton M: Orthopaedic Examination, Evaluation and Intervention, p 1054 (Fig. 23-14). New York, McGraw-Hill 2004.*)

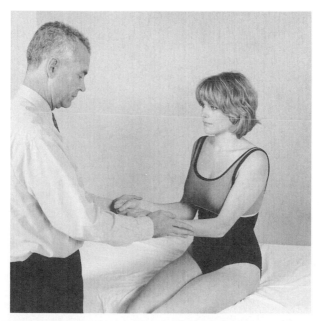

FIG. 14-6 Resisted shoulder external rotation. (*Reproduced with permission from Dutton M: Orthopaedic Examination, Evaluation and Intervention, p 1055 (Fig. 23-15). New York, McGraw-Hill 2004.*)

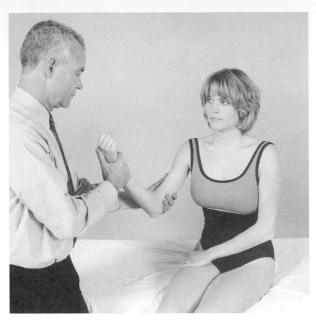

FIG. 14-7   Resisted elbow flexion. (*Reproduced with permission from Dutton M: Orthopaedic Examination, Evaluation and Intervention, p 1055 (Fig. 23-16). New York, McGraw-Hill 2004.*)

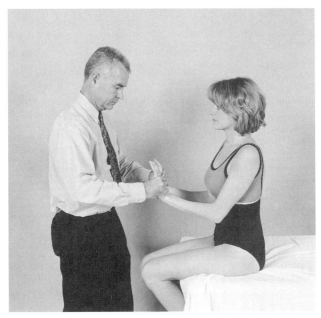

FIG. 14-8   Resisted wrist extension. (*Reproduced with permission from Dutton M: Orthopaedic Examination, Evaluation and Intervention, p 1055 (Fig. 23-17). New York, McGraw-Hill 2004.*)

Shoulder Internal Rotation (C6) The clinician asks the patient to put the arms by the sides, with the elbows flexed to 90° and forearms in neutral. The clinician applies an outward force to the forearms (Figure 14-9).

Elbow Extension (C7) The patient is seated with his or her elbow flexed to about 90°. The clinician stands behind the patient and tests the triceps by grasping the patient's forearms and attempting to flex his or her elbows (Figure 14-10).

Wrist Flexion (C7) The clinician asks the patient to place the arms by the sides, with the elbows flexed to 90° and the forearms, wrists, and fingers in neutral. The clinician applies an upward force to the palm of the patient's hands (Figure 14-11).

Thumb Extension (C8) The patient extends his or her thumb just short of full ROM. The clinician stabilizes the proximal interphalangeal joint of the thumb with one hand, and applies an isometric force into thumb flexion with the other (Figure 14-12).

Hand Intrinsics (T1) The patient is asked to squeeze a piece of paper between the fingers while the clinician tries to pull it away (Figure 14-13).

Muscle Length Testing

Upper Trapezius The patient is positioned supine. The patient's head is maximally flexed, inclined to the contralateral side, and ipsilaterally rotated (Figure 14-14). While stabilizing the head, the clinician depresses the shoulder

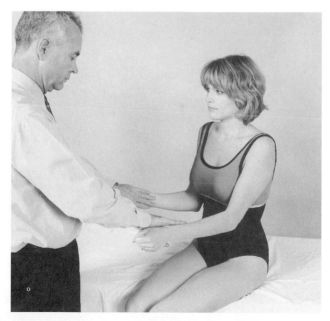

FIG. 14-9 Resisted shoulder internal rotation. (*Reproduced with permission from Dutton M: Orthopaedic Examination, Evaluation and Intervention, p 1055 (Fig. 23-18). New York, McGraw-Hill 2004.*)

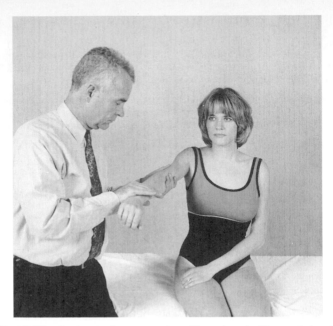

FIG. 14-10 Resisted elbow extension. (*Reproduced with permission from Dutton M: Orthopaedic Examination, Evaluation and Intervention, p 1056 (Fig. 23-19). New York, McGraw-Hill 2004.*)

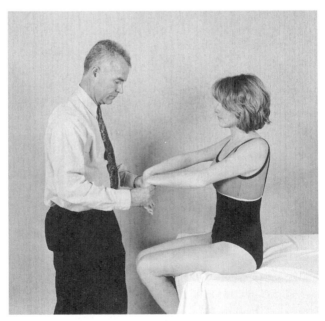

FIG. 14-11 Resisted wrist flexion. (*Reproduced with permission from Dutton M: Orthopaedic Examination, Evaluation and Intervention, p 1056 (Fig. 23-20). New York, McGraw-Hill 2004.*)

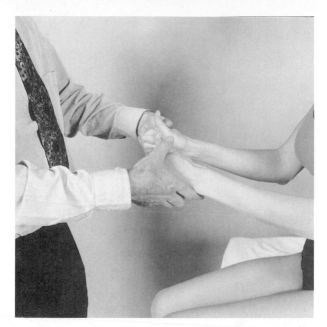

FIG. 14-12 Resisted thumb extension. (*Reproduced with permission from Dutton M: Orthopaedic Examination, Evaluation and Intervention, p 1056 (Fig. 23-21). New York, McGraw-Hill 2004.*)

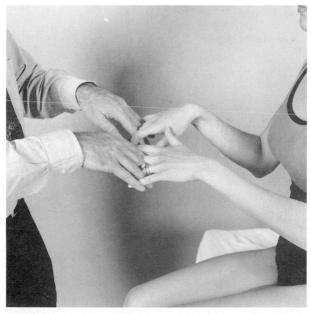

FIG. 14-13 Strength test for finger adductors (hand intrinsics). (*Reproduced with permission from Dutton M: Orthopaedic Examination, Evaluation and Intervention, p 1056 (Fig. 23-22). New York, McGraw-Hill 2004.*)

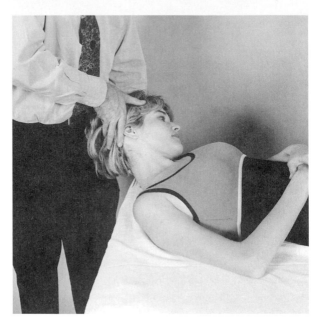

FIG. 14-14   Muscle length test of upper trapezius. (*Reproduced with permission from Dutton M: Orthopaedic Examination, Evaluation and Intervention, p 1058 (Fig. 23-27). New York, McGraw-Hill 2004.*)

distally. A normal finding is free movement of about 45° of rotation, with a soft motion barrier. Tightness of this muscle results in a restriction in the ROM and a hard barrier.

Levator Scapulae   A quick test to determine the extensibility of the levator involves positioning the patient in erect sitting. The patient is asked to side bend the head and to use one hand to stabilize (Figure 14-15). The patient is asked to raise his or her arm out to the side as far as possible (Figure 14-15). An evaluation is made as to the amount of restriction and tension, and whether pain is reproduced. The test is repeated on the other side for comparison.

Sternocleidomastoid   The patient is positioned supine with the clinician standing behind. From this position, the clinician palpates the clavicular and sternal origins of the sternocleidomastoid with the thumb and index finger. Starting from the neutral position, the clinician induces side-flexion of the neck to the contralateral side, and extension of the neck (Figure 14-16). The clinician then rotates the patient's head and neck toward ipsilateral side.

Scalenes   The patient is positioned supine, with the clinician behind. The clinician fixates the shoulder girdle with one hand and with the other hand bends the head to the contralateral side (Figure 14-17). The normal ROM should be about 45°.

Neurologic Examination

The neurologic examination is performed to assess the normal conduction of the central and peripheral nervous systems, and to help rule out such conditions

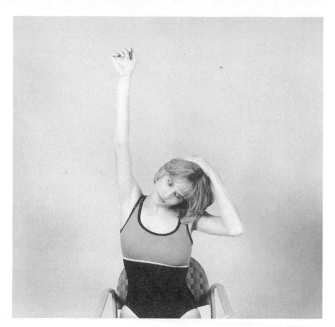

FIG. 14-15 Muscle length test of levator scapulae. (*Reproduced with permission from Dutton M: Orthopaedic Examination, Evaluation and Intervention, p 1058 (Fig. 23-28). New York, McGraw-Hill 2004.*)

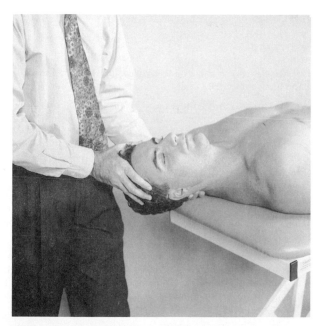

FIG. 14-16 Muscle length test of sternocleidomastoid. (*Reproduced with permission from Dutton M: Orthopaedic Examination, Evaluation and Intervention, p 1059 (Fig. 23-30). New York, McGraw-Hill 2004.*)

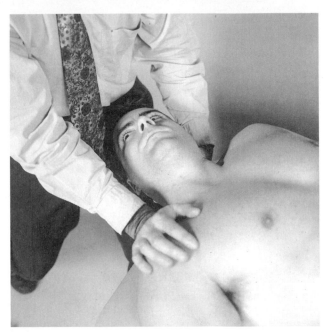

FIG. 14-17   Muscle length test of scalenes. (*Reproduced with permission from Dutton M: Orthopaedic Examination, Evaluation and Intervention, p 1059 (Fig. 23-31). New York, McGraw-Hill 2004.*)

as brachial neuritis and thoracic outlet syndrome. The tests for the thoracic outlet syndrome are described under *Special Tests*.

Sensory (Afferent System)   The sensory examination can usually be eliminated from an otherwise straightforward presentation of neck pain. The wide variation of dermatomal innervation and the subjectivity of the test make the sensory examination less useful than motor or reflex testing. However, if the differential diagnosis of upper-limb dysesthesias includes a peripheral nerve entrapment, then checking for a sensory loss in a peripheral nerve distribution is useful.

The clinician instructs the patient to say "yes" each time he or she feels something touching the skin. The clinician notes any hypo- or hyperesthesia within the distributions. Light touch of hair follicles is used throughout the whole dermatome followed by pinprick in the area of hypoesthesia. Remember that there is normally no C1 dermatome!

Deep Tendon Reflexes   Absent or decreased reflexes are not necessarily pathologic, especially in athletes who have well-developed muscles. Having the patient perform an isometric contraction such as squeezing the knees together during testing can often increase upper-limb reflexes. The following reflexes should be checked for differences between the two sides:

- C5-6: Brachioradialis (Figure 14-18)
- C6: Biceps (Figure 14-19)
- C7: Triceps (Figure 14-20)

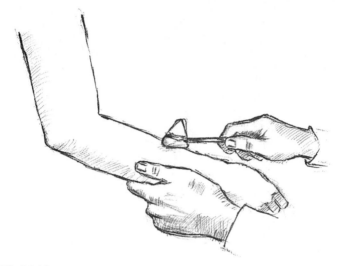

FIG. 14-18   Brachioradialis DTR.

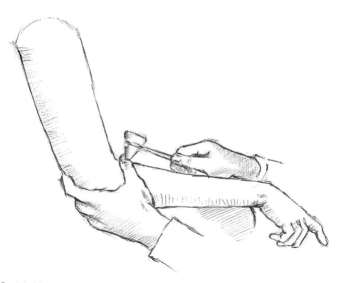

FIG. 14-19   Biceps DTR.

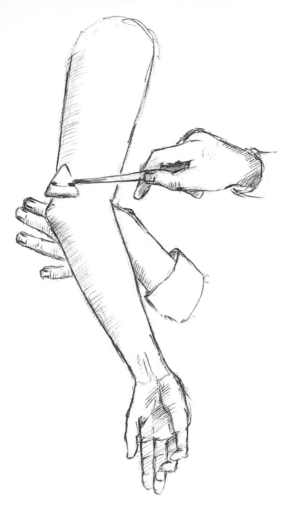

FIG. 14-20 Triceps DTR.

Spinal Cord Reflexes

- Hoffman's (Figure 14-21)
- Babinski (Figure 14-22)
- Lower limb tendon reflexes (Achilles, patellar)

Segmental Palpation

The spinous processes and the interspinous ligaments from C2 through T1 are usually palpable during the assessment of flexion and extension. C7 is usually the longest spinous process, being referred to as the vertebra prominens, although the spinous process of either C6 or T1 might be quite long as well. Exquisite bony tenderness may indicate a fracture; interspinous pain may be

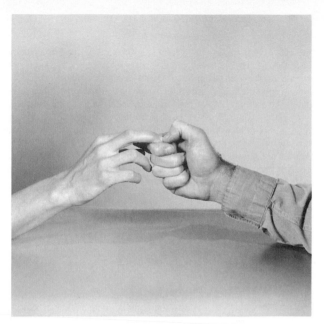

FIG. 14-21 Hoffman's reflex testing. (*Reproduced with permission from Dutton M: Orthopaedic Examination, Evaluation and Intervention, p 1060 (Fig. 23-35). New York, McGraw-Hill 2004.*)

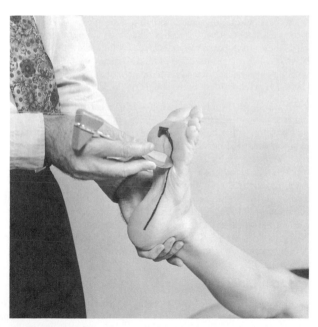

FIG. 14-22 Babinski. (*Reproduced with permission from Dutton M: Orthopaedic Examination, Evaluation and Intervention, p 1060 (Fig. 23-36). New York, McGraw-Hill 2004.*)

consistent with a ligament sprain, which is confirmed by pain in the same area during neck flexion. The facet articulations are approximately a thumb's breadth to either side of the spinous process. Point tenderness here, especially with extension and rotation to the same side, suggests that the patient has facet joint pain. Finally, the surrounding soft tissues of the neck and shoulder girdle should be palpated. Trigger points of the paraspinal and shoulder girdle regions will refer pain to a more distal area. Tender points may indicate a localized muscle strain, in which case contraction of the muscle containing the tender point should cause pain. An area that is tender to palpation but not painful during muscle contraction may represent pain referred from some other area. These patterns can also be identified during range-of-motion testing.

Differing Philosophies

The next stage in the examination process depends on the clinician's background. For those clinicians heavily influenced by the muscle energy techniques of the osteopaths,[42] position testing is used to determine which segment to focus on. Other clinicians omit the position tests and proceed to the combined motion and passive physiologic tests.

Position Testing   The patient is positioned in sitting and the clinician stands behind the patient. Using the thumbs, the clinician palpates the articular pillars of the cranial vertebra of the segment to be tested. The patient is asked to flex the neck, and the clinician assesses the position of the cranial vertebra relative to its caudal neighbor and notes which articular pillar of the cranial vertebra is the most dorsal. A dorsal left articular pillar of the cranial vertebra relative to the caudal vertebra is indicative of a left rotated position of the segment in flexion.[42]

The patient is asked to extend the joint complex, while the clinician assesses the position of the C4 vertebra relative to C5 by noting which articular pillar is the most dorsal. A dorsal left articular pillar of C4 relative to C5 is indicative of a left rotated position of the C4-5 joint complex in extension.[42]

This test may also be performed with the patient supine. However, in sitting one can better observe the effect of the weight of the head on the joint mechanics.

Passive Physiologic Intervertebral Mobility Testing   To test the intersegmental mobility of the midcervical region, the patient's neck is placed in the neutral position of the head on the neck, and the neck on the trunk. Once in this position, lateral glides are performed, beginning at C2 and progressing inferiorly. The lateral glides are usually tested in one direction before repeating the process on the other side. These lateral glides result in a relative side bending of the cervical spine in the opposite direction to the glide. Each spinal level is glided laterally to the left and right, while the clinician palpates for muscle guarding, ROM, end-feel, and the provocation of symptoms. Lateral glides are performed as far inferiorly as possible.

Following this procedure, the areas where a restricted glide was found are targeted, and repetition of the lateral glides is performed in the extended and then flexed positions.

Cervical Stress Tests

Depending on the irritability of the segment, a variety of tests can be used to assess for instability. It is worthwhile starting gently with segmental palpation and gentle posterior-anterior pressures before progressing to other techniques. The patient is positioned in supine and the following tests are performed to examine segmental stability.

Posterior-Anterior Spring Test For anterior stability testing, the clinician places the thumbs over the posterior aspects of the transverse processes of the inferior vertebra of the segment being tested. The vertebra is then pushed anteriorly, and the clinician feels for the quality and quantity of movement. A rotational component can be added to the test by applying force on only one of the transverse processes.

For posterior stability testing, the thumbs are placed on the anterior aspect of the superior vertebra, and the index fingers are on the posterior aspect (neural arch) of the inferior.[43] The inferior vertebra is then pushed anteriorly on the superior one, producing a relative posterior shear of the superior segment.

To keep this test comfortable, the thumbs must be placed under (posterior) to the sternocleidomastoid, rather than over it, and merely function to stabilize the maneuver, exerting no pushing force.

Transverse Shear The transverse shear test should not be confused with the lateral glide tests previously mentioned. The lateral glide tests are used to assess joint motion, whereas the transverse shear test assesses the stability of the segment. While motion is expected to occur in the lateral glide test, no motion should be felt to occur with the transverse shear test.[44]

The inferior segment is stabilized and the clinician attempts to translate the superior segment transversely using the soft part of the metacarpophalangeal (MCP) joint of the index finger.[43] The end-feel should be a combination of capsular, and slightly springy. The test is then reversed so that the superior segment is stabilized and the inferior segment is translated under it.

The test is repeated at each segmental level and for each side.

Distraction and Compression The patient is supine and the clinician stands at the patient's head. The clinician cups the patient's occiput in one hand and rests the anterior aspect of the ipsilateral shoulder on the patient's forehead. The other hand stabilizes at a level close to the base of the neck.[43] A traction-compression-traction force is applied. The clinician notes the quality and quantity of motion.

Pain reproduced with compression suggests the presence of:

- IVD herniation
- A vertebral end plate fracture
- A vertebral body fracture
- Acute arthritis or joint inflammation of a zygapophyseal joint
- Nerve root irritation, if radicular pain is produced

A reproduction of pain with cervical distraction suggests the presence of:

- A spinal ligament tear
- A tear or inflammation of the annulus fibrosis
- Muscle spasm
- Large disk herniation
- Dural irritability (if nonradicular arm, or leg pain is produced)

Functional Assessment Tests

The neck disability index (NDI) is a patient survey instrument (see *Orthopaedic Examination, Evaluation, and Intervention*, p 217). Overall, no instrument is known to be significantly more advantageous than the NDI for the neck. The NDI is a revision of the Oswestry Index and is designed to measure the level of activity of daily living reduction in patients with neck pain. The NDI has been widely researched and validated,[45] and the test/retest reliability has been found to be 0.89.[45]

Special Tests

Temporomandibular Joint Screen As the TMJ can refer pain to this region, the clinician is well advised to rule out this joint as the cause for the patient's symptoms.

The patient is asked to open and close the mouth, and to laterally deviate the jaw as the clinician observes the quality and quantity of motion, and notes any reproduction of symptoms (see *Orthopaedic Examination, Evaluation, and Intervention*, Chapter 24).

Lhermitte's Symptom or "Phenomenon" This is not so much a test, as a symptom described as an electric shock-like sensation that radiates down the spinal column into the upper or lower limbs when flexing the neck. It can also be precipitated by extending the head, coughing, sneezing, or bending forward or by moving the limbs.[19] Lhermitte's symptom and abnormalities in the posterior part of the cervical spinal cord on MRI are strongly associated.

Spurling's Test The Spurling test (foraminal compression test) is useful to evaluate nerve root irritability. The patient's cervical spine is placed in extension and the head rotated toward the affected shoulder. An axial load is then placed on the spine. Reproduction of radicular type pain to the ipsilateral side is a positive test and indicates an irritation of the nerve root. If this maneuver causes only local pain, the discomfort is probably related to irritation of the facet or other posterior element, making a nerve-root process less likely.

Brachial Plexus Tests

- *Stretch test.* This test is similar to the straight leg raise for the lower extremity as it stretches the brachial plexus. The patient is positioned in sitting. The patient is asked to side bend the head to the uninvolved side and to extend the shoulder and elbow on the involved side. Pain and paresthesia along the involved arm is indicative of a brachial plexus irritation.
- *Compression test.* The patient is positioned in sitting. The patient is asked to side bend the head to the uninvolved side. The clinician applies firm pressure to the brachial plexus by squeezing the plexus between the thumb and fingers. Reproduction of shoulder or upper arm pain is positive for mechanical cervical lesions.[46]
- *Tinel's sign.* The patient is positioned in sitting. The patient is asked to side bend the head to the uninvolved side. The clinician taps along the trunks of the brachial plexus using the fingertips. Local pain indicates a cervical plexus lesion. A tingling sensation in the distribution of one of the trunks may indicate a compression or neuroma of one or more trunks of the brachial plexus.[47]

Upper Limb Tension Tests The upper limb tension tests are equivalent to the straight leg raise test in the lumbar spine, and are designed to put stress on the neuromeningeal structures of the upper limb. Each test begins by testing the normal side first. Normal responses include:

- Deep stretch or ache in the cubital fossa
- Deep stretch or ache into the anterior or radial aspect of forearm and radial aspect of hand
- Deep stretch in the anterior shoulder area

- Sensation felt down the radial aspect of the forearm
- Sensation felt in the median distribution of the hand

Positive findings include:

- Production of patient's symptoms
- A sensitizing test in the ipsilateral quadrant alters the symptoms.

Thoracic Outlet Tests   When performing thoracic outlet syndrome tests, evaluation for either the diminution or disappearance of pulse or reproduction of neurologic symptoms indicates a positive test. However, the aim of the tests should be to reproduce the patient's symptoms rather than to obliterate the radial pulse, as more than 50 percent of normal, asymptomatic individuals will exhibit obliteration of the radial pulse during classic provocative testing.[48]

A baseline pulse should be established first, before performing the respective test maneuvers.

- *Adson's vascular test.* The patient extends his or her neck, turns the head toward the side being examined, and takes a deep breath (Figure 14-23). This test, if positive, tends to implicate the scalenes because this test increases the tension of the anterior and middle scalenes, and compromises the interscalene triangle.[49]
- *Allen's pectoralis minor test.* The Allen test increases the tone of the pectoralis minor muscle. The shoulder of the seated patient is positioned in 90°

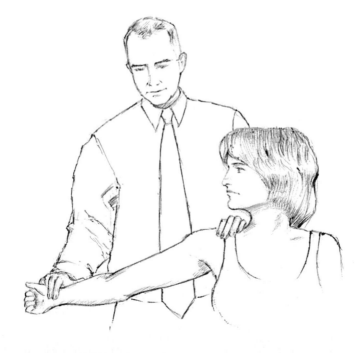

FIG. 14-23   Adson's test.

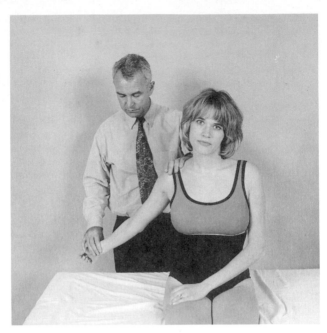

FIG. 14-24 Costoclavicular test. (*Reproduced with permission from Dutton M: Orthopaedic Examination, Evaluation and Intervention, p 1060 (Fig. 23-48). New York, McGraw-Hill 2004.*)

of glenohumeral abduction, 90° of glenohumeral external rotation, and 90° of elbow flexion on the tested side. While the radial pulse is monitored, the patient is asked to turn his or her head away from the tested side. This test, if positive, tends to implicate pectoralis tightness as the cause for the symptoms.

- *Costoclavicular.* During this test, the shoulders are drawn back- and down-ward in an exaggerated military position to reduce the volume of the costo-clavicular space (Figure 14-24).
- *Hyperextension maneuver.* The patient is positioned in sitting on the edge of a table. The clinician grasps the arm on the symptomatic side, passively depresses its shoulder girdle and then pulls the arm down toward the floor, while palpating the radial pulse. The patient is asked to extend the head and to turn away from the tested side. A positive test for thoracic outlet syndrome (TOS) is indicated if there is an absence or diminishing of the pulse.
- *Roos test.*[50] The patient is positioned in sitting. The arm is positioned in 90° of shoulder abduction and 90° of elbow flexion. The patient is asked to perform slow finger clenching for 3 minutes. The radial pulse may be reduced or obliterated during this maneuver, and an infraclavicular bruit may be heard. If the patient is unable to maintain the arms in the start position for 3 minutes or reports pain heaviness or numbness and tingling, the test is considered positive for TOS on the involved side. This test is also referred to as the Hands-up test or the elevated arm stress test (EAST).
- *Overhead test.* The overhead exercise test is useful to detect thoracic outlet arterial compression. The patient elevates both arms overhead, and then

rapidly flexes and extends the fingers. A positive test is achieved if the patient experiences heaviness, fatigue, numbness, tingling, blanching, or discoloration of a limb within 20 seconds.[49]

- *Hyperabduction maneuver (Wright Test).*[51] This test is considered by many to be the best provocative test for thoracic outlet compression caused by compression in the costoclavicular space. The patient is asked to take a deep breath, while the clinician passively abducts and externally rotates the patient's arm.
- *Passive shoulder shrug.* This simple, but effective test is used with patients who present with TOS symptoms to help rule out thoracic outlet syndrome. The patient is seated with his or her arms folded and the clinician stands behind. The clinician grasps the patient's elbows and passively elevates the shoulders up- and forward. This position is maintained for 30 seconds. Any changes in the patient's symptoms are noted. The maneuver has the affect of slackening the soft tissues and the plexus.

DIAGNOSTIC IMAGING

Diagnostic testing is most useful when it affects the intervention. However, if a patient does not progress as expected, diagnostic testing is indicated because the intervention strategy may need to change.

Radiographs

Plain radiographs of the cervical spine should be done with a history of significant trauma involving a direct blow to the neck or head. The basic evaluation includes anteroposterior (A-P), lateral, right and left oblique, and A-P odontoid views. Lateral flexion and extension views can help evaluate ligament stability.

An equivocal bony abnormality or persistent pain out of proportion to the clinical scenario may warrant a computed tomography scan. In most other painful conditions, including mild radiculopathy (motor strength $^4/_5$ or greater), radiographs can be delayed until after a trial of conservative treatment. However, if at 4 to 6 weeks no significant improvement is apparent, the basic plain radiographic evaluation should be done to evaluate for anatomic structures or abnormalities that may be delaying healing.

MRI

Magnetic resonance imaging (MRI) is useful to evaluate for a mechanical compression that may be causing radiculopathy. MRI, however, shows only anatomy and gives no information about the physiologic process that may be causing pain. Correlating the images with the history and physical examination, therefore, establishes whether MRI pathology is clinically relevant. In mild cases of radiculopathy, MRI is not usually needed initially because most patients improve with conservative care. If, however, the patient's weakness progresses, pain is intractable, or 6 to 8 weeks of conservative intervention bring no improvement, an MRI is useful to identify the anatomic lesion.

Needle Electromyography and Nerve Conduction

Needle electromyography (EMG) is useful in evaluating the physiologic state of nerves and muscles in a patient who has upper-limb weakness and is not improving with therapy. EMG can help indicate whether an injured nerve is stable or actively denervating, or whether reinnervation has occurred. It can also help distinguish between nerve root lesions and brachial plexopathy. EMG abnormalities, though, may not be seen for up to 21 days after onset of injury or symptoms, making it less useful in early stages.

EXAMINATION CONCLUSIONS—THE EVALUATION

Following the examination, and once the clinical findings have been recorded, the clinician must determine a specific diagnosis or a working hypothesis, based on a summary of all the findings. This diagnosis can be structure related (medical diagnosis), or a diagnosis based on the preferred practice patterns as described in the *Guide to Physical Therapist Practice*.[52]

REFERENCES

1. Bland JH: Diagnosis of thoracic pain syndromes. In Giles LGF, Singer KP (eds): Clinical Anatomy and Management of the Thoracic Spine, pp 145–156. Oxford, Butterworth-Heinemann, 2000.
2. Maigne J-Y: Cervicothoracic and thoracolumbar spinal pain syndromes. In Giles LGF, Singer KP (eds): Clinical Anatomy and Management of the Thoracic Spine, pp 157–168. Oxford, Butterworth-Heinemann, 2000.
3. Jull GA: Physiotherapy management of neck pain of mechanical origin. In Giles LGF, Singer KP (eds): Clinical Anatomy and Management of Cervical Spine Pain, pp 168–191. London, Butterworth-Heinemann, 1998.
4. Hardin J Jr: Pain and the cervical spine. Bull Rheum Dis 2001;50:1–4.
5. Meadows J: A Rationale and Complete Approach to the Sub-Acute Post-MVA Cervical Patient. Calgary, AB, Swodeam Consulting, 1995.
6. McKenzie RA: The Cervical and Thoracic Spine: Mechanical Diagnosis and Therapy. Waikanae, NZ, Spinal Publications, 1990.
7. Grieve G: Common patterns of clinical presentation. In Grieve GP (ed): Common Vertebral Joint Problems, pp 283–302. London, Churchill Livingstone, 1988.
8. Aptaker RL: Neck pain: Part 1: Narrowing the differential. Phys Sports Med 1996;24:26–38.
9. Dvorak J: Epidemiology, physical examination, and neurodiagnostics. Spine 1998;23:2663–2673.
10. Bush K, Hillier S: Outcome of cervical radiculopathy treated with periradicular/ epidural corticosteroid injections: a prospective study with independent clinical review. Eur Spine J 1996;5:319–325.
11. Dwyer A, Aprill C, Bogduk N: Cervical zygapophyseal joint pain patterns: a study from normal volunteers. Spine 1990;15:453.
12. Aprill C, Dwyer A, Bogduk N: Cervical zygapophyseal joint pain patterns II: a clinical evaluation. Spine 1990;15:458–461.
13. Magarey ME: Examination of the cervical and thoracic spine. In Grant R (ed): Physical Therapy of the Cervical and Thoracic Spine, pp 109–144. New York, Churchill Livingstone, 1994.
14. Maigne J-Y, Maigne R, Guerin-Surville H: Upper thoracic dorsal rami: anatomic study of their medial cutaneous branches. Surg Radiol Anat 1991;13:109–112.
15. Bogduk N, Valencia F: Innervation and pain patterns of the thoracic spine. In Grant R (ed): Physical Therapy of the Cervical and Thoracic Spine, pp 77–88. Melbourne, Churchill Livingstone, 1994.
16. Jull G, Bogduk N, Marsland A: The accuracy of manual diagnosis for cervical zygapophyseal joint pain syndromes. Med J Aust 1988;148:233–236.
17. Hohl M: Soft-tissue injuries of the neck in automobile accidents. J Bone Joint Surg 1974;56A:1675–1682.
18. Jamieson DRS, Ballantyne JP: Unique presentation of a prolapsed thoracic disk: Lhermitte's symptom in a golf player. Neurology 1995;45:1219–1221.
19. Kanchandani R, Howe JG: Lhermitte's sign in multiple sclerosis: a clinical survey and review of the literature. J Neurol Neurosurg Psychiatry 1982;45:308–312.

20. Ventafridda V, et al.: On the significance of Lhermitte's sign in oncology. J Neurooncol 1991;10:133–137.
21. Cyriax J: Textbook of Orthopaedic Medicine, Diagnosis of Soft Tissue Lesions, 8th ed. London, Bailliere Tindall, 1982.
22. Meadows J: Orthopedic Differential Diagnosis in Physical Therapy. New York, McGraw-Hill, 1999.
23. Jull GA, Treleaven J, Versace G: Manual examination: Is pain a major cue to spinal dysfunction? Aust J Physiother 1994;40:159–165.
24. Foreman SM, Croft AC: Whiplash Injuries: The Cervical Acceleration/Deceleration Syndrome. Baltimore, MD, Williams & Wilkins, 1988.
25. Bogduk N: Cervical causes of headache and dizziness. In Grieve GP (ed): Modern Manual Therapy of the Vertebral Column, pp 289–302. New York, Churchill Livingstone, 1986.
26. Radanov B, et al.: Factors influencing recovery from headache after common whiplash. Br Med J 1993;307:652–655.
27. Bradley JP, Tibone JE, Watkins RG: History, physical examination, and diagnostic tests for neck and upper extremity problems. In Watkins RG (ed): The Spine in Sports. St Louis, MO, Mosby, 1996.
28. Herkowitz HN: Syndromes related to spinal stenosis. In Weinstein JN, Rydevik B, Sonntag VKH (eds): Essentials of the Spine, pp 179–193. New York, Raven, 1995.
29. Walsh R, Nitz AJ: Cervical spine. In Wadsworth C (ed): Current Concepts of Orthopedic Physical Therapy—Home Study Course. La Crosse, WI, Orthopedic Section, APTA, 2001.
30. Jull GA, Janda V: Muscle and Motor control in low back pain. In Twomey LT, Taylor JR (eds): Physical Therapy of the Low Back: Clinics in Physical Therapy, p 258. New York, Churchill Livingstone, 1987.
31. Richardson CA, et al.: Therapeutic Exercise for Spinal Segmental Stabilization in Low Back Pain. London, Churchill Livingstone, 1999.
32. Janda V: Muscle strength in relation to muscle length, pain and muscle imbalance. In Harms-Ringdahl K (ed): Muscle Strength, p 83. New York, Churchill Livingstone, 1993.
33. Janda V: Muscles, motor regulation and back problems. In Korr IM (ed): The Neurological Mechanisms in Manipulative Therapy, p 27. New York, Plenum, 1978.
34. Sahrmann SA: Diagnosis and Treatment of Movement Impairment Syndromes. St Louis, MO, Mosby, 2001.
35. White AA, Sahrmann SA: A movement system balance approach to management of musculoskeletal pain. In Grant R (ed): Physical Therapy for the Cervical and Thoracic Spine, p 347. Edinburgh, Churchill Livingstone, 1994.
36. Gossman MR, Sahrmann SA, Rose SJ: Review of length-associated changes in muscle. Phys Ther 1982;62:1799–1808.
37. Dvorak J, et al.: Age and gender related normal motion of the cervical spine. Spine 1992;17:S393–S398.
38. Cocchiarella L, Andersson GBJ (eds): Guides to the Evaluation of Permanent Impairment, 5th ed. Chicago, American Medical Association, 2001.
39. Toole J, Tucker S: Influence of head position upon cerebral circulation. Arch Neurol 1960;2:616–623.
40. Jacob G, McKenzie R: Spinal therapeutics based on responses to loading. In Liebenson C (ed): Rehabilitation of the Spine: A Practitioner's Manual, pp 225–252. Baltimore, MD, Williams & Wilkins, 1996.
41. Ehrhardt R, Bowling RW: Treatment of the cervical spine. In APTA Orthopedic Section—Physical Therapy Home Study Course. 1996.
42. Mitchell FL, Moran PS, Pruzzo NA: An Evaluation and Treatment Manual of Osteopathic Muscle Energy Procedures. Manchester, MO, Mitchell, Moran & Pruzzo, 1979.
43. Lee DG: A Workbook of Manual Therapy Techniques for the Upper Extremity. Delta, BC, Canada, Delta Orthopaedic Physiotherapy Clinics, 1989.
44. Pettman E: Stress tests of the craniovertebral joints. In Boyling JD, Palastanga N (eds): Grieve's Modern Manual Therapy: The Vertebral Column, pp 529–538. Edinburgh, Churchill Livingstone, 1994.

45. Vernon H, Mior S: The neck disability index: a study of reliability and validity. J Manip Physiol Ther 1991;14:409–415.

46. Uchihara T, Furukawa T, Tsukagoshi H: Compression of brachial plexus as a diagnostic test of a cervical cord lesion. Spine 1994;19:2170–2173.

47. Landi A, Copeland S: Value of the Tinel sign in brachial plexus lesions. Ann R Coll Surg Engl 1979;61:470–471.

48. Selke FW, Kelly TR: Thoracic outlet syndrome. Am J Surg 1988;156:54–57.

49. Nichols AW: The thoracic outlet syndrome in athletes. J Am Board Fam Prac 1996;9:346–355.

50. Roos DB: Congenital anomalies associated with thoracic outlet syndrome. J Surg 1976;132:771–778.

51. Wright IS: The neurovascular syndrome produced by hyperabduction of the arms. Am Heart J 1945;29:1–19.

52. Guide to physical therapist practice. Phys Ther 2001;81:S13–S95.

OVERVIEW

In the thoracic spine, protection and function of the thoracic viscera take precedence over segmental spinal mobility (see *Orthopaedic Examination, Evaluation, and Intervention*, pp 1239–1249). Although historically the thoracic spine has not enjoyed the same popularity and attention of other regions of the spine, it can be a significant source of local and referred pain. Differential diagnosis of the various causes of thoracic symptoms is often difficult due to the proximity of the thoracic joints to vital organs, the complicated anatomy, and biomechanics and function of the region. Each thoracic vertebra is involved in at least six articulations. In addition, the posterior thoracic muscles, spinous processes, anterior and posterior longitudinal ligaments, vertebral bodies, zygapophyseal and costotransverse joints, inferior articular process, pars interarticularis, intervertebral disk, nerve root, joint meniscus, and dura mater are all capable of producing pain in this region.[1]

EXAMINATION

The thoracic spine is less commonly implicated in musculoskeletal pain syndromes than the lumbar and cervical spines. However, when pain arises from the thoracic spinal joints, it demonstrates considerable overlap and can refer symptoms to distal regions including the groin, pubis, and lower abdominal wall. The thoracic spine is a common source of systemic pain and the phenomenon of referred pain from viscera poses more diagnostic difficulties in the thoracic spine than in any other region of the vertebral column (Figure 15-1).[1] The algorithm outlined in Figure 15-2 can serve as a guide to the examination of the thoracic spine and ribs (see *Orthopaedic Examination, Evaluation, and Intervention*, pp 1255–1267).

History

The history should include the chief complaints and a pain drawing. The patient should be asked to point to the area of pain. Determining the specific location of tenderness can provide some clues as to the cause as many of the thoracic structures are superficial (Figure 15-3). If the patient has difficulty localizing the pain, the clinician should suspect referred pain as the source. Further clues as to the cause can be provided by determining whether the symptoms are reported to be provoked or alleviated with movement or posture, respiration, eating or drinking, or exertion.

The patient is asked to describe the quality of the symptoms. Thoracic nerve root pain is often sharp, stabbing, and severe, although it can also have a burning quality. Nerve pain is usually referred in a sloping band along an intercostal space.[2] Vascular pain and visceral pain are often described as being poorly localized and achy. Visceral pain tends to be dull, and may be accompanied by nausea and sweating. To help differentiate between visceral pain and musculoskeletal pain, the clinician should focus on the relationship of specific movements or activities. Any information regarding the onset, as well

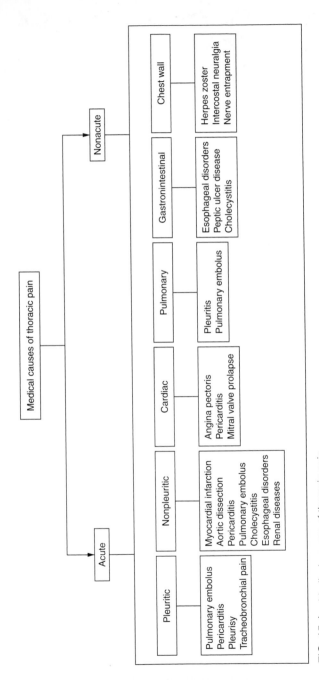

FIG. 15-1 Medical causes of thoracic pain.

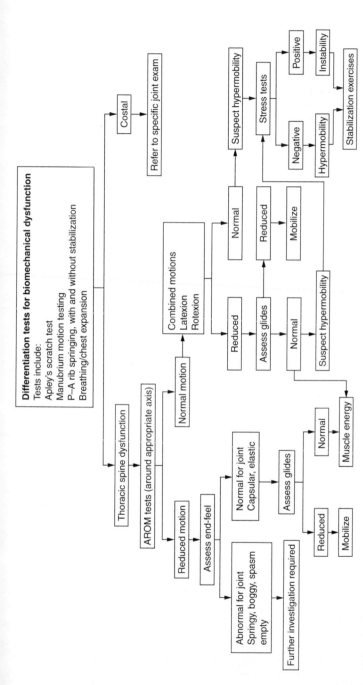

Differentiation tests for biomechanical dysfunction
Tests include:
Apley's scratch test
Manubrium motion testing
P–A rib springing, with and without stabilization
Breathing/chest expansion

Thoracic spine dysfunction

Costal

Refer to specific joint exam

AROM tests (around appropriate axis)

Normal motion

Reduced motion

Combined motions
Latexion
Rotexion

Assess end-feel

Normal

Reduced

Suspect hypermobility

Stress tests

Abnormal for joint
Springy, boggy, spasm
empty

Normal for joint
Capsular, elastic

Assess glides

Reduced

Mobilize

Normal

Suspect hypermobility

Negative

Positive

Hypermobility

Instability

Further investigation required

Assess glides

Muscle energy

Stabilization exercises

Reduced

Mobilize

Normal

FIG. 15-2   Algorithm for examination of thoracic spine and ribs.

461

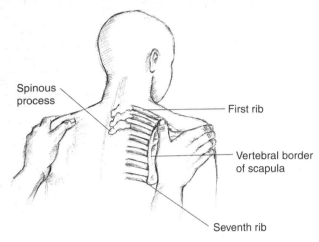

FIG. 15-3   Palpable structures of the thoracic spine.

as aggravating factors, is important, especially if the pain only appears during certain positions or movements, which would suggest a musculoskeletal lesion. Pulling and pushing activities typically worsen thoracic symptoms. Deep breathing or arm elevation tends to aggravate a rib dysfunction. Aggravation of pain by coughing, sneezing, or deep inspiration tends to implicate the costovertebral joint.[3] Chronic problems in this area tend to result from postural dysfunctions.

A sudden onset of pain related to trauma could indicate a fracture, muscle strain, or ligament sprain.

Systems Review

As alluded to, thoracic symptoms may originate from just about all of the viscera. Complicating the diagnosis is that both visceral and somatic afferent nerves transmit pain messages from a peripheral stimulus and converge on the same projection neurons in the dorsal horn. In addition, the thoracolumbar outflow of the autonomic nervous system has its location here. Stimulation of this outflow can lead to the presence of facilitated segments, and trophic changes in the skin of the periphery.[4]

Finally, systemic illnesses such as rheumatoid arthritis and malignancy must be included in the differential diagnosis (Table 15-1).

Nonmusculoskeletal causes of thoracic pain include, but are not limited to:[5]

- A dissecting aortic aneurysm
- A myocardial infarction
- Intercostal neuralgia
- Pleural irritation. When the tissues of irritated pleura are stretched, chest pain can result. This pain can be increased both by breathing, as well as by trunk movements, a situation that could lead the clinician to believe that the problem is musculoskeletal.
- Tumor

TABLE 15-1 Symptoms and Possible Causes

Indication	Possible condition
Severe bilateral root pain in elderly	Neoplasm (The most common areas for metastasis are lung, breast, prostate, and kidney.)
Wedging/compression fracture	Osteoporotic (estrogen deficiency) or neoplastic fracture
Onset–offset of pain unrelated to trunk movements	Ankylosing spondylitis, visceral
Decreased active motion contralateral side flexion painful with both rotations full	Neoplasm
Severe chest wall pain without articular pain	Visceral
Spinal cord signs/symptoms	Spinal cord pressure or ischemia
Pain onset related to eating or diet	Visceral

Questions should be asked with regard to bowel and bladder function, upper and lower extremity numbness, tingling, or weakness, and visual or balance disorders. These symptoms may indicate compromise to the spinal cord, cauda equina, or central nervous system (CNS).

Questions must also be asked about unexplained weight loss, fever, chills, and night pain. These symptoms are often associated with cancer or systemic disease or both, although night pain may just be because the patient has an increased and fixed kyphosis, and needs a softer bed to accommodate the deformity.[6]

Tests and Measures

Observation

The patient should be suitably disrobed to expose as much of this region as is necessary. As a quick orientation to the relationship of the bony structures (see Figure 15-3), the clinician should confirm the following:

- The spine of the scapula is level with the spinous process of T3.
- The inferior angle of the scapula is in line with the T7-9 spinous processes.
- The medial border of the scapula is parallel with the spinal column and about 5 centimeters lateral to the spinous processes.
- The iliac crests are level and symmetrical. One crest higher than the other could suggest a leg length discrepancy, an iliac rotation, or both.
- The shoulder heights are level. A normal variant is that individuals carry their dominant shoulder slightly lower than the nondominant side.
- The smoothness of the thoracic curve.
- *The degree of thoracic kyphosis.* As elsewhere in the spine, posture has an important influence on the available range of motion of the neighboring joints. Conversely, changes in the lumbar posture, such as an excessive lordosis, and changes in the cervical spine such as those rendered by a forward head position, can affect the thoracic spine.
- *Pelvic heights.* A significant leg length discrepancy (greater than 1/2 an inch) can alter the lateral curvature of the spine, and result in compensation.
- *The amount of lateral curvature of the thoracic spine.* Two terms, scoliosis and rotoscoliosis, are used to describe the lateral curvature of the spine. Scoliosis is the older term and refers to an abnormal side bending of the spine, but gives

no reference to the coupled rotation that also occurs. Rotoscoliosis is a more detailed definition, used to describe the curve of the spine by detailing how each vertebra is rotated and side-flexed in relation to the vertebra below.

Scoliosis is never normal, although most cases are idiopathic, manifesting in the preadolescent years.[7,8] An abnormal lateral thoracic curve is described as being structural or functional, and can produce a fixed deformity or a changeable adaptation, respectively, with the rib hump occurring on the convex side of the curve. Persistent scoliosis during forward bending (Adam's sign) is indicative of a structural curve.

- *Chest wall shape.* On the anterior aspect of the thoracic region, the clinician should look for evidence of deformity.
  - *Barrel chest.* A forward and upward projecting sternum increases the anterior-posterior diameter. The barrel chest results in respiratory difficulty, stretching of the intercostal and anterior chest muscles, and adaptive shortening of the scapular adductor muscles.
  - *Pigeon chest.* A forward and downward projecting sternum, which increases the anterior-posterior diameter. The pigeon chest results in a lengthening of the upper abdominal muscles and an adaptive shortening of the upper intercostal muscles.
  - *Funnel chest.* A posterior projecting sternum secondary to an outgrowth of the ribs.[9] The funnel chest results in adaptive shortening of the upper abdominals, shoulder adductors, pectoralis minor and intercostal muscles, and lengthening of the thoracic extensors, and middle and upper trapezius.
- The motion of the ribs during quiet breathing
- Asymmetry in muscle bulk, prominence, or length
- Any lesions, swellings, or scars on the back and chest. This is a common area for the characteristic lesion pattern of herpes zoster (shingles), which follows the course of the affected nerve.

Gait

The analysis of the patient's gait pattern can provide valuable information as to whether his or her condition originates in the spine or lower extremities, and discloses gross weakness of the muscles that affect gait.[10] For example, a decreased arm swing during gait can indicate stiffness of the thoracic segments.

Palpation of the Thoracic Spine

The spinous processes of the thoracic vertebrae are readily palpated (see Figure 15-3), as they are not covered by muscle or thick connective tissue.[10] The landmarks outlined in Table 15-2 may be helpful to determine the segmental level involved.

The spinous processes have varying degrees of obliquity and if they are used as landmarks, this obliquity must be understood and exploited. The areas of spinous process obliquity may be divided into four regions by the so-called "rule of threes" (Figure 15-4).[11]

- *First group of three spinous processes (T1-3).* These spinous processes are level with vertebral body of the same level.
- *Second group of three spinous processes (T4-6).* These spinous processes are level with the disk of the inferior level. This can be estimated at about three finger breadths.
- *Third group of three spinous processes (T7-9).* These spinous processes are level with the vertebral body of the level below.

TABLE 15-2 Anterior and Posterior Palpation Points

Anterior aspect	Posterior aspect
• Suprasternal notch	• Spinous and their associated transverse processes
• Sternomanubrial angle	• T2—level with base of spine of scapula
• Xiphoid process	• Spinal gutter (rotatores)
• Infrasternal angle	• Erector spinae
• Sternochondral junctions	• Rib angles
• Costal cartilage	• Rib shafts
	• Rib shafts and rib joint line of costotransverse joint
	• C6—locate the largest spinous process at the base of the neck, have patient extend their neck. The first spinous process to move anteriorly under your finger is C6.

- The fourth group of three spinous processes reverse the obliquity:
  - T10 is level with the vertebral body of the vertebra below (same as T7-9)
  - T11 is level with the disk of the inferior vertebra (same as T6)
  - T12 is level with its own vertebral body (same as T3)

Palpation of the soft tissues of the region is important. The clinician should note the presence of any tenderness, temperature changes, and muscle spasm.

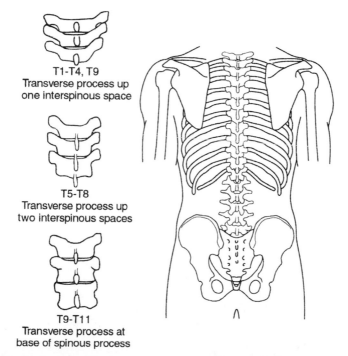

T1-T4, T9
Transverse process up
one interspinous space

T5-T8
Transverse process up
two interspinous spaces

T9-T11
Transverse process at
base of spinous process

FIG. 15-4   The rule of threes. (*Reproduced with permission from Dutton M: Orthopaedic Examination, Evaluation and Intervention, p 1258 (Fig. 26-10). New York, McGraw-Hill 2004.*)

A comparison should be made between the firmness and tenderness of the paravertebral muscles, and their relationship from side to side.

Screening Tests

A few simple screening tests can help differentiate between a rib dysfunction, and a thoracic joint dysfunction.

Rib Spring Test   The patient is positioned in prone and the clinician stands on one side of the patient. Reaching over the patient, the clinician spreads the length of the thumb over the right rib in question and applies a posterior-anterior force. This is the equivalent of a left rotation of the thoracic spine. The clinician then repeats the posterior-anterior force on the rib, except this time, he or she blocks the rotation of the thoracic spine by placing the ulnar border of his or her other hand over a group of left transverse processes. Pain produced with this maneuver implicates the rib as the thoracic spine is stabilized.

Thoracic Spring Test   The patient is positioned as above. Spring testing in a posterior-anterior direction is applied with the palm of the hand with the elbows locked over the spinous processes of the thoracic spine. These spring tests are provocative for pain, but may also be used for a gross assessment of mobility.

Reflex Hammer Test   The patient is prone and the clinician uses a reflex hammer to tap over each spinous process. If tenderness is encountered, especially with a history of trauma to the area, a fracture must be ruled out.

Neck Flexion   The patient is seated and is asked to fully flex the neck. Neck flexion in this position stretches the dura of the cervical and thoracic regions. Pain with neck flexion may suggest such diagnoses as dural irritation or meningitis.

Chest Expansion Measurement   A decreased expansion can highlight the presence of ankylosing spondylitis. It can also be the result of diaphragm palsy (C4), intercostal weakness, pulmonary (pleura) problems, old age, a rib fracture, or a chronic lung condition. Respiratory excursion is measured at three levels using a tape measure placed circumferentially around the chest: at the level of the axilla, the xiphoid level, and at 10th rib level. Comparisons are made between the measurements taken at the position of maximum expiration and the measurement taken at full inspiration. The normal difference between inspiration and expiration is 3 to 7.5 centimeters (1 to 3 inches).[12]

T1-2 Dural Stretch   The patient is seated and is asked to protract and retract the shoulders. Scapular approximation pulls on the thoracic extent of the dura mater via the first and second thoracic nerves.[10] A positive response of symptom reproduction should lead the clinician to suspect a postural dysfunction, an upper thoracic disk protrusion, or a space-occupying lesion, such as a tumor.[13]

Deep Breathing and Flexion   This test can be used for patients who complain of pain with thoracic flexion. The patient is seated with the thoracic spine positioned in neutral. The patient is asked to inhale fully and then to flex the thoracic spine until the pain is felt. At this point, the patient maintains the position of flexion and slowly exhales. If further flexion can be achieved after exhalation, the source of the pain is likely to be the ribs rather than the thoracic spine.[14]

Active Motion Testing

Active range of motion tests are used to determine the osteokinematic function of two adjacent thoracic vertebrae during active motions, to determine which joints are dysfunctional and the specific direction of motion loss.[15] Active range of motion is initially performed globally, looking for abnormalities, such as asymmetrical limitations of motion. A specific examination is then performed on any region that appeared to have either excessive or reduced motion. Various techniques are used to correctly assess each area of the thoracic spine.

Movement restriction of the upper thoracic spine may be secondary to pain or due to adaptive shortening of connective tissue or muscle.[16] Physiologic movement in the thoracic spine decreases with age. Midthoracic hypomobilities are the most common thoracic presentation,[17] with the movement restrictions being more common in the sagittal and frontal planes, particularly extension and side bending.[16] Most of the trunk rotation below the level of C2 occurs in the thoracic spine.

The clinician should look for capsular or noncapsular patterns of restriction, pain, and painful weakness (possible fracture or neoplasm) (Figure 15-5). The capsular pattern of the thoracic spine appears to be symmetrical limitation of rotation and side bending, extension loss, and least loss of flexion. Joint capsular lesions demonstrate a capsular pattern as equal and grossly severe limitation of movement in every direction.[10] With an asymmetrical impairment, such as trauma, the capsular pattern appears to be an asymmetrical limitation of rotation and side bending, extension loss, and a lesser loss of flexion.

The motions of flexion (Figure 15-6), extension (Figure 15-7), rotation (Figure 15-8), and side bending (Figure 15-9) are assessed. Overpressure applied at the end of the available range of motion is used to take the joint from its physiologic barrier to its anatomic barrier. During overpressure, an increase in resistance to motion should be felt. The end-feels should be noted.

Because of the length of the spine in this region, it is important to ensure that all parts of the thoracic spine are involved in the range of movement testing. Motion in the thoracic spine requires a synchronous movement between the intervertebral and zygapophyseal joints, and the rib articulations. Thus, the presence of joint dysfunction or degeneration, or structural changes in the spinal curvature, will influence the amount of available range of motion and the pattern of these coupled motions.[18]

The inclinometer techniques recommended by the American Medical Association are used to objectively measure thoracic motion.[19]

Inspiration/Expiration The motions of the ribs are palpated during breathing. If a rib stops moving in relation to the other ribs during inspiration, it is classified as a *depressed rib*.[11,20] If a rib stops moving in relation to the other ribs during expiration, it is classified as an *elevated rib*.[11,20] Due to the interrelationship of all the ribs, if a depressed rib is implicated, it is usually the most superior depressed rib that causes the most significant dysfunction. In contrast, if an elevated rib is implicated, it is usually the most inferior restricted rib that causes the most significant dysfunction.[11,20]

Resisted Testing

Resistance applied at the point of over pressure can give the clinician an indication as to the integrity of the musculotendinous units of this area. Resistance is applied at the end range of flexion, extension, rotation, and side bending, while the clinician looks for the reproduction of pain, evidence of weakness, or painful weakness. Pain that is exacerbated with motion, but not with resisted isometric contraction suggests a ligamentous lesion.[15]

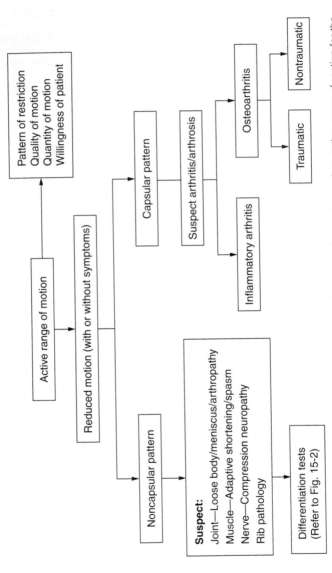

FIG. 15-5 Examination sequence in the presence of symptom-free or incomplete active range of motion for the thoracic spine.

The figure shows the following flowchart:

Active range of motion →

Reduced motion (with or without symptoms) →

- Pattern of restriction
- Quality of motion
- Quantity of motion
- Willingness of patient

Branches into:

Noncapsular pattern

Suspect:
- Joint—Loose body/meniscus/arthropathy
- Muscle—Adaptive shortening/spasm
- Nerve —Compression neuropathy
- Rib pathology

→ Differentiation tests (Refer to Fig. 15-2)

Capsular pattern → **Suspect arthritis/arthrosis**

Branches into:
- Inflammatory arthritis
- Osteoarthritis
  - Traumatic
  - Nontraumatic

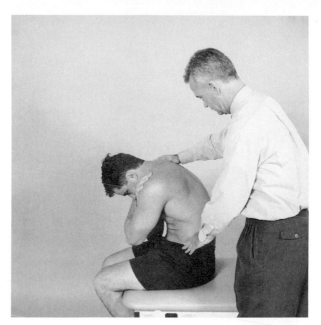

FIG. 15-6 Active thoracic flexion. (*Reproduced with permission from Dutton M: Orthopaedic Examination, Evaluation and Intervention, p 1261 (Fig. 26-16). New York, McGraw-Hill 2004.*)

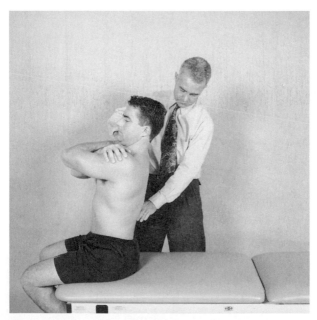

FIG. 15-7 Active thoracic extension. (*Reproduced with permission from Dutton M: Orthopaedic Examination, Evaluation and Intervention, p 1261 (Fig. 26-17). New York, McGraw-Hill 2004.*)

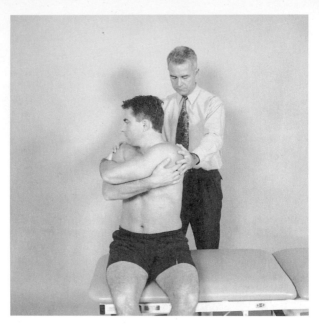

FIG. 15-8   Active thoracic rotation. (*Reproduced with permission from Dutton M: Orthopaedic Examination, Evaluation and Intervention, p 1262 (Fig. 26-18). New York, McGraw-Hill 2004.*)

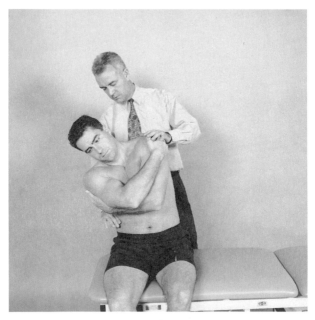

FIG. 15-9   Active thoracic side bending. (*Reproduced with permission from Dutton M: Orthopaedic Examination, Evaluation and Intervention, p 1262 (Fig. 26-19). New York, McGraw-Hill 2004.*)

Static Postural Testing

Thoracic pain of a postural origin is difficult to provoke with active motion and resistive testing. McKenzie recommends placing the patient in a position for approximately 3 minutes to load the structures sufficiently to provoke postural pain.[2,21]

Differing Philosophies

The next stage in the examination process depends on the clinician's background. For those clinicians heavily influenced by the muscle energy techniques of the osteopaths, position testing is used to determine which segment to focus on. Other clinicians omit the position tests and proceed to the combined motion and passive physiologic tests.

Position Testing–Spinal The vertebrae may be tested for positional symmetry. If an *e*xtended, *r*otated, *s*ideflexed (ERS) or *f*lexed, *r*otated, *s*ideflexed (FRS) is present, passive mobility testing will definitively diagnose the movement impairment. The upper thoracic joints (C7-T4) can be assessed using cervical techniques. The following techniques can be used for the T4-12 levels.

- *Example T7-8.* The patient is positioned in sitting with the clinician standing behind the patient. Using the thumbs, the clinician palpates the transverse processes of the T7 vertebra. The joint is tested in the following manner:
  - The joint complex is flexed and an evaluation is made as to the position of the T7 vertebra relative to T8 by noting which transverse process is the most posterior. A posterior left transverse process of T7 relative to T8 is indicative of a left rotated position of the T7-8 complex in flexion.
  - The joint complex is extended and an evaluation is made as to the position of the T7 vertebra in relation to T8 by noting which transverse process is the most posterior. A posterior left transverse process of T7 relative to T8 is indicative of a left rotated position of the T7-8 joint complex in extension.

Once a segment has been localized by one of the above techniques, the arthrokinematics of the segment can be tested using the following passive mobility tests, which incorporate specific symmetrical or asymmetrical motions. Care in the interpretation of the passive mobility tests is important, as local tenderness in the thoracic region is common, especially over the spinous processes owing to the proximity of the dorsal rami over the apex of these bony prominences.[18,22]

Passive Mobility Testing The upper thoracic joints (C7-T4) can be assessed using cervical techniques. For the T4-12 levels, the following techniques can be used.

- *Flexion of the zygapophyseal joints.* The patient is seated at the end of the table with his or her arms folded and hands resting on the shoulders (Figure 15-10). The clinician stands by the side of the patient, and reaches around the front of the patient with one arm and hand. The clinician then applies a slight pressure with the sternum against the patient's shoulder so that the patient is gently squeezed. Using the other hand to monitor intersegmental motion between the spinous processes, the clinician flexes the thoracic spine (see Figure 15-10). The quantity and quality of motion is noted and is compared with the levels above and below.
- *Extension of the zygapophyseal joints.* The patient sits against the raised end of the treatment table with his or her arms folded, and with the superior

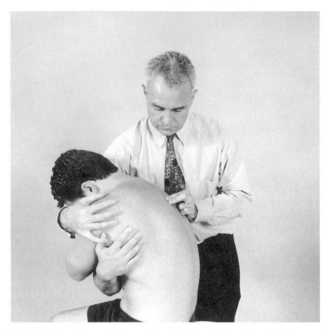

FIG. 15-10   Passive mobility testing—flexion. (*Reproduced with permission from Dutton M: Orthopaedic Examination, Evaluation and Intervention, p 1264 (Fig. 26-21). New York, McGraw-Hill 2004.*)

segment of the joint to be treated over the edge of the table (Figure 15-11). The clinician stands to the side of the patient. With one arm, the clinician supports the patient's head, neck, and upper thoracic spine, with the tip of the monitoring finger in contact with the spinous process of the superior segment of the joint being treated. With the other hand, the clinician grasps the patient's contralateral shoulder and exerts a slight pressure in a superior-posterior direction, which produces a distraction at the joint being treated. While maintaining the distraction, the thoracic spine is extended by pushing gently with the hand that is behind the patient's back and applying the extension force through the clinician's sternum on the lateral aspect of the patient's shoulder (see Figure 15-11). The quantity and quality of motion is noted and is compared with the levels above and below.

Combined Motions of the Zygapophyseal Joints   The patient is seated with one hand on top of one of the shoulders and the other hand under the opposite axilla. The clinician stands to the side of the patient. While palpating the interspinous spaces or the transverse processes of each level with one hand, the clinician wraps the other arm around the front of the patient, under his or her crossed arms, resting the hand on the patient's contralateral shoulder. Crouching slightly, the clinician then places his or her anterior shoulder region against the lateral aspect of the patient's shoulder. Side bending and rotation of the patient's thoracic spine is then performed away from the clinician (Figure 15-12) as the clinician lifts with his or her body. The palpating hand palpates the concave side of the curve.

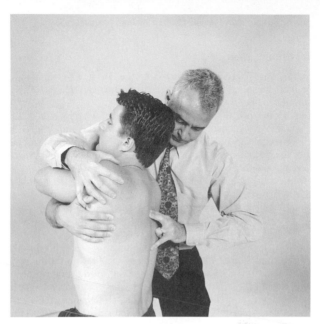

FIG. 15-11 Passive mobility testing—extension. (*Reproduced with permission from Dutton M: Orthopaedic Examination, Evaluation and Intervention, p 1264 (Fig. 26-22). New York, McGraw-Hill 2004.*)

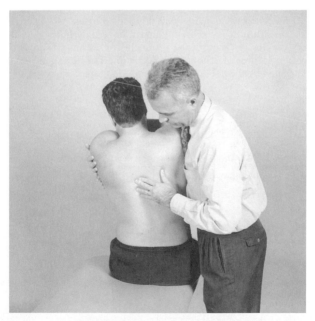

FIG. 15-12 Passive mobility testing—side bending or rotation. (*Reproduced with permission from Dutton M: Orthopaedic Examination, Evaluation and Intervention, p 1264 (Fig. 26-23). New York, McGraw-Hill 2004.*)

Costal Examination

As mentioned, it is well worth postponing the costal (rib) examination until after the thoracic spinal joints have been examined and treated, or the testing of which proved negative.

All the ribs move with complex combinations of what is often described as "pump handle," "bucket handle," and/or caliper motion. Pump handle (anterior) motion is analogous to flexion/extension, bucket handle (lateral rib) motion is analogous to adduction/abduction, and caliper motion is analogous to internal and external rotation.

The first rib has an equal proportion of pump and bucket handle motion, while the sternal ribs have a greater proportion of pump handle motion. Ribs 8 through 10 have a greater proportion of bucket handle motion.

Palpation of the Ribs

The first rib is located 45° medially to the junction of the posterior scalene and trapezius (see Figure 15-3). Palpation of the first rib during respiration can detect the presence of asymmetry. Palpation of the first rib can also be performed during the active motions of cervical rotation and side bending test in patients with suspected brachialgia. The clinician passively rotates the patient's cervical spine away from the involved side. From this position, the neck is side bent as far as is comfortable, moving the ear to the chest. A restriction occurring in the second part of the test indicates a positive test for brachialgia. The transverse processes are roughly level with their own body. The costal cartilages of the second rib articulate with the junction between the sternum and manubrium. The remainder of the ribs should be palpated (Table 15-3). Surface landmarks can be used to locate the other ribs. For example, the fifth rib passes directly under, or slightly inferior to, the male mammary nipples. To palpate the rib angles of the interscapular ribs, the shoulders are positioned in horizontal adduction. The rib angles of 3 through 10 can then be felt about 1–2 inches lateral to the spinous processes.

TABLE 15-3 Rib Dysfunctions

Dysfunction	Rib angle	Intercostal space	Anterior rib	Thoracic findings
Anterior subluxation	Less prominent	Tender	More prominent	—
Posterior subluxation	More prominent	Tender	Less prominent	—
External rib torsion	Prominent and tender superior border	Wide above, narrow below	—	ERS, ipsilateral at the level above
Internal rib torsion	Prominent and tender inferior border	Narrow above, wide below	—	FRS, contralateral at the level above

Source: Ellis JJ, Johnson GS: Myofascial considerations in somatic dysfunction of the thorax. In Flynn TW (ed): The Thoracic Spine and Rib Cage: Musculoskeletal Evaluation and Treatment, pp 211–262. Boston, MA, Butterworth-Heinemann, 1996.

When palpating anteriorly, on the sternum, a rib dysfunction will be highlighted by the presence of asymmetry, and should be compared with the posterior findings. A prominent rib angle on the back and a depression of that rib at the sternum would indicate a posterior subluxation, the reverse occurring in an anterior subluxation, while a rib that is prominent both anteriorly and posteriorly indicates single-rib torsion.

Passive Mobility Examination of Ribs 2–10

Bucket and Pump Handle Motion   For rib elevation, the over pressure is applied by grasping the patient's arm above the elbow and rocking the arm into hyperabduction for the lower ribs ("bucket") and flexion for the upper seven ribs ("pump").

Neurologic Tests

A neurologic deficit is very difficult to detect in the thoracic spine. In this region, one dermatome may be absent with no loss of sensation.[23]

Sensation should be tested over the abdomen; the area just below the xiphoid process is innervated by T8, the umbilicus area is innervated by T10, and the lower abdominal region, level with the anterior superior iliac spines, is innervated by T12.[6] Too much overlap exists above T8 to make sensation testing reliable.

Because of the proximity and vulnerability of the spinal cord in this region, long tract signs (Babinski, Oppenheim, clonus, deep tendon reflexes) should be routinely assessed. A number of tests have been devised to help assess the integrity of the neurologic system in this area.

Beevor's Sign (T7-12)   The patient is positioned in supine, with the knees flexed, and both feet flat on the bed. The patient is asked to raise the head against resistance, coughs or attempts to sit up with the hands resting behind the head.[24] The clinician observes the umbilicus for motion, which should remain in a straight line. If it deviates diagonally, this suggests a weakness in the diagonally opposite set of three abdominal muscles. If it moves distally, weak upper abdominal muscles are suggested, while if it moves proximally this suggests weak lower abdominal muscles. For example, if the umbilicus moves upward and to the right, the muscles in the lower left quadrant must be weak. The weakness may be caused by spinal nerve root palsy, in this case the tenth, eleventh, and twelfth thoracic nerves on the left.[25]

Slump Test   This neurodynamic mobility test is described in Chapter 3.

Abdominal Cutaneous Reflex   To test the abdominal cutaneous reflex, deep stroking over the abdominal muscles is performed using the handle of a reflex hammer. Etching diagonal lines around the patient's umbilicus tests each quadrant. Symmetry of skin rippling or umbilicus displacement or both is observed for.

Lhermitte's Symptom   This impairment is usually considered as a lesion to the cervical spinal cord, and is associated with demyelination, prolapsed cervical disk, neck trauma, or subacute combined degeneration of the cord. Since the denticulate ligaments immobilize the thoracic cord, flexion will produce only limited stretching of the cord, and thus fewer excursions. The Lhermitte's symptom may be present in the thoracic spine with compression of the thoracic cord by metastatic malignant deposits,[26] impairments of the thoracic vertebrae,[27] and thoracic spinal tumor.[28]

Brown-Séquard Syndrome This syndrome is characterized by an ipsilateral flaccid segmental palsy, an ipsilateral spastic palsy below the impairment, and an ipsilateral anesthesia and loss of proprioception, and loss of appreciation of the vibration of a tuning fork (dysesthesia). Contralateral discrimination of pain sensation and thermoanesthesia may be present and are both noted below the impairment. If a neurologic impairment is suspected, the clinician must first exclude a neoplastic process, infectious process or fracture, and then consider a disk protrusion. A nondiskal disorder of the thoracic spine could include a neurofibroma. Some of the signs to help confirm its presence are:

- The patient reports preferring to sleep sitting up.
- The pain, which slowly increases over a period of months, is felt mainly at night and is uninfluenced by activities.
- The patient reports a band-shaped area of numbness that is related to one dermatome.
- The patient reports the presence of pins and needles in one or both feet, or reports any other sign of cord compression.

Functional Outcomes

As yet, there are no specific measures for functional loss and disability in patients with a thoracic dysfunction. Until such time, the reader is recommended to use the neck disability index (NDI) for those dysfunctions that originate above the level of the T4 disk, and the Roland-Morris disability scale[29,30] for pain originating below the T4 disk level.[31]

Imaging Studies

Thoracic spine injuries are difficult to detect on chest radiographs, and dedicated thoracic spine radiographs should be obtained if a fracture is suspected. Lateral radiographs show details of the vertebral bodies in profile, the intervertebral foramen, and the spinous processes. Oblique radiographs show the zygapophyseal joints. Three types of fractures are recognized in the thoracic spine:

1. *Wedge compression.* This type involves the anterior two-thirds of the vertebral body and is a stable fracture.
2. *Sagittal slice.* This type of fracture consists of an anterior fracture/dislocation with compression of the vertebral body below. This injury is unstable and is frequently associated with neurologic compromise.
3. *Posterior dislocation.* This type usually results from a high-energy force and is an unstable injury.

Computed tomography (CT), especially MD (multidetector) CT, is currently the most effective method for examining the extent of the bony injury in the spine. In conjunction with sagittal reconstruction, CT is very useful in demonstrating retropulsed fragments and spinal canal compromise.

MRI is the imaging modality of choice in patients with a suspected neurologic deficit.

EXAMINATION CONCLUSIONS—THE EVALUATION

Following the examination, and once the clinical findings have been recorded, the clinician must determine a specific diagnosis or a working hypothesis, based on a summary of all the findings. This diagnosis can be structure related (medical diagnosis) or a diagnosis based on the preferred practice patterns as described in the *Guide to Physical Therapist Practice*.[32]

REFERENCES

1. Bogduk N, Valencia F: Innervation and pain patterns of the thoracic spine. In Grant R (ed): Physical Therapy of the Cervical and Thoracic Spine, pp 77–88. Melbourne, Churchill Livingstone, 1994.
2. Lyu RK, et al.: Thoracic disk herniation mimicking acute lumbar disk disease. Spine 1999;24:416–418.
3. Murtagh JE, Kenna CJ: Back Pain and Spinal Manipulation, 2nd ed. Oxford, Butterworth-Heinemann, 1997.
4. Lewit K: Chain reactions in disturbed function of the motor system. J Manual Med 1987;3:27.
5. Grieve GP: Common Vertebral Joint Problems. New York, Churchill Livingstone, 1981.
6. Meadows J: Orthopedic Differential Diagnosis in Physical Therapy. New York, McGraw-Hill, 1999.
7. Bradford S: Juvenile kyphosis. In Bradford DS, et al. (eds): Moe's Textbook of Scoliosis and Other Spinal Deformities, p 347. Philadelphia, PA, WB Saunders, 1987.
8. McKenzie RA: Manual correction of sciatic scoliosis. N Z Med J 1972;76:194–199.
9. Sutherland ID: Funnel chest. J Bone Joint Surg 1958;40B:244–251.
10. Bland JH: Diagnosis of thoracic pain syndromes. In Giles LGF, Singer KP (eds): Clinical Anatomy and Management of the Thoracic Spine, pp 145–156. Oxford, Butterworth-Heinemann, 2000.
11. Mitchell FL, Moran PS, Pruzzo NA: An Evaluation and Treatment Manual of Osteopathic Muscle Energy Procedures. Manchester, MO, Mitchell, Moran & Pruzzo, 1979.
12. Moll JMH, Wright V: Measurement of spinal movement. In Jayson MIV (ed): The Lumbar Spine and Back Pain, pp 93–112. New York, Grune and Stratton, 1981.
13. Winkel D, Matthijs O, Phelps V: Thoracic spine. In Winkel D, Matthijs O, Phelps V (eds): Diagnosis and Treatment of the Spine, pp 389–541. Maryland, Aspen, 1997.
14. Evjenth O, Gloeck C: Symptom localization in the spine and extremity joints. Minneapolis, OPTP, 2000.
15. Lawrence DJ, Bakkum B: Chiropractic management of thoracic spine pain of mechanical origin. In Giles LGF, Singer KP (eds): Clinical Anatomy and Management of Thoracic Pain, pp 244–256. Oxford, Butterworth-Heinemann, 2000.
16. Singer KP, Edmondston SJ: Introduction: the enigma of the thoracic spine. In Giles LGF, Singer KP (eds): Clinical Anatomy and Management of Thoracic Spine Pain. Oxford, Butterworth-Heinemann, 2000.
17. Maigne R: Diagnosis and Treatment of pain of Vertebral Origin. Baltimore, MD, Williams & Wilkins, 1996.
18. Edmondston SJ, Singer KP: Thoracic spine: anatomical and biomechanical considerations for manual therapy. Man Ther 1997;2:132–143.
19. Cocchiarella L, Andersson GBJ (eds): Guides to the Evaluation of Permanent Impairment, 5th ed. Chicago, American Medical Association, 2001.
20. Stoddard A: Manual of Osteopathic Practice. New York, Harper & Row, 1969.
21. McKenzie RA: The Cervical and Thoracic Spine: Mechanical Diagnosis and Therapy. Waikanae, NZ, Spinal, 1990.
22. Maigne J-Y, Maigne R, Guerin-Surville H: Upper thoracic dorsal rami: anatomic study of their medial cutaneous branches. Surg Radiol Anat 1991;13:109–112.
23. Magee DJ: Cervical spine. In Magee DJ (ed): Orthopedic Physical Assessment, pp 34–70. Philadelphia, PA, WB Saunders, 1992.
24. Post M: Physical Examination of the Musculoskeletal System. Chicago, Year Book Medical Publishers, 1987.

25. Hoppenfeld S: Orthopedic Neurology—A Diagnostic Guide to Neurological Levels, pp 97–98. Philadelphia, PA, JB Lippincott, 1977.
26. Ventafridda V, et al.: On the significance of Lhermitte's sign in oncology. J Neurooncol 1991;10:133–137.
27. Ongerboer de Visser BW: Het teken van Lhermitte bij thoracale wervelaandoeningen. Ned Tijdschr Geneeskd 1980;124:390–392.
28. Broager B: Lhermitte's sign in thoracic spinal tumour. Personal observation. Acta Neurochir (Wien) 1978;106:127–135.
29. Hudson-Cook N, Tomes-Nicholson K, Breen A: A revised Oswestry disability questionnaire. In Roland M, Jenner J (eds): Back Pain: New Approaches to Rehbilitation and Education, pp 187–204. New York, Manchester University Press, 1989.
30. Roland M, Morris R: A study of the natural history of back pain, part I: the development of a reliable and sensitive measure of disability of low back pain. Spine 1986;8:141–144.
31. Flynn TW: Thoracic spine and chest wall. In Wadsworth C (ed): Current Concepts of Orthopedic Physical Therapy—Home Study Course. La Crosse, WI, Orthopaedic Section, APTA, 2001.
32. Guide to physical therapist practice, Phys Ther 2001;81:S13–S95.

16 | The Lumbar Spine

OVERVIEW

The low back can be the source of pain for many conditions, both serious and benign. Given the numerous causes and types of low back pain (LBP), it is imperative that any clinician examining and treating the lumbar spine has a sound understanding and knowledge of the anatomy and biomechanics (see *Orthopaedic Examination, Evaluation, and Intervention*, pp 1154–1170).

EXAMINATION

Low back pain can arise from both local and distal structures (Table 16-1). The Agency for Health Care Policy and Research (AHCPR) has grouped back pain into three categories: potentially serious spinal conditions, sciatica, and nonspecific back symptoms.[1,2]

- *Potentially serious spinal conditions.* These conditions, suggested by characteristic findings from the history and physical examination (Table 16-2), include spinal tumor, infection, fracture, and the cauda equina syndrome.[3] The seriousness of these conditions obviates the need for immediate for further investigation and referral as they require an intervention directed at the underlying condition.[3] Fortunately, these secondary causes of LBP are much less frequent than the other two categories.
- *Sciatica.* Back-related lower extremity symptoms suggest nerve root compromise. Sciatica is often debilitating but, in most cases, the symptoms abate with conservative intervention.
- *Nonspecific back symptoms.* These include those patients with primary complaints of back pain that suggest neither nerve root compromise nor a serious underlying condition.[3] Conditions in this category include mechanical causes and typically respond well to a conservative approach.

The physical examination of the lumbar spine must include a thorough assessment of the neuromuscular, vascular and orthopaedic systems of the hip, lower extremities, thoracic, low back, and pelvic regions.[4] Figure 16-1 depicts a simple algorithm for decision-making during the examination of the lumbar spine (also refer to *Orthopaedic Examination, Evaluation, and Intervention*, pp 1170–1199).

History

Correct diagnosis of LBP requires a careful history to determine whether the causes are mechanical, or secondary and more threatening. Examples of mechanical causes of low back symptoms include dysfunction of the musculoskeletal and ligamentous structures, including the disk, annulus, and zygapophyseal (facet) joints.[3]

The clinician should establish the chief complaint of the patient, in addition to the location, behavior, irritability, and severity of the symptoms. Although dysfunctions of the lumbar spine can be very difficult to diagnose, the history can provide some very important clues (see *Orthopaedic Examination, Evaluation, and Intervention*, pp 1170–1172). To aid in the provisional diagnosis, the clinician should determine the following:

TABLE 16-1 Causes of Low Back Pain

Condition	Clinical findings
Nonspecific back pain (mechanical back pain, facet joint pain, osteoarthritis, muscle sprains, spasms)	No nerve root compromise, localized pain over lumbosacral area
Sciatica (herniated disk)	Back-related lower extremity symptoms and spasm in radicular pattern, positive straight leg raising test
Spine fracture (compression fracture)	History of trauma, osteoporosis, localized pain over spine
Spondylolysis	Affects young athletes (gymnastics, football, weight lifting); pain with spine extension; oblique radiographs show defect of pars interarticularis
Malignant disease (multiple myeloma), metastatic disease	Unexplained weight loss, fever, abnormal serum protein electrophoresis pattern, history of malignant disease
Connective tissue disease (systemic lupus erythematosus)	Fever, increased erythrocyte sedimentation rate, positive for antinuclear antibodies, scleroderma, rheumatoid arthritis
Infection (disk space, spinal tuberculosis)	Fever, parenteral drug abuse, history of tuberculosis or positive tuberculin test
Abdominal aortic aneurysm	Inability to find position of comfort, back pain not relieved by rest, pulsatile mass in abdomen
Cauda equina syndrome	Urinary retention, bladder or bowel incontinence, saddle anesthesia, severe and progressive weakness of lower extremities
Hyperparathyroidism	Insidious, associated with hypercalcemia, renal stones, constipation
Ankylosing spondylitis (morning stiffness)	Mostly men in their early 20s, positive for HLA-B27 antigen, positive family history, increased erythrocyte sedimentation rate
Nephrolithiasis	Colicky flank pain radiating to groin, hematuria, inability to find position of comfort

Source: Bratton RL: Assessment and management of acute low back pain. Am Fam Phys 1999;60:2299–2308.

- The patient's age
- The patient's occupation
- *The mechanism of injury.* The forces applied to the lumbar spine and intervertebral disk (IVD) vary according to the task or position of the body.

    The onset of the symptoms, how long the patient has had the problem, and whether they have had similar episodes in the past. Low back disorders may be acute, chronic, or recurrent.
- *The location of the pain at present.* Back pain may be localized centrally, unilaterally, or bilaterally. Determining the location of the pain can provide some clues as to the cause (Figure 16-2).
- *The type and behavior of symptoms.* Questions related to the type and behavior of symptoms can help determine the structure involved and the stage of healing. It is important to determine whether the condition is improving or worsening. Constant pain indicates an inflammatory process.

TABLE 16-2 Differential Diagnosis of Low Back Pain

Primary mechanical derangements	Ligamentous strain
	Muscle strain or spasm
	Facet joint disruption or degeneration
	Intervertebral disk degeneration or herniation
	Vertebral compression fracture
	Vertebral end-plate microfractures
	Spondylolisthesis
	Spinal stenosis
	Diffuse idiopathic skeletal hyperostosis
	Scheuermann's disease (vertebral epiphyseal aseptic necrosis)
Infection	Epidural abscess
	Vertebral osteomyelitis
	Septic discitis
	Pott's disease (tuberculosis)
	Nonspecific manifestation of systemic illness
	Bacterial endocarditis
	Influenza
Neoplasia	Epidural or vertebral carcinomatous metastases
	Multiple myeloma, lymphoma
	Primary epidural or intradural tumors
Metabolic disease	Osteoporosis
	Osteomalacia
	Hemochromatosis
	Ochronosis
Inflammatory rheumatologic disorders	Ankylosing spondylitis
	Reactive spondyloarthropathies (including Reiter's syndrome)
	Psoriatic arthropathy
	Polymyalgia rheumatica
Referred pain	Abdominal or retroperitoneal visceral process
	Retroperitoneal vascular process
	Retroperitoneal malignancy
	Herpes zoster

Source: Heffernan JJ: Low back. In Noble J, et al. (eds): Textbook of Primary Care Medicine, pp 1026–1040. St Louis, MO, Mosby, 1996.

Steadily increasing pain, especially in elderly patients may indicate malignancy.[5] Pain that is gradually expanding and increasing is associated with a lesion that is increasing in size such as a neuroma or neoplasm.[5] Pain with movement or sustained positions suggests a mechanical cause of pain.[6]

- *Whether there is a diurnal or nocturnal variation in the symptoms.* Complaints of morning stiffness may indicate an IVD lesion, osteoarthritis, ankylosing spondylitis, or Scheuermann's disease.
- *Activities that have been found to aggravate or relieve the symptoms* (Table 16-3). Classically, the symptoms of lumbar canal stenosis begin or worsen with the onset of ambulation or by standing, and are promptly relieved by sitting or lying down.[3] The symptoms of vascular and neurogenic claudication are also provoked with activity (Table 16-4).

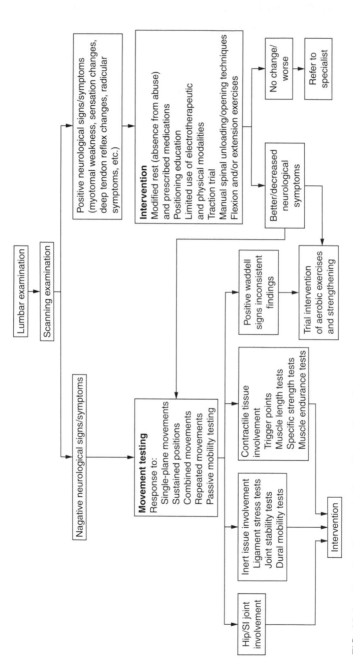

FIG. 16-1 Algorithm for examination of the lumbar spine.

482

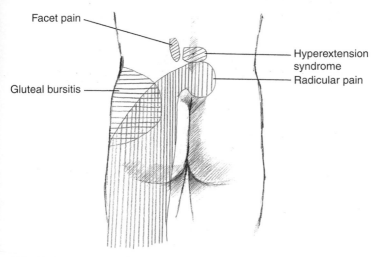

FIG. 16-2 Pain location and possible causes.

- The patient's sleeping position (Table 16-5).
- *The patient's general health and past medical history.* This includes checking for a family propensity for rheumatoid arthritis, IVD lesions,[7] diabetes, osteoporosis, and vascular disease.
- The affect the symptoms have on the patient's work, daily activities, and recreational pursuits
- *Whether the patient is taking any medications.* Pain medications can mask symptoms. If the patient reports taking pain medication prior to the examination, the clinician may not get a true response to pain from the patient.

Systems Review

It must always be remembered that pain can be referred to the lumbar area from pathologies in other regions. For example, reports of pain in the upper lumbar region could suggest the possibility of aortic thrombosis, neoplasm, dental caries, chronic appendicitis,[8] ankylosing spondylitis, or visceral disease (Table 16-2).

TABLE 16-3 Relieving Positions or Movements

Relieving position or movement	Probable cause
Flexion	Facet joint involvement
	Low back strain
	Lateral stenosis
Extension	Disk involvement
	Nerve root irritation (disk herniation)
Rest	Neurogenic claudication

TABLE 16-4 Differentiating the Causes of Claudication

Vascular claudication	Neurogenic claudication	Spinal stenosis
Pain[a] is usually bilateral	Pain is usually bilateral, but may be unilateral	Usually bilateral pain
Occurs in the calf (foot, thigh, hip, or buttocks)	Occurs in back, buttocks, thighs, calves, feet	Occurs in back, buttocks, thighs, calves, feet
Pain consistent in all spinal positions	Pain decreased in spinal flexion	Pain decreased in spinal flexion
	Pain increased in spinal extension	Pain increased in spinal extension
	Pain increased with walking	Pain increased with walking
Pain brought on by physical exertion (e.g., walking)	Pain decreased by recumbency	Pain relieved with pro-longed rest (may persist hours after resting)
Pain relieved promptly by rest (1–5 minutes)		Pain decreased when walking uphill[a]
Pain increased by walking uphill		
No burning or dysesthesia	Burning and dysesthesia from the back to the buttocks and leg(s)	Burning and a numbness present in lower extremities
Decreased or absent pulses in lower extremities	Normal pulses	Normal pulses
Color and skin changes in feet	Good skin nutrition	Good skin nutrition
Cold, numb, dry, or scaly skin		
Poor nail and hair growth		
Affects ages from 40 to over 60	Affects ages from 40 to over 60	Peaks in the seventh decade
		Affects men primarily

[a]Pain associated with vascular claudication may also be described as an "aching," "cramping," or "tired" feeling.
Source: Goodman CC, Snyder TEK. Differential Diagnosis in Physical Therapy. Philadelphia, PA, WB Saunders, 1990.

The clinician should determine whether there has been any recent and unexplained weight loss, night pain that is unrelated to movement, and any changes in bowel and bladder dysfunction (see *Orthopaedic Examination, Evaluation, and Intervention,* p 1172). In addition, any one of the findings listed in Table 16-6 may indicate the presence of a serious pathology.

TABLE 16-5 Preferred Sleeping Positions and Potential Diagnosis

Preferred sleeping position	Potential diagnosis
Sidelying with hips and knees flexed	Lumbar canal stenosis
	Lumbar hyperextension syndrome
	Spondylolisthesis
Prone or supine with legs straight	IVD pathology

TABLE 16-6 Red Flags for Acute Low Back Pain

History	Physical examination
Cancer	Saddle anesthesia
Unexplained weight loss	Loss of anal sphincter tone
Immunosuppression	Major motor weakness in lower extremities
Prolonged use of steroids	Fever
Intravenous drug use	Vertebral tenderness
Urinary tract infection	Limited spinal range of motion
Pain that is increased or unrelieved by rest	Neurologic findings persisting beyond 1 month
Fever	
Significant trauma related to age (e.g., fall from a height or motor vehicle accident in a young patient, minor fall or heavy lifting in a potentially osteoporotic or older patient or a person with possible osteoporosis)	
Bladder or bowel incontinence	
Urinary retention (with overflow incontinence)	

Source: Bigos S et al.: Acute low back problems in adults. Clinical Practice Guideline No. 14. Rockville, MD, Agency for Health Care Policy and Research, 1994.

Tests and Measures

Observation

Observation involves an analysis of the entire patient as to how they move, and respond in addition to the positions they adopt (see *Orthopaedic Examination, Evaluation, and Intervention*, pp 1172–1174). Good posture is subjective and highly variable as it is based on what the clinician believes to be correct. Although spinal alignment provides some valuable information, a positive correlation has not been made between abnormal alignment and pain.[9,10] For example a lateral curvature of the spine (scoliosis) may be functional or may indicate underlying muscle spasm or neurogenic involvement.

The clinician should note any external manifestations of pain, including an abnormal stance. The patient's posture and gait should be examined for sciatic list, which is indicative of disk herniation.

The skin should be inspected for the presence of any cutaneous signs of occult spinal dysraphisms. Occult spinal dysraphisms, or occult spina bifida, are failures in the complete closure of the neural (vertebral) arches, which often have external signs indicating their presence. These signs may include patches of hair, nevi, hemangiomas, or dimples on the lower back in the midline.

Palpation

Palpation of the lumbar spine area should be performed in a systematic manner, and should be performed in conjunction with palpation of the pelvic area, which is described in Chapter 17. The clinician should move superiorly from the L5 spinous process, carefully palpating each segmental level. Evidence of tenderness, altered temperature, muscle spasm, or abnormal alignment during palpation can highlight an underlying impairment.

Posterior Aspect Palpation of the posterior aspect of the lumbar spine is best achieved by placing the patient in a relaxed prone position, or bent over the treatment table.

The clinician moves the index and middle finger quickly down the spine feeling for any abnormal projections or asymmetries of the spinous processes. Any alterations in the alignment of the spinous processes in a posterior-anterior direction, particularly at the L4-5 or L5-S1 segmental level may indicate the presence of a spondylolisthesis.[11] Specific pain elicited with posterior-anterior pressure over the segment serves as further confirmation. Asymmetry of the spinous processes in a posterior-anterior direction may also indicate wedging of a vertebral body or a complete loss of two adjacent IVD spaces.[12] Absence of a spinous process may be associated with spina bifida. Side-to-side alterations in the spinous process may indicate the presence of a rotational asymmetry of the vertebra.[13]

The supraspinous and interspinous ligaments should be palpated. The ligament is usually supple, springy, and nontender. Because this ligament is the most superficial of the spinal ligaments and farthest from the axis of flexion, it has a greater potential for sprains.[14]

Palpation of the transverse processes of T12 and L5 present difficulties. That of L3 is easy to feel, being usually the longest of all transverse processes; it is usually possible to feel those of L1, L2, and L4. That of L5 is covered by the posterior ilium.[15]

The lumbar zygapophyseal joints of each motion segment are located approximately 2 to 3 centimeters (0.8 to 1.2 inches) lateral from the spinous processes. Patients with localized tenderness over the zygapophyseal joints without other root tension signs or neurologic signs may have zygapophyseal joint pain.[16] This can be confirmed if the patient responds well to intra-articular joint injections or to blocks of the medial branches of the dorsal rami.[16,17]

A well-localized and tender point at the gluteal level of the iliac crest, 8 to 10 centimeters from the midline, may indicate the presence of Maigne's syndrome.[18] Maigne's syndrome is characterized by sacroiliac joint, low lumbar, and gluteal pain, with occasional referral to the thigh, laterally or posteriorly.

Normally the skin can be rolled over the spine and gluteal region with ease. Tightness or pain produced with the skin rolling may indicate some underlying pathology.[19] The source of the signs and symptoms is an irritation of the medial cutaneous branch of dorsal rami of the T12 or L1 spinal nerves as it passes through a fibro-osseous tunnel at the iliac crest.[18]

Anterior Aspect The inguinal area, located between the anterior superior iliac spine and the symphysis pubis should be carefully palpated for evidence of tenderness, which may be indicative of a hernia, abscess, sprain of the inguinal ligament, or an infection if the lymph nodes are swollen and tender.

In some patients, the anterior aspect of the vertebral bodies may be palpable with the patient positioned in supine with the hips flexed and feet flat on the bed. Tenderness of the anterior aspect of the vertebral bodies over the anterior longitudinal ligament may indicate the presence of an anterior instability.[20]

Active Movement Testing

Normal active motion (Table 16-7) involves fully functional contractile and inert tissues, and optimal neurologic function.[21–25] Because active range of motion of the lumbar spine demonstrates considerable variability between individuals, the evaluation of the quantity of spinal range of motion has limited diagnostic use. Instead, more emphasis should be placed on the quality of motion and

TABLE 16-7 Normal Active Range of
Motion of the Lumbar Spine

Flexion	40–60°
Extension	20–35°
Side bending	15–20°
Axial rotation	3–18°

the symptoms provoked. However, the direction of the available pain-free range of motion may be helpful in planning the intervention. The capsular pattern for the lumbar spine is normal trunk flexion, a decrease in lumbar extension with rotation and side bending equally limited bilaterally.[26]

A good view of the spine is essential during motion testing and the patient should be disrobed appropriately. When standing, the patient performs flexion (Figure 16-3A), extension (Figure 16-3B), and side bending to both sides (Figure 16-3C and D). If these motions fail to reproduce the symptoms,

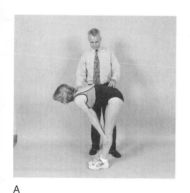

A

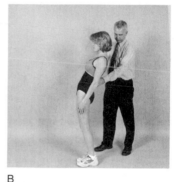

B

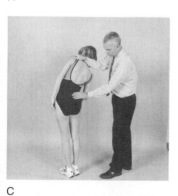

C

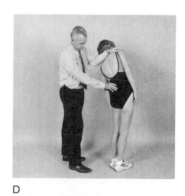

D

FIG. 16-3 Active range of motion of the lumbar spine: (A) flexion, (B) extension, (C) right side bending, (D) left side bending. (*Reproduced with permission from Dutton M: Orthopaedic Examination, Evaluation and Intervention, p 1176 (Fig. 25-21A-D). New York, McGraw-Hill 2004.*)

combined motions are introduced (see *The Six-Position Test*). At the end of each of the active motions, passive over pressure is applied to assess the end-feel, and resistance tests are performed with the muscles in the lengthened positions. The clinician should consider having the patient remain at the end range of each of the motion tests for 10–20 seconds, if sustained positions were reported to increase the symptoms.

If repetitive or combined motions were reported in the history to increase the symptoms, McKenzie[27] advocates the use of sustained or repeated movements of the spine in an attempt to affect nuclear position. These movements are performed to either peripheralize the symptoms, lateral from the midline, or distally down the extremity, or to ideally centralize the symptoms to a point more central or near midline. During the active motions, the clinician notes the following:

- The affect the movement has on the natural curves of the spine
- The presence of any deviations during or at the end of range
- The provocation and distribution of symptoms
- Any gross limitations of motion
- Any compensatory motions

The Six-Position Test

The six-position test is a screening tool that the author has found to be particularly useful with the acute patient in helping to determine the position of comfort for the patient, and for focusing the examination and intervention (see *Orthopaedic Examination, Evaluation, and Intervention*, pp 1178–1180). The patient is positioned in the following positions:

- Supine with the hips and knees extended
- Supine in the hook lying position, with the hips and knees flexed, and feet flat on the bed
- Supine with both knees held against the chest
- Supine with one knee held against the chest and the other leg lying on the bed with the hip and knee extended
- Prone lying with the legs straight
- Prone lying with passive knee flexion applied by the clinician

The results from these tests should provide the clinician with information on the affect of pelvic tilting in a non-weight-bearing position has on the symptoms. If anterior pelvic tilting appears to aggravate the patient's symptoms, initial positions and exercises that promote posterior pelvic tilting are advocated. If posterior pelvic tilting appears to aggravate the patient's symptoms, initial positions and exercises that promote an anterior pelvic tilt are advocated. If both anterior and posterior pelvic tilting appear to aggravate the patient's condition, the patient may not benefit from physical therapy.

Muscle Strength

Key Muscle Testing　　The key muscle tests are used as part of the lower quarter scanning examination as they examine the integrity of the neuromuscular junction and the contractile and inert components of the various muscles (Table 16-8).[26] With the isometric tests, the contraction should be held for at least 5 seconds to demonstrate any weakness. If the clinician suspects weakness, the test is repeated two to three times to assess for muscle fatigability, which could indicate spinal nerve root compromise.

TABLE 16-8 Key Muscles of the Lumbar Quarter
Scanning Examination

'Myotome'	Key muscle tested
L1-2	Hip flexion
L3-4	Knee extension
L4	Ankle dorsiflexion
L5	Great toe extension
L5-S1	Hip extension
	Great toe extension
S1-2	Plantar flexion
	Knee flexion
S3	Intrinsic muscles of the foot (except abductor hallucis)

The larger muscle groups, such as the quadriceps, hip extensors, and calf muscles must be tested by repetitive resistance against a sufficient load to sufficiently stress the muscle–nerve components, usually through full weight bearing.

- *Standing up on the toes (S1-2).* The patient raises both heels off the ground (Figure 16-4). The key muscles tested during this maneuver are the plantar flexors. These are difficult muscles to fatigue, so the patient should perform 20 heel raises unilaterally with arms resting on the clinician's shoulders.

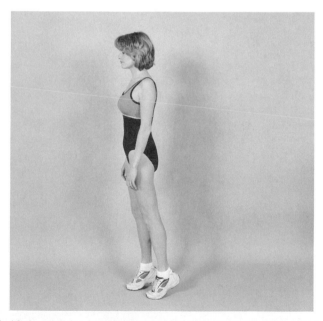

FIG. 16-4   Standing up on toes. (*Reproduced with permission from Dutton M: Orthopaedic Examination, Evaluation and Intervention, p 1181 (Fig. 25-25). New York, McGraw-Hill 2004.*)

- *Unilateral squat while supported (L3-4).* The patient performs unilateral squats while supported. The key muscles being tested during this maneuver are the quadriceps and hip extensors. Neurologic weakness of the quadriceps (L3-4) is relatively rare and often suggests a nondiscogenic lesion such as a neoplasm, especially if the weakness is bilateral.[28]
- *Heel walking (L4).* The patient walks toward, or away from, the clinician while weight bearing through his or her heels (Figure 16-5). The key muscles being tested during this maneuver are the dorsi-flexors (L4). About 40% of IVD lesions affect this level, about an equal amount as those that affect the L5 root.[29]
- *Hip flexion (L1-2).* The patient is seated on the edge of a table. The patient's hip is actively raised off the treatment table to about 30°–40° of flexion. The clinician then applies a resisted force proximal to the knee, into hip extension (Figure 16-6), ensuring that the heel of the patient's foot is not contacting the examining table. Both sides are tested for comparison. An inability to raise the thigh off the table indicates palsy. Palsy at this level should always serve as a red flag, as IVD protrusions at this level are rare, but this is a common site for metastasis.[30] Painful weakness of hip flexion may indicate the presence of a fractured transverse process, metastatic invasion, acute spondylolisthesis, acute segmental articular dysfunction, a major contractile lesion of the hip flexors (rare), or hip joint pathology.
- *Knee extension (L3-4).* The patient is seated. The clinician positions the patient's knee in 25°–35° of flexion and then applies a resisted flexion force at the mid-distal shaft of the tibia (Figure 16-7). Both sides are tested

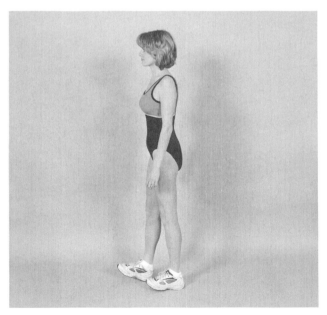

FIG. 16-5 Heel walking. (*Reproduced with permission from Dutton M: Orthopaedic Examination, Evaluation and Intervention, p 1182 (Fig. 25-27). New York, McGraw-Hill 2004.*)

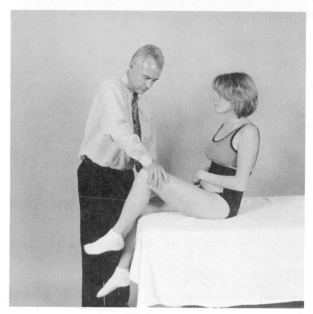

FIG. 16-6 Resisted hip flexion. (*Reproduced with permission from Dutton M: Orthopaedic Examination, Evaluation and Intervention, p 1182 (Fig. 25-28). New York, McGraw-Hill 2004.*)

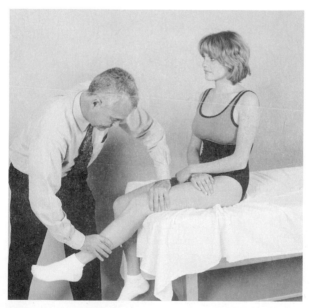

FIG. 16-7 Resisted knee extension. (*Reproduced with permission from Dutton M: Orthopaedic Examination, Evaluation and Intervention, p 1183 (Fig. 25-29). New York, McGraw-Hill 2004.*)

for comparison. An alternate position for testing knee extension can be performed in prone. The patient's leg is positioned in about 120° of knee flexion taking care to do this passively. The clinician rests the superior aspect of his or her shoulder against the dorsum of the patient's ankle and a superior force is applied while the clinician grips the edges of the examining table. Both sides are tested for comparison.

- *Hip extension (L5-S1)*. The patient is prone. The patient's knee is flexed to 90° and the thigh is lifted slightly off the examining table by the clinician, while the other leg is stabilized. A downward force is applied to the patient's posterior thigh while the clinician ensures that the patient's thigh is not in contact with the table. Both sides are tested for comparison.
- *Knee flexion (S1-2)*. The patient is prone. The patient's knee is flexed to 90° and an extension isometric force is applied just above the ankle (Figure 16-8). Both sides are tested for comparison.
- *Great toe extension (L5)*. The patient is supine. The patient is asked to hold both big toes in a neutral position and the clinician applies resistance to the nails of both toes (Figure 16-9) and compares the two sides.
- *Ankle eversion (L5-S1)*. The patient is supine. The patient is asked to place the feet at 0° of plantar and dorsiflexion relative to the leg. A resisted force is applied to move each foot into inversion by the clinician (Figure 16-10) and a comparison is made.

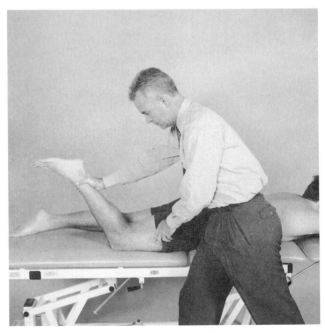

FIG. 16-8 Resisted knee flexion. (*Reproduced with permission from Dutton M: Orthopaedic Examination, Evaluation and Intervention, p 1183 (Fig. 25-30). New York, McGraw-Hill 2004.*)

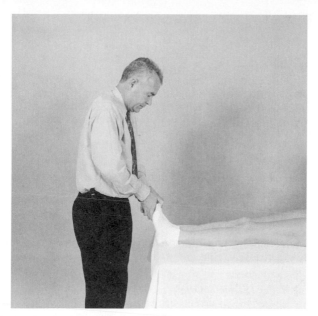

FIG. 16-9 Resisted great toe extension. (*Reproduced with permission from Dutton M: Orthopaedic Examination, Evaluation and Intervention, p 1183 (Fig. 25-31). New York, McGraw-Hill 2004.*)

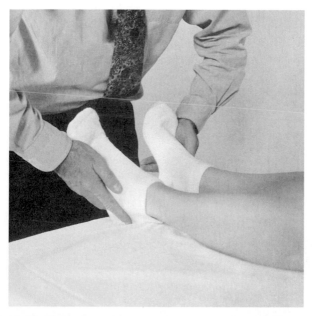

FIG. 16-10 Resisted ankle eversion. (*Reproduced with permission from Dutton M: Orthopaedic Examination, Evaluation and Intervention, p 1183 (Fig. 25-32). New York, McGraw-Hill 2004.*)

Core Stability The term *core* when used with reference to the lumbar spine, describes a point from where the center of gravity for all movement is initiated.[31–35] The static and dynamic structures of the core serve to maintain postural alignment and dynamic equilibrium during functional activities (see *Orthopaedic Examination, Evaluation, and Intervention,* pp 1183–1186).[36] Thus, it is important to examine the core musculature for weakness and adaptive shortening. Of the core muscles, the rectus abdominis has a tendency to become weak, and the quadratus lumborum has a tendency to become adaptively shortened and overactive.[37]

Deep Tendon Reflexes

The reflexes should be assessed and graded accordingly, with any differences between the two sides noted. The tendon should be struck directly once the patient's muscles and tendons are relaxed.

Patella Reflex (L3) The patient is positioned in sitting with the legs hanging freely. Alternatively, both knees can be supported in flexion with the patient positioned in supine (Figure 16-11).

Hamstring Reflex (Semimembranosus: L5, S1 and Biceps Femoris: S1-2) The patient is positioned in prone with the knee flexed and the foot resting on a pillow. The clinician places a thumb over the appropriate tendon and taps the thumbnail with the reflex hammer to elicit the reflex.

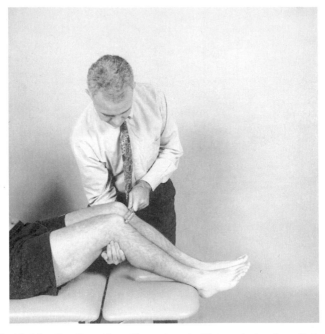

FIG. 16-11 Patellar reflex. (*Reproduced with permission from Dutton M: Orthopaedic Examination, Evaluation and Intervention, p 1186 (Fig. 25-37). New York, McGraw-Hill 2004.*)

Achilles Reflex (S1-2)   The patient should be positioned so that the ankle is slightly dorsiflexed with passive overpressure (Figure 16-12).

Pathologic Reflexes

- Babinski
- Clonus
- Oppenheim

Sensory Testing

The clinician checks the dermatome patterns of the nerve roots, as well as the peripheral sensory distribution of the peripheral nerves (see *Orthopaedic Examination, Evaluation, and Intervention*, pp 68–69). Dermatomes vary considerably between individuals.

Differing Philosophies

The next stage in the examination process depends on the clinician's background. For those clinicians heavily influenced by the muscle energy techniques of the osteopaths, position testing is used to determine which segment to focus on. Other clinicians omit the position tests and proceed to the combined motion and passive physiologic tests.

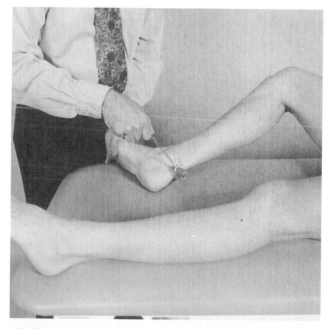

FIG. 16-12   Achilles reflex. (*Reproduced with permission from Dutton M: Orthopaedic Examination, Evaluation and Intervention, p 1187 (Fig. 25-38). New York, McGraw-Hill 2004.*)

Position Testing Position testing is performed with the patient positioned in three positions: neutral (Figure 16-13), flexion (Figure 16-14), and extension (Figure 16-15). The transverse processes are then layer palpated. The findings and possible causes for the position testing are outlined in Tables 16-9 and 16-10.

Combined Motion Testing The combined motion tests of the lumbar spine are used to detect biomechanical impairments. Although combined motion tests do not provide information as to which segment is at fault, they may provide information as to which motion or position reproduces the pain (see *Orthopaedic Examination, Evaluation, and Intervention*, p 1178).[38]

Combined motions can be performed as repetitive motions or as sustained positioning.

Passive Physiologic Intervertebral Mobility Testing [39,40] These tests are most effectively carried out if the combined motion tests locate a hypomobility, or if the position tests are negative, rather than as the entry tests for the lumbar spine (see *Orthopaedic Examination, Evaluation, and Intervention*, pp 1187–1190). Judgments of stiffness made by experienced physical therapists examining patients in their own clinics have been found to have poor reliability.[41]

The passive physiologic movement tests are performed into:

- Flexion
- Extension
- Rotation
- Side bending

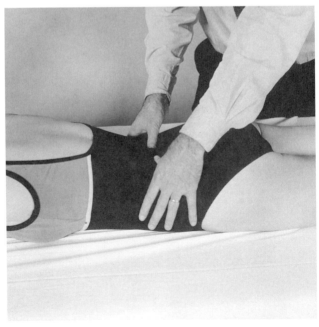

FIG. 16-13 Position testing in neutral. (*Reproduced with permission from Dutton M: Orthopaedic Examination, Evaluation and Intervention, p 1187 (Fig. 25-39). New York, McGraw-Hill 2004.*)

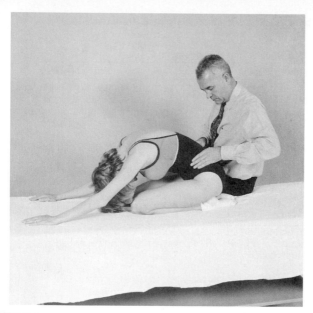

FIG. 16-14   Position testing in flexion. (*Reproduced with permission from Dutton M: Orthopaedic Examination, Evaluation and Intervention, p 1187 (Fig. 25-40). New York, McGraw-Hill 2004.*)

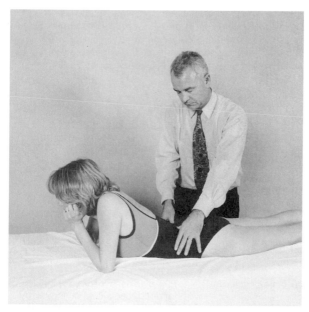

FIG. 16-15   Position testing in extension. (*Reproduced with permission from Dutton M: Orthopaedic Examination, Evaluation and Intervention, p 1188 (Fig. 25-41). New York, McGraw-Hill 2004.*)

TABLE 16-9 Causes and Findings of an ERSL

Causes of an ERSL	Associated findings
Isolated left joint flexion hypomobility	PPIVM and PPAIVM tests in the right flexion quadrant are reduced
Tight left extensor muscles	PPIVM test in the right flexion quadrant is decreased, while the PPAIVM is normal
Arthrosis/-itis left joint/ Capsular pattern	PPIVM and PPAIVM tests are equally reduced in the right flexion and left flexion quadrants
Fibrosis left joint	PPIVM and PPAIVM tests equally reduced in the right and left flexion quadrants
Right posterior-lateral disk protrusion	PPIVM tests in the right extension quadrant reduced with a springy end-feel. Both flexion quadrants appear normal

ERSL = extended, rotated, side flexed left; PPIVM = passive physiological intervertebral motion; PPAIVM = passive physiological accessory intervertebral motion.

The adjacent spinous processes of the segment are palpated simultaneously, and movement between them is assessed as the segment is passively taken through its physiologic range.

Unfortunately, the passive physiologic intervertebral mobility tests do not completely exclude such intersegmental impairments as minor end range asymmetrical hypomobilities or hypermobilities, because the application of side bending or rotation in neutral does not fully flex or extend the zygapophyseal joints, nor is it possible to fully flex or extend both zygapophyseal joints simultaneously. In order to completely flex a particular joint, the opposite joint has to move out of the fully flexed position by utilizing side bending, and allowing the increased superior glide of the superior

TABLE 16-10 Causes and Findings for an FRSR

Causes of an FRSR	Associated findings
Isolated left joint extension hypomobility	PPIVM and PPAIVM tests in the left extension quadrant are reduced
Tight left flexor muscles	PPIVM test in the left extension quadrant is decreased PPAIVM test is normal
Arthrosis/-itis left joint/ capsular pattern	PPIVM and PPAIVM tests in the right flexion quadrant are more reduced than in the left extension quadrant
Fibrosis left joint	PPIVM and PPAIVM tests equally reduced in the right flexion and left extension quadrants
Left posterior-lateral disk protrusion	PPIVM tests in the left extension quadrant are reduced with a springy end-feel. Both flexion quadrants are normal

FRSR = flexed, rotated, side flexed right; PPIVM = passive physiological intervertebral motion; PPAIVM = passive physiological accessory intervertebral motion.

zygapophyseal joint on the opposite joint. The findings and possible causes for the passive physiologic intervertebral mobility testing (PPIVM) are outlined in Tables 16-9 and 16-10.

Passive Physiologic Accessory Intervertebral Mobility Test

Passive physiologic accessory intervertebral mobility tests (PPAIVM) investigate the degree of linear or accessory glide that a joint possesses, and are used on segmental levels where there is a possible hypomobility, to help determine if the motion restriction is articular, periarticular, or myofascial in origin (see *Orthopaedic Examination, Evaluation, and Intervention*, pp 1191–1192). In other words, they assess the amount of joint motion, as well as the quality of the end-feel. The motion is assessed, in relation to the patient's body type and age and the normal range for that segment, and the end-feel is assessed for:

- Pain
- Spasm/hypertonicity
- Resistance
- Spinal locking techniques may be used to help localize these techniques to the specific level, or to a specific side of the segment (see *Orthopaedic Examination, Evaluation, and Intervention*, pp 932–935).

The findings and possible causes for the PPAIVM are outlined in Tables 16-9 and 16-10.

Functional Assessment Tools

The functional assessment tools used for this region are outlined in *Orthopaedic Examination, Evaluation, and Intervention*.

Special Tests

Neurodynamic Mobility Testing   These include the straight leg raise (SLR) test, slump test, the Bowstring tests, the double SLR and the prone knee flexion test (see *Orthopaedic Examination, Evaluation, and Intervention*, Chapter 12). The SLR test should be a routine test during the examination of the lumbar spine among patients with sciatica or pseudoclaudication. A leg elevation of less than 60° is abnormal, suggesting compression or irritation of the nerve roots if associated with symptoms in a dermatomal distribution. A positive test reproduces the symptoms of sciatica, with pain that radiates below the knee, not merely back or hamstring pain.[42] Ipsilateral straight-leg raising has sensitivity but not specificity for a herniated IVD, whereas crossed straight-leg raising is insensitive but highly specific.[42]

H and I Tests   These are biomechanical tests for the spine, testing both the range and the function of the joint complex using combined motions.[28,39,43] The tests get their name from the pattern produced by the motions that make up each test, and are used to detect biomechanical impairments in the chronic or subacute stages of healing.

The *H* test involves the patient initiating with side-flexion of the lumbar spine, followed by extreme forward flexion of the lumbar spine. From this position, the patient maintains the side-flexion, and moves into extreme extension of the lumbar spine. The test is then repeated using side-flexion to the other side, and repeating the flexion and extension motions while maintaining the side-flexion.

The *I* test involves the patient initiating with extreme forward flexion of the lumbar spine, before moving into side-flexion of the lumbar spine. From this position the patient side-flexes the trunk to the other side. The test is then repeated using extreme extension and side-flexion to both sides, and the range of motion and end-feels are compared.

Posterior-Anterior Pressures Posterior-anterior pressures, advocated by Maitland,[44] are applied over the spinous, mammillary, and transverse processes of this region. The clinician should apply the posterior-anterior force in a slow and gentle fashion using the index and middle finger of one hand, while monitoring the paravertebrals with the other hand.

While these maneuvers are capable of eliciting pain, restricted movement, and muscle spasm, they are fairly nonspecific in determining the exact level involved or the exact cause of the symptoms, and have been found to have poor inter-rater reliability in the absence of corroborating clinical data.[45]

Imaging Studies

Plain radiographs are not recommended for the routine evaluation of acute LBP within the first month unless a finding from the history and clinical examination raises concern (Table 16-11). A major diagnostic problem with LBP is that many anatomic abnormalities seen on imaging tests including myelography, computed tomography (CT), and magnetic resonance imaging (MRI) are common in healthy individuals.[46,47] However, if red flags suggest cauda equina syndrome or progressive major motor weakness, the prompt use of CT, MRI, myelography, or combined CT and myelography is recommended.[2] In the absence of red flags after 1 month of symptoms, it is reasonable to obtain an imaging study if surgery is being considered.

Laboratory Studies

Laboratory tests generally are not necessary in the initial evaluation of LBP. However, if tumor or infection is suspected, the physician may order a complete blood cell count and erythrocyte sedimentation rate. Other blood studies, such as testing for HLA-B27 antigen (present in ankylosing spondylitis) and serum protein electrophoresis (results abnormal in multiple myeloma), are performed as warranted.[3]

TABLE 16-11 Selective Indications for Radiography in Acute Low Back Pain

- Age >50 years
- Significant trauma
- Neuromotor deficits
- Unexplained weight loss (10 pounds in 6 months)
- Suspicion of ankylosing spondylitis
- Drug or alcohol abuse
- History of cancer
- Use of corticosteroids
- Temperature ≥37.8°C (100.0°F)
- Recent visit (within 1 month) for same problem and no improvement
- Patient seeking compensation for back pain

Sources: Bigos S, et al.: Acute low back problems in adults. Clinical Practice Guideline No. 14. Rockville, MD, Agency for Health Care Policy and Research, 1994.
Deyo RA, Diehl AK: Lumbar spine films in primary care: Current use and effects of selective ordering criteria. J Gen Intern Med 1986;1:20–25.

TABLE 16-12 Reduced Movement

Myofascial	Joint/pericapsular
Cause	
Muscle shortening (scars, contracture, adaptive)	Capsular or ligamentous shortening caused by:
	Scars
	Adaptation to a chronically shortened position
	Joint surface adhesions
Findings	
Reduced movement or hypomobility may have an insidious or sudden onset. The presence or absence of pain depends on the level of chemical and/or mechanical irritation of the local nociceptors, which in turn is a function of the stage of healing. Pain is usually aggravated with movement and alleviated with rest.	Reduced movement or hypomobility may have an insidious or sudden onset. The presence or absence of pain depends on the level of chemical and/or mechanical irritation of the local nociceptors, which in turn is a function of the stage of healing. Pain is usually aggravated with movement and alleviated with rest.
Negative scan	Negative scan
PPIVM and PAIVM Findings:	*PPIVM and PAIVM Findings*:
Reduced gross PPIVM but PPAIVM normal	Reduced gross PPIVM and PPAIVM
Intervention:	*Intervention*:
Muscle relaxation techniques	Joint mobilizations at specific level
Transverse frictions	
Stretches	

Pericapsular/arthritis	Disk protrusion
Cause	
Degenerative or degradative changes	Cumulative stress
	Low-level but prolonged overuse
	Sudden macrotrauma
Findings	
Negative scan	Positive scan
Reduces gross PPIVM in all directions except flexion	Key muscle fatigable weakness
Active motion restricted in a capsular pattern (decreased extension and equal limitation of rotation and side-flexion)	Hyporeflexive DTRs
	Sensory changes in dermatomal distribution
	Subjective complaints of radicular pain
PPIVM and PAIVM Findings:	*PPIVM and PAIVM Findings*:
Reduced gross PPIVM, but PPAIVM normal	Reduced gross PPIVM and PPAIVM
Intervention:	*Intervention*:
Capsular/muscle stretching	1. Traction
Active exercises/PREs	2. Active exercises in to spinal extension
Anti-inflammatory modalities if necessary	Positioning
Joint protection techniques	

EXAMINATION CONCLUSIONS—THE EVALUATION

Following the examination, and once the clinical findings have been recorded, the clinician must determine a specific diagnosis or a working hypothesis, based on a summary of all the findings. This diagnosis can be structure related (medical diagnosis), or a diagnosis based on the preferred practice patterns as described in the *Guide to Physical Therapist Practice*.[48] Tables 16-12 and 16-13 summarize the typical findings in a patient with a biomechanical diagnosis, highlighting both the similarities and the differences between each.

TABLE 16-13 Excessive Movement

Hypermobility	Instability
Causes	
Cumulative stress caused by neighboring hypomobility	Sudden macrotrauma (ligamentous)
Low-level but prolonged overuse	Hypermobility allowed to progress (ligamentous)
Sudden macrotrauma that is not enough to produce instability	Degeneration of interposing hyaline or fibrocartilage (articular)
Findings	
Subjective complaints of "catching." Good days and bad days. Symptoms aggravated with sustained positions	Subjective complaints of "catching." Good days and bad days. Symptoms aggravated with sustained positions
Negative scan	Negative scan
PPIVM Findings:	*PPIVM Findings*:
Increase in gross PPIVM with pain at end range	Increase in gross PPIVM with pain at end range
	Presence of nonphysiologic movement (positive stress test)
	Recurrent subluxations
Intervention:	*Intervention*: falls into three areas:
Educate the patient to avoid excessive range	• Global stabilization
Take stress off joint (mobilize hypomobility)	Educate patient to stay out of activities likely to take him or her into the instability
Anti-inflammatory modalities if necessary	Total body neuromuscular movement pattern re-education
Stabilize if absolutely necessary	Work or sports conditioning and rehabilitation
	• Local stabilization
	Muscular splinting of the region (lifting techniques, twisting on feet, chin tucking when lifting)
	Bracing with supports (collars, corsets, splints, and braces)
	Regional neuromuscular movement pattern re-education
	Segmental stabilization
	Proprioceptive neuromuscular facilitation (PNF) and active exercises to the segment

REFERENCES

1. Bigos S, et al.: Acute low back problems in adults. Clinical Practice Guideline No. 14. Rockville, MD, Agency for Health Care Policy and Research, 1994.
2. Bigos S, et al.: Acute Low Back Problems in Adults. AHCPR Publication 95–0642. Rockville, MD, Agency for Health Care Policy and Research, Public Health Service, U.S. Department of Health and Human Services, 1994.
3. Bratton RL: Assessment and management of acute low back pain. Am Fam Physician 1999;60:2299–2308.
4. Jermyn RT: A nonsurgical approach to low back pain. JAOA 2001;101 (Suppl):S6–S11.
5. Ombregt L, et al.: In Ombregt L (ed): A System of Orthopaedic Medicine. London, WB Saunders, 1995.
6. Donelson R: The McKenzie approach to evaluating and treating low back pain. Orthop Rev 1990;19:681–686.
7. Matsui H, et al.: Familial predisposition, clustering for juvenile lumbar disk herniation. Spine 1992;17:1323–1328.
8. Drezner JA, Harmon KG: Chronic appendicitis presenting as low back pain in a recreational athlete. Clin J Sport Med 2002;12:184–186.
9. Biering-Sorenson F: Low back trouble in a general population of 30-, 40-, 50- and 60-year-old men and women: study design, representiveness and basic results. Dan Med Bull 1982;29:289–299.
10. Magora A: Investigation of the relation between low back pain and occupation: 4. physical requirements: bending, rotation, reaching and sudden maximal effort. Scand J Rehabil Med 1973;5:186–190.
11. Nachemson A, Bigos SJ: The low back. In Cruess RL, Rennie WRJ (eds): Adult Orthopaedics, pp 843–938. New York, Churchill Livingstone, 1984.
12. Ombregt L, et al.: Clinical examination of the lumbar spine. In Ombregt L, et al. (eds): A System of Orthopaedic Medicine, pp 577–611. London, WB Saunders, 1995.
13. Sahrmann SA: Diagnosis and Treatment of Movement Impairment Syndromes. St Louis, MO, Mosby, 2001.
14. Kapandji IA: The Physiology of the Joints, the Trunk and Vertebral Column. New York, Churchill Livingstone, 1991.
15. Bourdillon JF: Spinal Manipulation, 3rd ed. London, Heinemann, 1982.
16. Fukui S, et al.: Distribution of referred pain from the lumbar zygapophyseal joints and dorsal rami. Clin J Pain 1997;13:303–307.
17. Robert CM, Thomas H, Tery T: Facet joint injection and facet nerve block: a randomized comparison in 86 patients with chronic low back pain. Pain 1992; 49:325–328.
18. Maigne R: Diagnosis and Treatment of pain of Vertebral Origin. Baltimore, MD, Williams & Wilkins, 1996.
19. Greenman PE: Principles of Manual Medicine, 2nd ed. Baltimore, MD, Williams & Wilkins, 1996.
20. O'Sullivan PB: Lumbar segmental "instability": clinical presentation and specific stabilizing exercise management. Man Ther 2000;5:2–12.
21. Allbrook D: Movements of the lumbar spinal column. J Bone Joint Surg 1957;39B:339–345.
22. Ng JK, et al.: Range of motion and lordosis of the lumbar spine: reliability of measurement and normative values. Spine 2001;26:53–60.
23. Pearcy M, Portek I, Shepherd J: Three-dimensional analysis of normal movement in the lumbar spine. Spine 1984;9:294–297.
24. Pearcy M, Tibrewal SB: Axial rotation and lateral bending in the normal lumbar spine measured by three-dimensional radiography. Spine 1984;9:582.
25. Troup JDG, Hood CA, Chapman AE: Measurements of the sagittal mobility of the lumbar spine and hips. Ann Phys Med 1967;9:308–321.
26. Cyriax J: Textbook of Orthopaedic Medicine, Diagnosis of Soft Tissue Lesions. 8th ed. London, Bailliere Tindall, 1982.

27. McKenzie RA: The Lumbar Spine: Mechanical Diagnosis and Therapy. Waikanae, NZ, Spinal Publication, 1981.
28. Meadows J: Orthopedic Differential Diagnosis in Physical Therapy. New York, McGraw-Hill, 1999.
29. Saal JA: Natural history and nonoperative treatment of lumbar disk herniation. Spine 1996;21:2S–9S.
30. Seichi A, et al.: Intraoperative radiation therapy for metastatic spinal tumors. Spine 1999;24:470–473, discussion 474–475.
31. Gracovetsky S, Farfan HF: The optimum spine. Spine 1986;11:543.
32. Gracovetsky S, Farfan HF, Helleur C: The abdominal mechanism. Spine 1985; 10:317–324.
33. Aaron G: The use of stabilization training in the rehabilitation of the athlete. In Sports Physical Therapy Home Study Course. La Crosse, WI, Sports Physical Therapy Section, APTA, 1996.
34. Panjabi M et al.: Spinal stability and intersegmental muscle forces. A biomechanical model. Spine 1989;14:194–199.
35. Panjabi MM: The stabilizing system of the spine. Part 1. Function, Dysfunction Adaption and Enhancement. J Spinal Disord 1992;5:383–389.
36. Clark MA: Integrated Training for the New Millenium. Thousand Oaks, CA, National Academy of Sports Medicine, 2001.
37. Vasilyeva LF, Lewit K: Diagnosis of muscular dysfunction by inspection. In Liebenson C (ed): Rehabilitation of the Spine: A Practitioner's Manual, pp 113–142. Baltimore, MD, Williams & Wilkins, 1996.
38. Edwards BC: Combined movements of the lumbar spine: examination and clinical significance. Aust J Physiother 1979;25(4).
39. Meadows, JTS: The principles of the Canadian approach to the lumbar dysfunction patient. In Management of Lumbar Spine Dysfunction—Independent Home Study Course. La Crosse, WI, APTA, Orthopedic Section, 1999.
40. Lee DG, Walsh MC: A Workbook of Manual Therapy Techniques for the Vertebral Column and Pelvic Girdle, 2nd ed. Vancouver, Nascent, 1996.
41. Maher C, Latimer J, Adams R: An investigation of the reliability and validity of posteroanterior spinal stiffness judgments made using a reference-based protocol. Phys Ther 1998;78:829–837.
42. Deyo RA, Weinstein JN: Low back pain. N Engl J Med 2001;344:363–370.
43. Dutton M: Manual Therapy of the Spine: An Integrated Approach. New York, McGraw-Hill, 2002.
44. Maitland G: Vertebral manipulation. Sydney, Butterworth, 1986.
45. Binkley J, Stratford PW, Gill C: Interrater reliability of lumbar accessory motion mobility testing. Phys Therapy Rev 1995;75:786–792, discussion 793–795.
46. Boden SD, et al.: Abnormal magnetic resonance scan of the lumbar spine in asymptomatic subjects: a prospective investigation. J Bone Joint Surg 1990;72A:403–408.
47. Weisel SE, et al.: A study of computer-assisted tomography, I: the incidence of positive CAT scans in an asymptomatic group of patients. Spine 1984;9:549–551.
48. Guide to physical therapist practice. Phys Ther 2001;81:S13–S95.

17 | **The Sacroiliac Joint**

OVERVIEW

The sacroiliac joint (SIJ), which serves as the point of intersection between the spinal and the lower extremity joints, is the least understood and, therefore, one of the most controversial and interesting areas of the spine. Most of this misunderstanding is derived from the joint's complicated anatomy and biomechanics (see *Orthopaedic Examination, Evaluation, and Intervention*, pp 1287–1298).

EXAMINATION

In most cases an examination of the pelvic joints is of little use if the lumbar spine and hip joints have not been previously cleared by examination or intervention, as both of these joints can refer pain to this area and may also profoundly affect the function of the SIJ.[1] In general, the SIJ can be the origin for unilateral pain with no referral below the knee, whereas irritation of a lumbar spinal nerve may cause radicular symptoms below the knee.[2] Given the questionable reliability and validity of the tests for this region, the diagnosis needs to be based on the results from a thorough history and a physical examination that includes both pain provocative tests and a biomechanical examination (see *Orthopaedic Examination, Evaluation, and Intervention*, pp 1298–1307). The algorithm depicted in Figure 17-1 should serve as a guide.

History

Sacroiliac joint problems can cause both local and referred pain. Determining the location of the pain can provide some clues as to the cause. The SIJ can refer pain to the posterior superior iliac spine (PSIS), iliac fossa, medial buttock, and the superior lateral and posterior thigh.[3] Pain may also be referred to the sacrum from a distant structure, including the contralateral sacrospinalis muscle,[4] the ipsilateral L3-S2 interspinous ligaments,[5] and the L4-5 facet joints.[6] Problems of a muscular nature can also cause SIJ pain (Table 17-1). It is well established that dysfunctional pelvic floor muscles can contribute to the symptoms of interstitial cystitis and the so-called urethral syndrome, which is urgency-frequency with or without chronic pelvic pain.[7–9] The symphysis pubis can also be a source of symptoms. Pubic symphysis dysfunction typically results in localized pain, or groin pain, which is aggravated by activities involving hip adductor or rectus abdominis muscles.[10]

The presence of the following findings suggests likely SIJ dysfunction:[11–14]

- A history of sharp pain awakening the patient from sleep on turning in bed
- Pain with walking, ascending or descending stairs, standing from a sitting position, or with hopping or standing on the involved leg
- A positive straight leg raise at, or near, the end of range (occasionally early in the range when hyperacute), pain reproduction, and sometimes limitation, on extension and ipsilateral side bending of the trunk.

Systems Review

Given the number of visceral organs in the vicinity of the SIJ and the capability of these organs to refer pain to the SIJ region, the clinician should determine the patient's past medical and surgical history to rule out any visceral

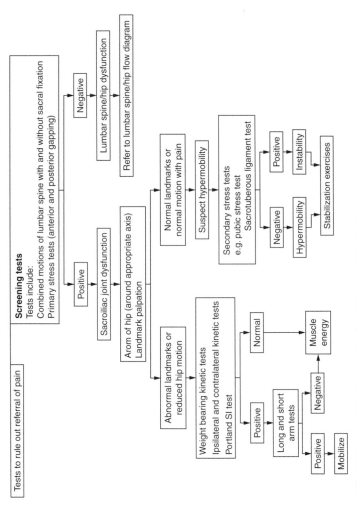

FIG. 17-1 Algorithm for examination of the sacroiliac joint.

TABLE 17-1 Muscles that Attach to the Sacrum, Ilium, or Both

• Latissimus dorsi	• External oblique	• Adductor magnus
• Erector spinae	• Internal oblique	• Rectus femoris
• Semimembranosus	• Transversus abdominis	• Quadratus lumborum
• Semitendinosus	• Rectus abdominis	• Pectineus
• Biceps femoris	• Pyramidalis	• Psoas minor
• Sartorius	• Gluteus minimus	• Adductor brevis
• Inferior gemellus	• Gluteus medius	• Adductor longus
• Multifidus	• Gluteus maximus	• Levator ani
• Obturator internus	• Quadratus femoris	• Sphincter urethrae
• Obturator externus	• Superior gemellus	• Superficial transverse
• Piriformis	• Gracilis	perineal
• Tensor fascia lata	• Iliacus	• Ischiocavernous
		• Coccygeus

sources for the symptoms. A Cyriax scanning examination should be performed on any patient who presents with an insidious onset of pelvic pain. The scanning examination, which includes the primary stress tests (anterior and posterior gapping—see *Primary Stress Tests*) can be used to detect sacroiliitis resulting from microtraumatic arthritis, macrotraumatic arthritis, or systemic arthritis (ankylosing spondylitis, Reiter's, etc.), or the more serious pathologies grouped under the *Sign of the Buttock* (see *Orthopaedic Examination, Evaluation, and Intervention*, p 244). Primary breast, lung, and prostate cancers are among the most common cancers to metastasize to the axial skeleton, including the pelvic ring.[15]

Tests and Measures

Observation

Observing the patient from the side, the clinician should observe the degree of tilt at the pelvis. The question of cause and effect should be raised. An anterior pelvic tilt causes an increase in the lumbar lordosis and thoracic kyphosis. The anterior pelvic tilt also results in a stretching of the abdominals, sacrotuberous, sacroiliac, and sacrospinous ligaments, and an adaptive shortening of the hip flexors. A posterior pelvic tilt results in a decrease in the lumbar lordosis and thoracic kyphosis, a stretching of the hip flexors and lower abdominals, and adaptive shortening of the hamstrings.

The bony landmarks are also observed from the front and back. A lateral pelvic tilt, where one iliac crest is higher than the other, may be caused by a scoliosis with ipsilateral lumbar convexity, a leg length discrepancy, or a shortening of the contralateral quadratus lumborum. This position results in adaptive shortening of the ipsilateral hip abductors and contralateral hip adductors, and weakness of the contralateral hip abductors.

An examination of overall posture is performed to check for the presence of asymmetry (see *Orthopaedic Examination, Evaluation, and Intervention*, p 1300).

Landmark Palpation

The palpation of landmarks is used to locate areas of tenderness. The various landmarks of the pelvis are palpated with the patient positioned in standing, sitting, and prone lying (Figures 17-2, 17-3). As pelvic landmark asymmetry is probably the norm, "positive findings" are to be expected.[16]

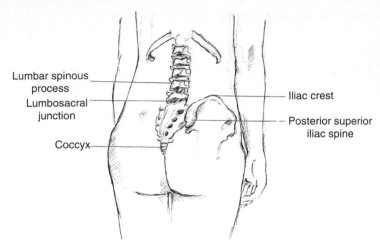

FIG. 17-2   Bony landmarks of the pelvis—posterior view.

An altered positional relationship within the pelvic girdle should only be considered positive if a mobility restriction of the SIJ or pubic symphysis or both is also found. The following landmarks or structures are palpated:

- *Iliac crest*. The iliac crests (see Figure 17-2) on both sides are located using the medial aspects of the index fingers. The crest heights should be level.

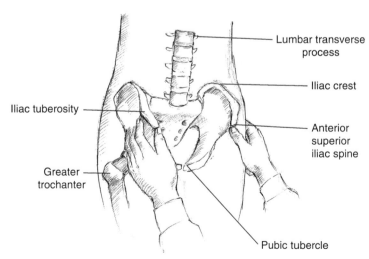

FIG. 17-3   Bony landmarks of the pelvis—anterior view.

- *Anterior superior iliac spine* (see Figure 17-3). The anterior superior iliac spines (ASIS) are located anteriorly to the iliac crests. An inferior ASIS relative to the other side may indicate a rotated innominate.[17] In supine, if the innominate is anteriorly rotated, the leg will be longer on that side, but shorter if it is posteriorly rotated.[17] Tenderness of the ASIS may indicate a "hip pointer" injury or injury to the inguinal ligament.

- *Posterior superior iliac spine.* These are located posteriorly to the iliac crests and approximately 1 inch beneath the dimples of the lumbar spine, and level with the S2 spinous process (see Figure 17-2). The clinician should hook the thumbs under the PSIS. A superior PSIS relative to the other side may indicate a rotated innominate.[17] Slightly medially and distal to the PSIS are the SIJs

- *Pubic symphysis and pubic tubercles.* The pubic tubercles (see Figure 17-3) are lateral to the pubic symphysis.

- *Thoracodorsal fascial attachments.*

- *Long dorsal ligament.*

- *Greater trochanter* (see Figure 17-3).

- *Ischial tuberosity and the sacrotuberous ligament (medial to the tuberosities).* The ischial tuberosity (see Chapter 10, Figure 10-4) serves as the attachment for the hamstrings and the sacrotuberous ligament. The ischial bursa is also located here. According to osteopathic doctrine, the sacrotuberous ligament is firm on the side of an anteriorly rotated innominate, and taut on the side of a posteriorly rotated innominate.[17] The patient is positioned in prone and the clinician stands at the patient's side. With the heel of the hands, the clinician locates the ischial tuberosities through the soft tissue at the gluteal folds. Then, with the thumbs, the clinician palpates the inferior-medial aspect of the ischial tuberosities. From this point, the clinician slides the thumbs superior-laterally and palpates the sacrotuberous ligament. The clinician then compares the relative tension between the left and right side.

- *Sacral sulcus/sacral base.* From the posterior inferior iliac spine, the clinician moves in a thumbs width, and then up a thumb width.

- *Inferior lateral angle (ILA).* These structures are level with the prominent part of the tail bone.

- *The L5 segment.* The clinician palpates medially along the iliac crest. L5 is usually level with the point at which the palpating finger begins to descend on the crest. The L5-S1 zygapophyseal joints are located halfway between the L5 spinous process and the ipsilateral posterior inferior iliac spine (see Figure 17-2).

- *Lumbosacral angle.* An increased or decreased lumbosacral angle on one side may indicate a rotated innominate. Although very difficult to measure without radiographs, the normal lumbosacral angle (the angle the sacrum makes with the lumbar spine) is approximately 140°.

- *S2.* S2 is normally level with the posterior inferior iliac spine.

Hip Range of Motion

Range of motion of the hip, including internal and external rotation, is performed to help rule out pain referred from the hip joint. Given the argued association between hip joint motion and innominate motion, a correlation exists between a loss of hip motion and a loss of innominate motion.[18–21] For example, if there is a loss of hip flexion compared to the uninvolved side, there should also be a loss of the posterior rotation of the innominate on the same side.

Lumbosacral Screening Tests

Two screening tests can be used to assess the overall function of the lumbopelvic complex, and if negative, would indicate that these regions are not the source of pain.

In the first test, the patient is asked to stand with the feet shoulder-width apart. Crouching behind the patient, the clinician locates the sacral sulcus and the contralateral ILA and places a thumb over each (e.g., the right sacral sulcus and the left ILA). The patient is asked to bend forward and then to rotate to the left while in full flexion. The patient is asked to bend backward and then to rotate to the left while bent backward. The test is then repeated using forward flexion and right rotation, and extension and right rotation. The clinician notes the quality and quantity of motion and whether any of the motions reproduce the patient's pain. Confirmation of the results of these tests can be produced by repeating the combined motions of the lumbar spine while stabilizing the sacrum using the heel of one hand. This fixation should restrict the motion occurring to just the lumbar spine and should therefore result in an absence of symptom reproduction if only the SIJ is involved.

In the second test, the patient places one foot on a chair and the other behind in the full lunge position. If the patient is able to achieve this position, the innominates are now in a relatively locked position. The clinician notes the quality and quantity of motion and whether achieving this position reproduced the patient's pain. Lumbar motion is then added by asking the patient to bend forward and then backward at the waist while in the lunge position. Again the clinician notes the quality and quantity of motion and whether any of the motions reproduce the patient's pain. A reproduction of the patient's symptoms with either the lumbar flexion or extension, or both, would suggest a lumbar spine dysfunction as the SIJ are locked. The test is then repeated but with the other foot placed on the chair.

Primary Stress Tests

Stress tests for the SIJ are divided into primary tests and secondary tests. The primary stress tests (anterior gapping test and posterior gapping test) are used to determine the presence of an inflammatory disorder such as sacroiliitis, systemic arthritis, and sacroiliac arthritis. A positive primary stress test is one that reproduces unilateral or bilateral sacroiliac pain, either anteriorly or posteriorly.[22] Although a positive test indicates the presence of inflammation, it does not give any information as to the cause. If either of the primary stress tests is positive in the older patient who has recently fallen, there is a possibility that a fracture of the pelvis exists.[23]

Anterior Gapping Test   The anterior gapping stress test is performed with the patient supine with the legs extended. The clinician stands to one side of the patient and, crossing his or her arms, places the palm of the hands on the patient's *ASIS*s (see Chapter 10, Figure 10-11). The clinician then applies a laterally directed force with both hands, thereby gapping the anterior aspect of the SIJ. The stress is maintained for 7–10 seconds, or until an end-feel is felt.

In addition to being sensitive for severe arthritis, this test and its posterior counterpart (see below) are also believed to be sensitive to ligament tears,[22] although they have been shown to be poorly reproducible.[24]

Posterior Compression Test   The patient is positioned in side lying and the clinician applies pressure to the lateral side of the ilium, thereby compressing the anterior aspect of the joint, and gapping its posterior aspect (see Chapter 10,

Figure 10-12). The posterior and interosseus ligaments are among the strongest in the body and are not usually torn by trauma, but may be attenuated by prolonged or repeated stress. This test is less sensitive for arthritis due to the reduced leverage available to the clinician. Thus, if it is positive, it indicates severe arthritis. This test also indirectly tests the ability of the sacrum to counternutate.

Leg Length Tests

These are usually performed as part of the bony landmark examination. Anatomic discrepancies in leg length can theoretically predispose patients to a pelvic or lumbar impairment or both. Posterior rotation of the innominate on the sacrum results in a decrease in leg length, as does an anterior rotation of the innominate on the contralateral side.[25] Although not exact measurements of leg length, these tests can highlight any significant asymmetries.

Prone Test   Chiropractors initially assess leg length with the patient prone. The comparative lengths of the legs are compared by observing the heels or medial malleoli. If a discrepancy is noted, the knees are flexed to 90° while maintaining a neutral hip rotation (neutral upright position), and the landmarks are reassessed to screen for a shortened tibia. The patient is then positioned in supine and the leg lengths are reassessed using the same landmarks. Finally, the leg lengths are assessed using the long sit test. Functional leg length inequality that is secondary to sacroiliac subluxation/dysfunction may reverse from the supine to sitting position, whereas anatomic leg length inequality or functional inequality secondary to dysfunction at other sites likely will not.[25]

Standing Leg Length Test   The iliac crest palpation and book correction (ICPBC) method for assessing leg length is used throughout many clinics. The patient stands with the feet shoulder-width apart. The clinician palpates the iliac crests, and compares the relative heights for asymmetry. The asymmetry identified is corrected using a book opened to the required number of pages. The iliac crest heights are reassessed. If the iliac crests are level, the thickness of the book correction is measured. One study with 34 healthy subjects found the ICPBC technique for measuring leg length discrepancy to be highly reliable and moderately valid when there is no history of pelvic deformity and the iliac crests can be readily palpated.[26]

Functional Leg Length   The patient stands with the feet shoulder-width apart. The clinician palpates the iliac crests, ASISs, and the PSISs, and compares the relative heights for asymmetry. The patient is then positioned with the subtalar joints in neutral, the toes pointing forward, and the knees fully extended. The same landmarks are reassessed. If the second position corrects any asymmetry found in the first position, the test is positive for a functional leg length discrepancy, and indicates that the leg is *structurally* normal but has abnormal joint mechanics.

Weight-Bearing Kinetic Tests

The kinetic tests, as a group, include both weight-bearing and non-weight-bearing tests. These tests are designed to assess the osteokinematics occurring at the SIJ during patient-generated movements. The tests assess the mobility of the innominate, the ability of the sacrum to flex (nutate) (ipsilateral test), and to side bend (contralateral test). As these movements are difficult to observe, bony landmarks are palpated during the movements. The tests for the right side are described.

Ipsilateral Flexion Kinetic Test (Gillet Test) The ipsilateral flexion kinetic test[27] assesses the mobility of the short arm of the auricular surface, and the ability of the ipsilateral innominate to posteriorly rotate. With the patient standing, the inferior aspect of the right posterior superior iliac spine is palpated with one thumb, while the left thumb palpates the median sacral crest (S2) directly parallel. The clinician then asks the patient to flex his or her right hip as far as is comfortable (Figure 17-4). The patient may steady himself or herself using a hand against a wall or similar stable object.

During this maneuver, the lumbar spine side-flexes to the left and rotates to the right. The clinician should feel the right innominate rotate posteriorly, and the median sacral crest (S2) of the sacrum rotate to the right.

A positive ipsilateral kinetic test is observed when the thumb on the inferior aspect of the posterior superior iliac spine moves cranially instead of caudally, and the patient hikes the right side of the pelvis, or leans excessively away from the tested side, indicating a dysfunction of the ipsilateral SIJ or the lumbar spine.

The test is repeated on the other side and the results compared.

Ipsilateral Extension Kinetic Test This test serves as a functional mobility test of the SIJ. The clinician palpates under the right PSIS with one thumb, and at the median sacral crest (S2) directly parallel with the opposite thumb (Figure 17-5). The patient extends the right hip with the knee extended into varying degrees of hip extension, while the clinician notes the superior-lateral displacement of the PSIS relative to the sacrum.

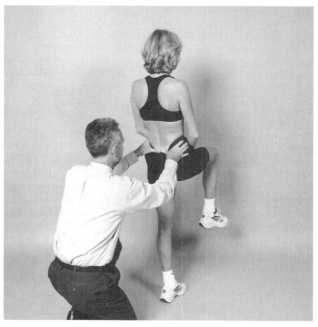

FIG. 17-4 The ipsilateral kinetic test. (*Reproduced with permission from Dutton M: Orthopaedic Examination, Evaluation and Intervention, p 1302 (Fig. 27-13). New York, McGraw-Hill 2004.*)

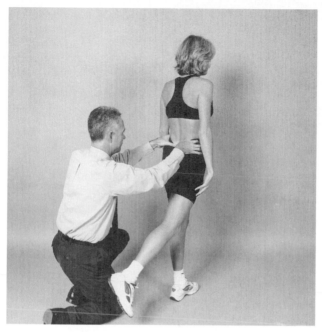

FIG. 17-5   Extension kinetic test. (*Reproduced with permission from Dutton M: Orthopaedic Examination, Evaluation and Intervention, p 1303 (Fig. 27-14). New York, McGraw-Hill 2004.*)

Both sides are tested. The right extension test examines the ability of the right innominate to anteriorly rotate, and the sacrum to left rotate (counternutate). The left extension test examines the ability of the left innominate to anteriorly rotate, and the sacrum to right rotate (counternutate).

- *Summary of findings.* The potential impairments within the pelvic girdle, which render the ipsilateral kinetic tests positive, include:[28]
    a. An anteriorly or posteriorly rotated innominate of the ipsilateral side (intra-articular or extra-articular in origin)
    b. An impairment of the pubic symphysis on the ipsilateral side
    c. An innominate flare on the ipsilateral side
    d. A subluxed innominate on the ipsilateral side (intra-articular in origin)

Contralateral Kinetic Test[28]   This test evaluates the mobility of the long arm of the auricular surface, and the ability of the sacrum to side bend to the opposite side of the hip flexion. With the patient standing, the clinician places the left thumb on the medial sacral crest of the sacrum (S2), and the right thumb on the left PSIS. The patient is asked to flex the left hip to 90° (Figure 17-6). During this movement, the left thumb, on the sacral crest, travels caudally initially because of the posterior rotation of the left innominate, which produces a right side bending and left rotation of the sacrum (conjunct rotation).

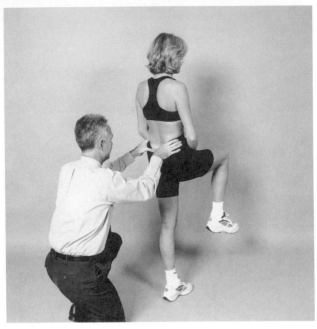

FIG. 17-6 The contralateral kinetic test. (*Reproduced with permission from Dutton M: Orthopaedic Examination, Evaluation and Intervention, p 1303 (Fig. 27-15). New York, McGraw-Hill 2004.*)

In addition, the lumbar vertebral bodies will rotate to the left due to the influence of the iliolumbar ligament on L5.

When the contralateral kinetic test is positive, the left thumb travels caudally or it does not move, indicating that the sacrum is unable to side bend.

- *Summary of findings.* The potential sacroiliac impairments that render the contralateral kinetic test positive include:[28]
  1. Sacral torsion
  2. Sacral nutation/counternutation

The ipsilateral and contralateral tests are evaluated on both sides for comparison.

Portland SI Test[29] The patient is asked to stand in a stride position with the right leg forward, and his or her weight equally distributed between both feet. The clinician stands behind the patient. The clinician places the right thumb on the posterior lateral position of the right sacrum at the level of S3. Pressure is applied through the right thumb to produce an anteromedial force 5° to the sagittal plane. Then the clinician places the thumb on the sacrum at the level of the right S1 and applies a pressure to produce an anterolateral force 20° to the sagittal plane. After completing the test on the right side, the patient is asked to change his or her stride position so that the left leg is now in a forward position with the weight evenly distributed between the two feet. The clinician then places the left thumb on the left lateral sacrum at the level of S3 and an anteromedial force is applied at 5° to the sagittal plane. Then, the clinician places the left thumb on the sacrum at the level of the left S1 and applies a pressure to produce an anterolateral force 20° to the sagittal plane. The clinician notes the differences between the two sides in the quality and quantity of motion.

Short-and Long-Arm Tests[30]

To confirm or refute the findings from the kinetic tests, the short- and long-arm tests, are performed.

Short-Arm Test   The short-arm test is designed to confirm or refute the findings of the ipsilateral kinetic tests. The following description is for a test of the left side of the sacrum. The patient lies supine with the legs straight, while the clinician stands on the left side of the patient. The clinician slides his or her right hand under the left side of the patient's lumbar spine, and palpates the left sacral base/sulcus with the index and long finger. With the left hand, the clinician grasps the anterior aspect of the patient's left innominate/ASIS. From this position, the clinician stabilizes the left sacral base/sulcus with the right hand, and pushes the left innominate down toward the bed, using the left hand. Some motion should be felt before a ligamentous end-feel is reached. A loss of motion compared to the contralateral side indicates dysfunction and confirms the findings of the ipsilateral kinetic test.

Long-Arm Test   The long-arm test is designed to confirm or refute the findings of the contralateral kinetic tests. The following description is for a test of the right side of the sacrum. The palpation and stabilization points are as for the short-arm test. The patient's right hip is flexed to about 45°. Using the heel of the right hand, the clinician pushes down the length of the flexed femur, while stabilizing the sacral base with the left hand. Again, slight motion should be felt (more than with the short arm) before a solid ligamentous end-feel is reached. There should be no pain. A loss of motion compared to the contralateral side indicates dysfunction and confirms the findings of the contralateral kinetic test.

Following the weight-bearing tests and the confirmatory long- and short-arm tests, the clinician should be able to determine the side of the lesion. Ideally, the patient's condition can be categorized into one of the following:

- One side of the sacrum is nutated while the ipsilateral innominate is posteriorly rotated. The pubic tubercle is superior on the side of the posteriorly rotated innominate.
- One side of the sacrum is counternutated while the ipsilateral innominate is anteriorly rotated. The pubic tubercle is inferior on the side of the anteriorly rotated innominate.
- One side of the sacrum is nutated while the ipsilateral innominate is anteriorly rotated. The pubic tubercle is inferior on the side of the anteriorly rotated innominate.
- One side of the sacrum is counternutated while the ipsilateral innominate is posteriorly rotated. The pubic tubercle is superior on the side of the posteriorly rotated innominate.

However, if the tests just described proved negative, further investigation is required in the form of the secondary stress tests and the special tests.

Secondary Stress Tests

Secondary stress tests of the SIJ are designed to selectively stress various tissues to determine whether those tissues are provoking the symptoms.

Pubic Stress Tests[31]   The patient is positioned in supine, and the clinician stands at the patient's side. With the heel of one hand, the clinician palpates the superior aspect of the superior ramus of one pubic bone, and with the heel of the other hand, palpates the inferior aspect of the superior ramus of the opposite pubic bone. Fixing one pubic bone, the clinician applies a slow, steady inferior-superior force to the other bone and, noting the quantity and end-feel of motion, as well as the reproduction of any symptoms, the clinician then switches hands and repeats the test so that both sides are stressed superiorly and inferiorly.

Sacrotuberous Ligament Stress Test   The performance and interpretation of this test rely on the patient having no hip joint pathology and full hip range of motion. The patient is positioned in supine. The clinician flexes and adducts the patient's hip by moving the patient's knee toward the opposite shoulder. This maneuver is reported in an otherwise normal hip joint to stretch the sacrotuberous ligament and to cause the sacrum to nutate.[32,33] This force is maintained for about 20 seconds, and any reproduction of symptoms is noted. Pain in the SIJs is considered a positive test, but this finding must be incorporated with other clinical findings such as palpation of the sacrotuberous ligament for tenderness, before drawing any conclusions.

Sacral Compression Test   The patient is positioned prone on a firm surface and the clinician stands at the patient's side. With one hand, the clinician palpates the inferior aspect of the sacrum in the midline and reinforces this hand with the other. The clinician then applies an anterior force to the apex of the sacrum, thus forcing the sacrum to counternutate. This force is maintained for about 20 seconds and the reproduction of symptoms is noted. This test is considered positive if pain is reproduced over the SIJs or the long dorsal sacroiliac ligament, or both.[34]

Rotational Stress Test[34]   The patient is positioned prone and the clinician stands at the patient's side. The clinician places a thumb over the transverse process of L5 on one side to stabilize the segment against rotation. The clinician uses the other hand to pull up the contralateral iliac crest from the bed, thereby inducing a rotational stress at the lumbosacral junction. Pain produced with this maneuver may indicate an iliolumbar ligament or anterior sacroiliac ligament tear, or a dysfunction of the lumbosacral junction, or both.

Special Tests

The Seated Flexion Test (Piedallu's Sign)   The patient is sitting with his or her legs over the end of the table and feet supported.[17] In this position, the innominate motion is severely abbreviated as the sitting position places the innominates near the end of their extension range. The test is performed as follows. Each PSIS is palpated with the thumb placed under it caudally. The patient then bends forward at the waist. Providing there is no impairment in the SIJ or the lower lumbar spine, as the patient bends forward, both thumbs should move cranially. If the joint is "blocked," it moves upward further in relation to the other side.[24] The test is purported to help distinguish between a sacroiliac lesion and an iliosacral lesion.[35–37]

The Long Sit Test The long sit test is used to indicate the direction of the rotation that the innominate has adopted, and is used in conjunction with the standing flexion test. After noting the side of the impairment obtained from the standing flexion test, the clinician observes whether the medial malleolus on that side moves distally or proximally during the long sit test. Rotation about a coronal axis, whose resultant movement leads to an increase in the length of a limb, is defined as extension. If it shortens the length of the limb, it is defined as flexion. Thus, if the apparent shorter leg becomes longer during the test, the innominate on that side is purportedly held in a posteriorly rotated malposition, while if the apparent longer leg becomes shorter during the test, the innominate on that side is allegedly held in an anteriorly rotated malposition.

The problems with this test involve the maneuver itself. To ask a patient who is in some degree of discomfort to rise off the bed from a supine position into a long-sit position without any twisting or use of the arms is unnecessarily painful. In addition, for the successful completion of the maneuver, the patient needs 90° of hip flexion/hamstring length.

Sign of the Buttock Test The patient lies supine and the clinician performs a passive unilateral straight leg raise. If there is a unilateral restriction, the clinician flexes the knee and notes whether the hip flexion increases. If the restriction was caused by the lumbar spine or hamstrings, hip flexion increases. If the hip flexion does not increase when the knee is flexed, it is a positive sign of the buttock test. The sign of the buttock is not a single sign as the name would suggest, but is a collection of signs indicating a serious pathology present posterior to the axis of flexion and extension in the hip. Among the causes of the syndrome are osteomyelitis, infectious sacroiliitis, and fracture of the sacrum/pelvis, septic bursitis, ischiorectal abscess, gluteal hematoma, gluteal tumor, and rheumatic bursitis. If the sign of the buttock is encountered, the patient must be immediately returned to the physician for further investigation.

Gaenslen's Test The patient is positioned in supine at the edge of the bed. The leg furthest from the edge of the bed (nontested leg) is flexed at the hip and knee, and held by the patient with both arms. The clinician stabilizes the pelvis and passively positions the upper leg (test leg) into hyperextension at the hip, so that it hangs over the edge of the table (Figure 17-7).[38] The clinician applies a further stretch to the test leg into hip extension and adduction. Pain with this maneuver is considered a positive test for an SIJ lesion, hip pathology, or an L4 nerve root lesion. The test also stresses the femoral nerve.

Yeoman's Test[39] This test is performed with the patient positioned in prone. The clinician stabilizes the sacrum with the palm of one hand. With the other hand, the clinician grasps the patient's distal thigh and extends the patient's hip (Figure 17-8). At the end of the available motion, the hip is hyperextended so that the innominate is forced into anterior rotation. A positive test produces pain over the SIJ. Other structures that are stressed with this maneuver include the lumbar spine, the hip joint, and the psoas muscle.

Patrick's (Faber or Figure-Four) Test The patient is positioned in supine. The test leg is positioned so that the sole of the foot rests against the side of the other knee (or on top of the knee of the opposite leg). This position flexes, abducts, and externally rotates the femur at the hip joint. The clinician slowly lowers the knee of the test leg toward the bed. At the end of available motion, the pelvis is stabilized, and overpressure is applied.

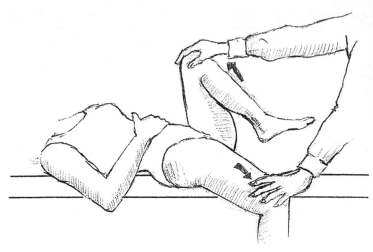

FIG. 17-7 Gaenslen's Test.

Pain with this maneuver indicates hip joint pathology, SIJ dysfunction, or an iliopsoas muscle spasm.[40]

Active Straight Leg Raise Test When performed passively, the straight leg raise test is usually associated as a test of neurodynamic mobility, or hamstring length. When performed actively, the straight leg raise test has been recommended as a disease severity scale for patients with posterior pelvic

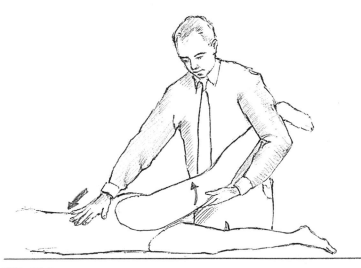

FIG. 17-8 Yeoman's test.

pain after pregnancy.[41–43] It seems that the integrity of the function to transfer loads between the lumbosacral spine and legs is tested by the active straight leg raise (ASLR) test.

EXAMINATION CONCLUSIONS—THE EVALUATION

Following the examination, and once the clinical findings have been recorded, the clinician must determine a specific diagnosis or a working hypothesis, based on a summary of all the findings. This diagnosis can be structure related (medical diagnosis), a biomechanical diagnosis (see Figure 17-1), or a diagnosis based on the preferred practice patterns as described in the *Guide to Physical Therapist Practice*.[44]

REFERENCES

1. Vleeming A, et al.: The role of the sacroiliac joints in coupling between spine, pelvis, legs and arms. In Vleeming A, et al. (eds): Movement, Stability and Low Back Pain, p 53. Edinburgh, Churchill Livingstone, 1997.
2. Hall H: A simple approach to back pain management. Patient Care 1992;15:77–91.
3. Fortin JD, et al.: Sacroiliac joint pain referral maps upon applying a new injection/arthrography technique. Part I: Asymptomatic volunteers. Spine 1994;19: 1475– 1482.
4. Kellgren JH: Observations on referred pain arising from muscle. Clin Sci 1938;3:175–190.
5. Kellgren JH: On the distribution of pain arising from deep somatic structures with charts of segmental pain areas. Clin Sci 1939;4:35–46.
6. McCall IW, Park WM, O'Brien JP: Induced pain referral from posterior lumbar elements in normal subjects. Spine 1979;4:441–446.
7. Weiss JM: Pelvic floor myofascial trigger points: manual therapy for interstitial cystitis and the urgency-frequency syndrome. J Urology 2001;166:2226–2231.
8. Raz S, Smith RB: External sphincter spasticity syndrome in female patients. J Urology 1976;115:443.
9. Lilius HG, Oravisto KJ, Valtonen EJ: Origin of pain in interstitial cystitis. Scand J Urol Nephrol 1973;7:150.
10. LaBan MM, et al.: Symphyseal and sacroiliac joint pain associated with pubic symphysis instability. Arch Phys Med Rehabil 1978;59:470–472.
11. Alderink GJ: The sacroiliac joint: review of anatomy, mechanics, and function. J Orthop Sports Phys Ther 1991;13(2):71–84.
12. DonTigny RL: Function and pathomechanics of the sacroiliac joint. A review. Phys Ther 1985;65(1):35–44.
13. Dreyfuss P, et al.: The value of medical history and physical examination in diagnosing sacroiliac joint pain. Spine 1996;21:2594–2602.
14. Schwarzer AC, Aprill CN, Bogduk N: The sacroiliac joint in chronic low back pain. Spine 1995;20:31–37.
15. Fornasier VL, Horne JG: Metastases to the vertebral column. Cancer 1975;36: 590–594.
16. Levangie PK: The association between static pelvic asymmetry and low back pain. Spine 1999;24:1234–1242.
17. Mitchell FL, Moran PS, Pruzzo NA: An Evaluation and Treatment Manual of Osteopathic Muscle Energy Procedures. Manchester, MO, Mitchell, Moran & Pruzzo, 1979.
18. Cibulka MT, et al.: Unilateral hip rotation range of motion asymmetry in patients with sacroiliac joint regional pain. Spine 1998;23:1009–1015.
19. Smidt GL, et al.: Sacroiliac kinematics for reciprocal straddle positions. Spine 1995;20:1047–1054.
20. Papadopoulos SM, McGillicuddy JE, Albers JW: Unusual cause of piriformis muscle syndrome. Arch Neurol 1990;47:1144–1146.

21. Vandertop WP, Bosma WJ: The piriformis syndrome. A case report. J Bone Joint Surg 1991;73A:1095–1097.
22. Cyriax J: Textbook of Orthopedic Medicine, Diagnosis of Soft Tissue Lesions, 8th ed. London, Bailliere Tindall, 1982.
23. Van Deursen LL, et al.: The value of some clinical tests of the sacroiliac joint. J Manual Med 1990;5:96–99.
24. Potter NA, Rothstein JM: Intertester reliability for selected clinical tests of the sacroiliac joint. Phys Ther 1985;65:1671.
25. Bergmann TF, Peterson DH, Lawrence DJ: Chiropractic Technique: Principles and Procedures. New York, Churchill Livingstone, 1993.
26. Hanada E, et al.: Measuring leg-length discrepancy by the "iliac crest palpation and book correction" method: reliability and validity. Arch Phys Med Rehab 2001;82: 938–942.
27. Gillet H, Liekens M: Belgian Chiropractic Research Notes, 10th ed. Brussels, 1973.
28. Fowler C: Muscle energy techniques for pelvic dysfunction. In Palastanga N, Boyling JD (eds): Grieve's Modern Manual Therapy: The Vertebral Column, pp 781–792. Edinburgh, Churchill Livingstone, 1986.
29. Fowler C: The Portland SI test. In NAIOMT Newsletter, vol. IX, issue 1, Spring 2004; p 1.
30. Lee DG: A Workbook of Manual Therapy Techniques for the Upper Extremity. Delta, BC, Canada, Delta Orthopaedic Physiotherapy Clinics, 1989.
31. Lee DG: A Workbook of Manual Therapy Techniques for the Upper Extremity, pp 58–79, 2nd ed. Delta, BC, DOPC, 1991.
32. Lee DG: The Pelvic Girdle: An Approach to the Examination and Treatment of the Lumbo-Pelvic-Hip Region, 2nd ed. Edinburgh, Churchill Livingstone, 1999.
33. Porterfield JA, DeRosa C: Mechanical Low Back Pain, 2nd ed. Philadelphia, PA, WB Saunders, 1998.
34. Lee DG: Clinical manifestations of pelvic girdle dysfunction. In Palastanga N, Boyling JD (eds): Grieve's Modern Manual Therapy: The Vertebral Column, pp 453–462. Edinburgh, Churchill Livingstone, 1994.
35. Fryette HH: Principles of Osteopathic Technique. Carmel, CA, Academy of Osteopathy, 1980
36. Hartman SL: Handbook of Osteopathic Technique, pp 135–143, 2nd ed. London, Unwin Hyman, 1990.
37. DiGiovanna EL, Schiowitz S: An Osteopathic Approach to Diagnosis and Treatment. Philadelphia, PA, JB Lippincott.
38. Hoppenfeld S: Physical examination of the hip and pelvis. In Physical Examination of the Spine and Extremities, p 143. East Norwalk, CT, Appleton-Century-Crofts, 1976.
39. Yeoman W: The relation of arthritis of the sacro-iliac joint to sciatica, with an analysis of 100 cases. Lancet 1928;2:1119–1122.
40. Evans RC: Illustrated Essentials in Orthopedic Physical Assessment. St Louis, MO, Mosby, 1994.
41. Mens JM, et al.: Validity of the active straight leg raise test for measuring disease severity in patients with posterior pelvic pain after pregnancy. Spine 2002;27: 196–200.
42. Mens JMA, et al.: Validity and reliability of the active straight leg raise test as diagnostic instrument in posterior pelvic pain since pregnancy. Spine 2001;26:1167– 1171.
43. Mens JMA, et al.: The active straight-leg-raising test and mobility of the pelvic joints. Eur Spine J 1999;8:468–473.
44. Guide to physical therapist practice. Phys Ther 2001;81:S13–S95.

Appendix | **Terminology**

Prefixes Indicating Location, Direction, and Tendency

Prefix	Meaning	Example
Ab-	From, away	Abnormal: away from normal
Ad-	To, near, toward	Adrenal: near the kidney
Ante-	Before	Antepartum: before delivery of child
Brady-	Slow	Bradycardia: slow heart beat
Brev-	Short	Brevity: brief in duration
Circum-	Around	Circumduction: circular movement of a limb
Co-	With, together	Cooperate: work together
Con-	With, together	Congenital: with birth
Contra-	Against	Contraindicated: not indicated
Counter-	Against	Counterirritant: against irritation
Dis-	Apart from	Dislocation: displacement of a body part
Ect-	Outside	Ectonuclear: outside the nucleus
End-	Within	Endocardium: membrane lining inner heart
Epi-	Upon, on top of	Epidermis: upon the skin
Ex-	Out from	Exhalation: breathe out
Hypo-	Under, lower	Hypodermic: under the skin
Hyper-	Above, higher	Hyperactive: higher level activity
Im-	Not	Immobile: not mobile
In-	Not	Incurable: not curable
Infra-	Under, below	Infrapatellar below the knee cap
Peri-	Around	Pericardium: sac around the heart
Post-	After	Postmortem: after death
Pre-	Before	Prenatal: before birth
Pro-	Before	Prognosis: foreknowledge
Super-	Above, on top	Superficial: lying on above, on top
Supra-	Lying on above, on top	Suprapubic: above the pubic bone
Sym-	With, together	Symphysis: an articulation in which the bony surfaces are connected by pads of fibrous cartilage
Syn-	With, together	Synarthrosis: union of bones
Trans-	Through, across	Transurethral: through the urethra

Prefixes Indicating Number and Measurement

Prefix	Meaning	Example
Uni-	One	Unicycle: one wheel
Mono-	One	Mononuclear: one nucleus
Bi-	Two	Bilateral: two sides
Bin-	Two	Binocular two eyes
Di-	Two	Dicephalic: two heads
Ter-	Three	Tertiary: the third part or stage
Tri-	Three	Trilobar: three lobes
Quadr-	Four	Quadriceps: muscle with four heads
Tetra-	Four	Tetracycline: a four ringed molecule
Poly-	Many	polydactyly—many digits (more than 5)
Oligo-	Few	oligosaccharide—few sugars linked together
Micro-	Small	microscope—equipment to view small things
Macro-	Large	macrophage—large eating cell
Mega-	Great, enormous	megadontia—huge teeth

Prefixes Denoting Organs, Structures, Things

Prefix	Meaning	Example
Acoust-	Sound	Acoustics: quality of sound
Aud-	Ear, hear	Audition: to hear someone
Abdomin/o-	Relating to the abdomen	Abdomen, abdominal
Acr/o-	Extremity, limbs	Acromegaly: abnormally large limbs
Blast/o-	Early, embryonic	Blastocyte: embryonic type cell
Aden/o-	Gland	Adenopathy: disease of a gland
Angi/o-	Vessel	Angiogram: picture of a vessel
Arthr/o-	Joint	Arthritis: inflammation of a joint
Bucc/o-	Cheek	Buccolabial: relating to cheek and lip
Cardi/o-	Heart	Cardiology: study of the heart
Corp-	Body	Corpus callosum: connecting body
Chondr/o-	Cartilage	Chondrocyte: cartilage cell
Cephal/o-	Head	Cephalic: relating to the head
Cyst/o-	Bladder	Cystoscopy: view of the bladder
Cyt/o-	Cell	Cytokinesis: cell movement
Dent/o-	Tooth	Dental: referring to teeth
Dermat/o-	Skin	Dermatitis: skin inflammation
Duoden/o-	Duodenum	Duodenal: relating to the duodenum
Encephal/o-	Brain	Encephalitis: brain inflammation
Gastr/o-	Stomach	Gastrointestinal: stomach and intestine
Hepat/o-	Liver	Hepatitis: liver inflammation
Gloss/o-	Tongue	Glossopathy: tongue disease
Glute-	Buttocks	Gluteus minimus: small buttocks muscle
Laryng/o-	Larynx	Laryngitis: larynx inflammation
My/o-	Muscle	Myocardium: heart muscle
Nephr/o-	Kidney	Nephrologist: one who studies kidneys
Neur/o-	Nerve	Neurosurgeon: surgeon of nervous system
Oste/o-	Bone	Osteocyte: bone cell
Ot/o-	Ear	Otitis media: middle ear inflammation
Ophthalm/o-	Eye	Exophthalmos: eyes bulge out
Path/o-	Disease	Pathological: relating to disease
Pneumon/o-	Lung	Pneumonia: condition of the lung
Rhin/o-	Nose	Rhinoplasty: reform the nose
Stomat/o-	Mouth, opening	Stomatitis: mouth inflammation
Thorac/o-	Chest or thorax	Thoracocentesis: puncture of the thorax

Suffixes Denoting Relations, Conditions, and Agents

Suffix	Meaning	Example
-ac	Related to	Cardiac: related to the heart
-ious	Related to	Contagious: communicable by contact
-ic	Related to	Pyloric: related to pyloric valve of stomach
-ism	Condition	Mutism: condition of being mute
-osis	Condition	Scoliosis: S-shaped condition of backbone
-tion	Condition	Constipation: constant blockage condition
-ist	Agent (a person)	Opthalmologist: eye doctor
-or	Agent	Operator
-er	Agent	Examiner
-ician	Agent	Physician

Suffixes Used for Surgical and Operative Terminology

Suffix	Meaning	Example
-centesis	To puncture	Amniocentesis: puncture the amnion (fluid)
-ectomy	To cut out and remove	Appendectomy: cut out and remove appendix
-ostomy	To cut and form opening	Colostomy: opening to drain the colon
-otomy	To cut or slice	Tracheotomy: cut the trachea
-pexy	To fix or repair	Gastropexy: repair the stomach
-plasty	To reform or repair	Rhinoplasty: reform the nose
-rraphy	To suture, sew	Arteriorrhaphy: suture an artery
-scopy	To view	Otoscope: instrument to view ear

Other Suffixes Used in Anatomy

Suffix	Meaning	Example
-algia	Pain	Neuralgia: nerve pain
-cide	Kill or destroy	Germicide: substance that kills germs
-emia	Of the blood	Cholesterolemia: cholesterol in the blood
-gram	Writing or record	Electrocardiogram: record of heart action
-graph	Recording instrument	Electrocardiograph: records the heart
-itis	Inflammation	Appendicitis: appendix inflammation
-ology	The study of	Ophthalmology: study of the eye
-oma	Tumor	Lymphoma: tumor of lymphatics
-orrhea	Flow	Menorrhea: flow during menstruation
-malacia	Soft	Osteomalacia: bone softening
-phasia	Speech	Dysphasia: slurred or blunted speech
-phobia	Fear	Arachnophobia: fear of spiders

Surgical Glossary

Procedure	Explanation
Allograft	A tissue transplanted to a different individual of the same species
Arthrodesis	The surgical fixation of a joint, usually performed to provide stability or relieve pain. The operation is designed to cause fusion of joint surfaces. It is sometimes performed after failed joint replacement surgery or after joint damage has occurred.
Arthrography	Radiographic examination of joints with intraarticular injection of contrast medium. General indications include demonstration of anatomical abnormalities, and verification of the intraarticular position of a needle tip, either for aspiration of joint fluid or injection of steroids.
Arthroplasty	The surgical reconstruction of a joint
Arthroplasty, girdlestone	A surgical procedure on the hip joint in which extensive debridement and resection of paraarticular bone are employed. Girdlestone arthroplasty is used in the treatment of infection after hip replacement.
Arthrotomy	Cutting into a joint
Autograft	A tissue transplanted from one part to another part of the same body
Bankart	A surgical technique for repair of recurrent anterior glenohumeral joint dislocations. In this technique, the anterior capsular mechanism is repaired using drill holes and sutures.
Brisement	Joint distention during arthrography of the glenohumeral joint. The brisement procedure may aid in the treatment of adhesive capsulitis. In this technique, larger and larger volumes of contrast material mixed with saline solution and lidocaine are instilled by a slow, intermittent injection.
Bristow–Helfet	A surgical procedure used to repair recurrent anterior glenohumeral joint dislocations. In this technique, the coracoid process with its attached tendons is transferred to the neck of the scapula.
Brostrom	A surgical procedure for correcting an acute injury to the lateral ligaments of the ankle involving restoration or reconstruction by shortening the ligaments and reattaching them.
Chemonucleolysis	The injection of a proteolytic enzyme (e.g., chymopapain) into the herniated nucleus pulposus of a disk
Cloward's	A surgical technique for removing cervical herniated discs, bony spurs, and osteophytes. Through an anterior approach, separating the trachea from the neck vessels and sternocleidomastoid muscle, the intervertebral disk is removed and the two adjacent bodies are fused with a bony or artificial graft.
Diskectomy	The surgical removal of all or part of a herniated intervertebral disk compressing a nerve root. When microscopic or visually aided surgical techniques are used, this procedure is referred to as microdiskectomy. The procedure can also be done through a small incision using indirect visualization (percutaneous diskectomy).
Diskcography	The injection of a water-soluble imaging material directly into the nucleus pulposus of a disk to assess the extent of disk damage and characterize the pain response

(Continued)

Surgical Glossary (*Continued*)

Procedure	Explanation
Displacement osteotomy	A surgical cutting of bone, usually performed to correct or reduce a deformity. In this procedure the distal fragment is shifted in position with respect to the proximal one.
Dorsal myelography	Radiographic examination of the thoracic spinal canal with intrathecal injection of contrast medium. The contrast medium, which today should be water-soluble and nonionic, is injected via lumbar puncture.
Eden–Hybinette	A technique used to treat recurrent dislocations of the anterior glenohumeral joint, in which a bone graft is placed in the anterior glenoid region.
Magnusson–Stack	A surgical procedure used in the correction of recurrent anterior glenohumeral joint dislocation. In this operation, the subscapularis tendon is transferred from the lesser tuberosity to the greater tuberosity.
Modified Weaver-Dunn	A ligament allograft and microsuture fixation of the clavicle to the scapula
Myelography	Radiographic examination of the spinal canal with intrathecal injection of contrast medium. The word myelo (Greek myelos: marrow) in this context refers to the spinal cord, but the procedure includes examination not only of the spinal cord, but also its nerve roots and the subarachnoid space.
Oudard	A type of bone graft operation for surgical treatment of recurrent glenohumeral joint dislocations. In this procedure, bone is grafted to the coracoid process.
Percutaneous vertebroplasty	Invasive procedure developed by French authors to consolidate collapsed osteoporotic vertebral bodies by percutaneous injection of acrylic cement within the vertebral body.
Putti–Platt	Type of surgical procedure used to correct recurrent dislocations of the glenohumeral joint. In this technique, the anterior capsule and subscapularis muscle are shortened.
Resection arthroplasty	Removal of one or both articular surfaces of a joint, usually as a salvage procedure after failure of a total joint replacement operation.
Rotator cuff patch	A surgical procedure to repair severely damaged rotator cuff tissue by inserting a collagen patch that combines with the patient's own tissue and enhances healing through minimally invasive surgery.
Trillat	A surgical technique for correction of recurrent anterior glenohumeral joint dislocations. In this procedure, an osteotomy is combined with displacement of the coracoid process.
Valgus osteotomy	A type of surgery performed in patients with osteoarthritis of the hip, in which a wedge of bone is removed from the femoral head. The procedure is also termed adduction osteotomy. This operation is used when the femoral head is not hemispherical and when adduction improves congruency.
Weaver-Dunn procedure	The use of a ligament (coracoacromial ligament) to reconstruct two other torn ligaments (coracoclavicular ligaments) that are typically torn in more severe acromioclavicular (AC) joint separations.

Fracture Eponyms

Body Region	Name	Description
Cervical spine	Hangman's	Bilateral fracture of pedicles of axis (C2)
	Jefferson	Burst fracture of atlas (C1)
	Teardrop	Avulsion of anteroinferior corner of cervical vertebral body by anterior ligament
Pelvis	Duverney's	Two vertical fractures involving one side of the pelvic ring
	Malgaigne	
Forearm	Essex-Lopresti	Comminuted fracture of radial head, dislocation of distal radioulnar joint
	Chisel	Incomplete fracture of radial head (intra-articular)
	Monteggia	Proximal ulnar fracture, dislocated radial head
	Piedmont	Closed fracture of radius at the junction of the middle and distal thirds, no associated ulnar fracture
	Galeazzi	Radial fracture, dislocated distal ulna
	Night stick	Fracture of the ulna. The second most common single bone forearm fracture, generally resulting from blunt forearm trauma
Wrist	Barton's	Intra-articular fracture of distal radius
	Colles'	Radial fracture in distal 2 centimeter, with or without ulnar styloid fracture. Involves dorsal displacement of distal fragment and "silver-fork" deformity
	Smith's	Fracture of the distal radius that occurs if the patient lands with the wrist in flexion
	Hutchinson's	See Chauffeur's fracture
	Chauffeur's	Radial styloid fracture due to direct blow and avulsion of the radial styloid process by the radial collateral ligament
Hand	Bennett's	Intra-articular fracture dislocation of the base of the first metacarpal
	Rolando's	Comminuted intra-articular fracture of the metacarpal base of the thumb
	Boxer's	Fracture of neck of fifth metacarpal
Leg	Segond	Vertical avulsion fracture of the proximal lateral tibia at the insertion of the lateral capsular ligament
	Maisonneuve	Fracture of the proximal third of the fibula
Ankle	Pilon/pestle	A comminuted fracture of the distal tibia
	Bosworth	Ankle fracture dislocation, characterized by the locking of the proximal fibular fragment behind the tibia
	Tillaux	Fracture of the lateral aspect of distal tibia
	Wagstaffe-LeForte	Avulsion fracture of the fibula
	Salter Harris	Various fractures of the distal tibia or fibula

(Continued)

Fracture Eponyms (*Continued*)

Body Region	Name	Description
Foot	Jones	Fracture of the base of the 5th metatarsal
	Aviator's	Fracture through the dome of the talus and fracture dislocation of the talus
	March	Stress or fatigue fracture of the metatarsals
	Beak	Extra-articular fracture of the calcaneal tuberosity

Index

Page numbers followed by italic *f* or *t* denote figures or tables, respectively.